W9-CBF-178

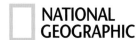

COMPLETE GUIDE TO
HERBS & SPICES

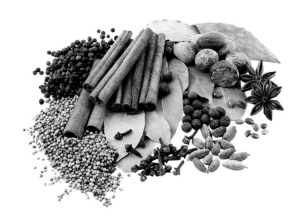

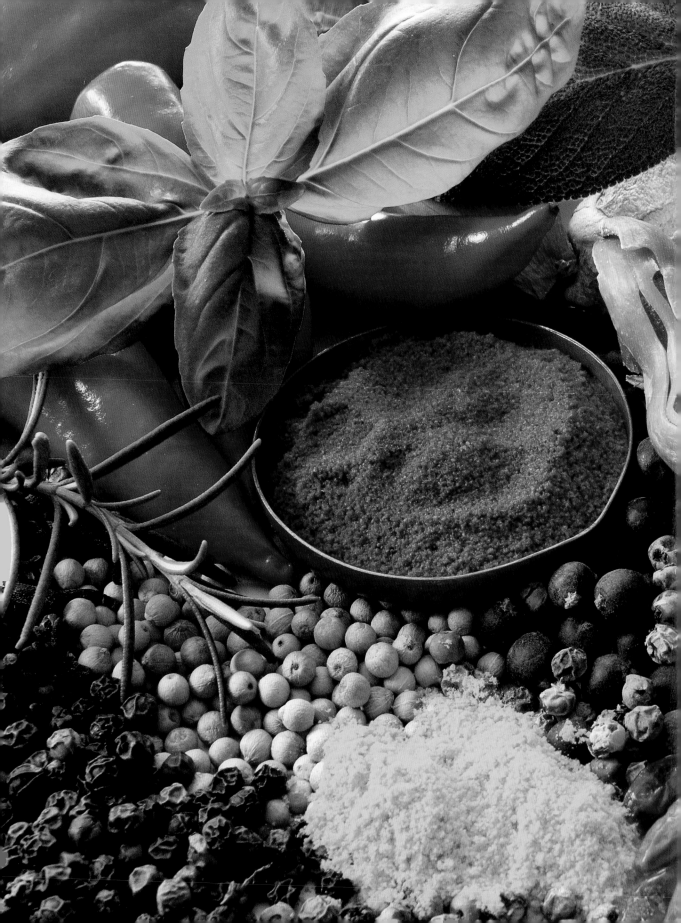

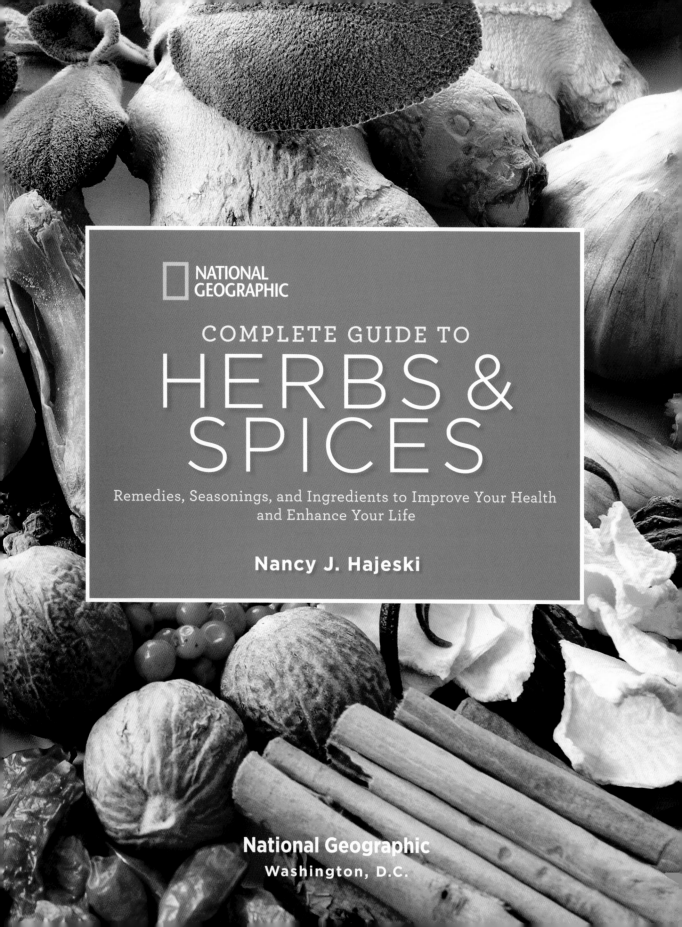

NATIONAL GEOGRAPHIC

COMPLETE GUIDE TO
HERBS &
SPICES

Remedies, Seasonings, and Ingredients to Improve Your Health
and Enhance Your Life

Nancy J. Hajeski

National Geographic
Washington, D.C.

CONTENTS

PART TWO: SPICES

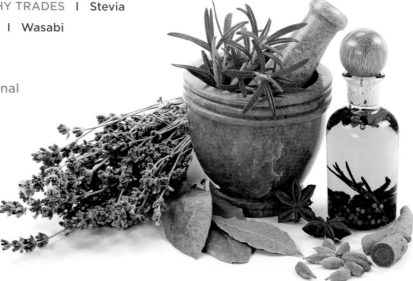

Herbs, Spices, and Seasonings

HEALTHY FLAVORS ARE ALWAYS IN STYLE

In spite of all the hardships they faced, early human hunter-gatherers clearly took the time to seek out herbs and other plants to season their meals. And they began doing so at least 500,000 years ago, based on herb seeds recently found in prehistoric cave dwellings. Since that time, herbs and spices have served us as culinary essentials; as objects of worship; as a means of offering worship by scenting the air or purifying a space; and as healing medicines for the body and uplifting tonics or calming balms for the spirit.

Herbs and spices add flavor, aroma, color, texture, and even nutrients to our meals, and both possess medicinal, aromatic, and cosmetic applications. Yet, there are several distinctions: The majority of herbs come from the green parts of a plant, the stem and leaves. Spices are typically derived from the seeds, flowers, fruit, bark, root, bulb, or rhizome of a tree or shrub. Herbs can be served either fresh or dried, while spices are almost always dried. Geographically, most herbs are found in temperate climates and make good garden plants. Spices require tropical climates to thrive or they need to be cultivated in greenhouses. Their exotic origins also make them more expensive than herbs.

So where do seasonings fit in? Their parameters are a bit more amorphous. According to the *Larousse gastronomique*, seasoning a dish is not the same as flavoring it. While herbs and spices are meant to blend with a recipe, some seasonings, such as mustard, garlic, onions, and horseradish, stand up to the other ingredients—and often win. The seasonings known as condiments began as salt, sugar, and pickles, and they soon became anything that was added by the diner after the meal was on the table.

HERBS

Herbs are hardy, often perennial, soft-stemmed plants that grow in temperate regions. With more intense flavors or aromas than regular vegetables or fruits, they are used in much smaller quantities. The Greeks and Roman began to catalog the names of various plants, including many herbs, around the fourth century B.C. Theophrastus recorded 500 names, Pliny the Elder, another 1,000. In the first century, Dioscorides, a Roman

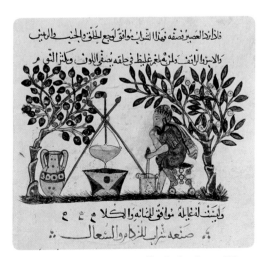

"Physician Preparing an Elixir," an illumination from a 13th-century Arabic manuscript of Dioscorides' famed *De Materia Medica,* written between A.D. 50 and 70. A Roman physician of Greek origin, Dioscorides was widely read for centuries.

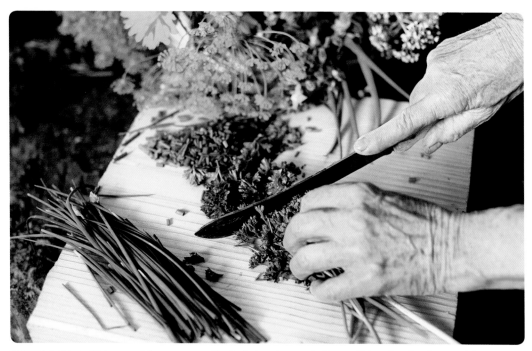

Whether used in cooking, as medicine, or as aromatics, herbs have been part of human history since time immemorial.

physician and author of *De Materia Medica,* further described 600 medicinal plants. Meanwhile, the Chinese had begun recording herbal names, including 365 medicinal plants, 3,500 years ago.

The name *herb* comes from the Old French *erbe* and appeared in English around the late 13th century, connoting both a plant without a woody stem and one that had medicinal or culinary value. The "h" appeared in the 1500s but was not pronounced until the 19th century—although Americans still pronounce the word as "urb."

Midwives and Healers

During the Middle Ages, there was little true medicine in Europe. Physicians believed that illness was caused by a buildup of bad humors—black bile, yellow bile, blood, and phlegm—and that only a course of bloodletting could help. These physicians had a low rate of success, especially with women facing childbirth. Yet, in most villages, there existed midwives, or natural healers, who successfully used herbs to treat a variety of ills. Their knowledge was passed down from one generation to the next, and many of their herbal applications are still in use today.

Among the medicinal herbs employed by these village healers, those known to be toxic, such as foxglove and deadly nightshade, were dispensed with great caution. Today, however, foxglove *(Digitalis purpurea)* furnishes us with a drug that can control heart rate. Deadly nightshade *(Atropa belladonna)* has been used in cases of cardiac arrest. (The name *belladonna,* or "beautiful lady," arose because women used it to dilate their pupils for a wide-eyed effect.) The volatile respiratory inhibitor hemlock *(Conium maculatum),* which Greek philosopher Socrates drank to commit suicide, is used as a sedative and antispasmodic.

A Trio of Uses

There are three categories of herbs: the *culinary herbs* that enhance the taste of dishes; the *medicinal herbs* that are used to cure illness and prevent disease; and the *aromatic herbs* that bring the soothing, pleasurable scents of the garden indoors. There are also crossovers—culinary herbs that have delightful scents and medicinal herbs that were first used as food additives.

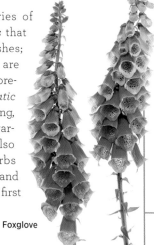

Foxglove

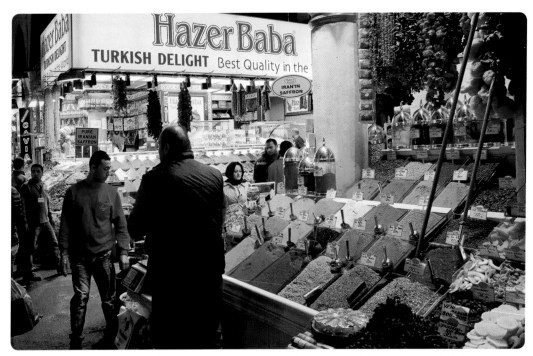

A spice stall at the Egyptian Bazaar, also known as the Spice Bazaar, in Istanbul, Turkey. Gateway cities like Istanbul—formerly Constantinople—and Venice, Italy, with strategic positions on the spice routes, profited from the lucrative trade in these products.

Since the 1960s, TV cooking programs and celebrity chefs have challenged American homemakers to experiment with new types of cuisine. One result of this kitchen revolution was that familiar dried culinary herbs like basil and parsley—those dusty, gray flakes in the spice rack—began appearing fresh and flavorful in supermarkets. Less familiar herbs, like cilantro and dill, also soon became staples. Today, specialty stores and Asian groceries offer hard-to-find exotics, and modern cooks no longer flinch at preparing Indian curry, pad thai, quesadillas, Cajun jambalaya, or French bouillabaisse—all dishes with herbal flavors as their essence.

A renewed focus on natural healing and holistic medicine began near the end of the 20th century, incorporating many traditional remedies made with medicinal herbs. At first, physicians and medical researchers scoffed at these "home cures"... until many of the herbs in question were shown to contain powerful antioxidants, including flavonoids, which help us improve our health and also have the potential to combat cancer, diabetes, high blood pressure, and heart disease.

As the new millennium dawned, many homeowners sought to create a well-balanced home environment and make their living spaces more inviting to guests and more relaxing for themselves. Aromatic herbs, in the form of essential oils, diffusers, incense, and potpourris, played a big part in this new attitude and soon became fixtures of the American lifestyle. The practice of aromatherapy—using essential oils through inhalation, ingestion, or massage—to treat medical conditions, also grew in popularity. And as more people experienced spiritual quests in their personal lives, perhaps emulating Asian or Native American rituals, they turned to aromatic herbs as aids to meditation and for purification ceremonies.

SPICES

Spices have a long and tumultuous history, one that is entwined with humankind's journey toward civilization, the expansion of trade, the rise of empires, and the growth of stable communities in remote regions. As merchants in the West sought exotic seasonings from the Near East and Far East, "spice roads" across Southern Asia opened up, creating flourishing market cities in many of the regions they passed through. Meanwhile, explorers like Columbus sought

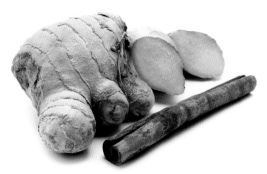
Ginger and cinnamon. These sweet, warm spices currently number among the five most popular flavorings in the world, along with the seasonings salt, pepper, and garlic.

Savory Spices

Savory spices have not gone out of style since the day a Neolithic hunter-gatherer living in what is now Switzerland sprinkled caraway seeds into the stew pot. Trusted favorites of modern cooks include paprika, black pepper, and saffron. Yet, novel flavorings have also been embraced as the farthest reaches of the globe are plumbed for their culinary secrets. Who knew, 30 years ago, that so many of us would be relishing the exotic notes of turmeric or cumin?

Seasonings

All spices and herbs are technically seasonings, but food experts use the label seasonings for certain flavorings that are added after a meal has been cooked—although some get used during the preparation process as well. In recent years, seasonings such as salt and sugar have been linked with high blood pressure, diabetes, and obesity, yet others such as garlic and ginger have been found to offer significant health advantages. Whatever seasoning or condiment it is that you are shaking onto your meals or stirring into your sauces, try to make healthy choices. There are a number of tasty substitutes, but if you *must* use real sugar or salt, remember to apply them in moderation. *Bon appétit!*

alternate trade routes to the spice-filled "Indies" by sailing in the opposite direction—and ended up discovering a new world of unfamiliar spices.

Culturally, the use of spices has been documented since the beginning of recorded history. They are mentioned in the *Epic of Gilgamesh,* the *Bhagavad Gita,* and the Old Testament. Archeologists have found traces of garlic-mustard seeds on pottery shards dating back six thousand years and remains of spices in Egyptian tombs that date back to 3000 B.C. The preservative quality of certain spices made them ideal for embalming, and, in some cultures, spices had strong affiliations with specific gods.

Medicinally, many spices are loaded with phytonutrients that offer protection from disease and boost the healing process. Though ingested in relatively small quantities, they still pack quite a wallop. Perhaps the best news for chefs is that Internet ordering gives instant access to fresh, hard-to-find spices and makes them just a few mouse clicks away.

Sweet Spices

For most home cooks in the 20th century, the sweet spices provided the familiar tastes of traditional holiday dishes: aniseed in Italian Christmas cookies, nutmeg and cinnamon in Twelfth Night wassail punch, cloves placed on Easter ham; cardamom in Swedish St. Lucia's day buns, ginger and allspice in Thanksgiving pumpkin pie, and vanilla or chocolate in birthday cake. Today's home cooks go beyond the familiar, eager to try the trendiest gourmet desserts touted by TV chefs—panna cottas, gelatos, crème brûlées, sandesh, macarons, and pavlovas—yet the sweet spices have never been more appreciated.

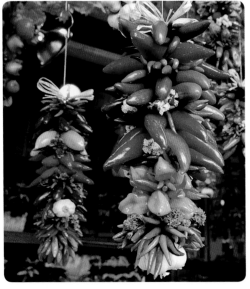
A bright mix of *Capsicum annuum* varieties strung with herbs and garlic hang at a Seattle market stall. Alliums—such as garlic, onions, and scallions—and the many varieties of capsicum peppers are making news for their potent health benefits.

About This Book

This book features 113 herbs, spices, and seasonings. It is divided into two parts—Herbs and Spices, and six chapters: Classic Culinary Herbs, Medicinal Herbs, Aromatic Herbs, Sweet Spices, Savory Spices, and Seasonings. Each chapter includes an introductory spread prior to the entries.

Each of the 113 herbs, spices, and seasonings is represented by one spread. The main heading on the entry page gives the mostly widely known of the common names of the plant, with its scientific name directly below. The main text then gives a brief overview of the entry, including its applications as a food source, medicine, and aromatic, plus any additional uses, such as in industry. The plant is then described in detail, and its habitat and commercial growing sites are covered. A brief history of the plant reveals its country of origin, its early applications, its cultural implications, and how its usage may have changed over the passing centuries. The etymology of its common and/or Latin name is often covered.

Text Headings

The entries share many of the same topical headings that contain specific information.

» **Culinary Uses** can cover cooking, storing, and purchasing guidelines; typical dishes prepared with the entry; and how cooks around the world utilize this herb, spice, or seasoning.

» **Medicinal Properties** explains how different cultures used the plant for preventing or curing ailments from ancient times up to the present. If applicable, there is also mention of any scientific studies that have corroborated the traditional medicinal uses of this plant and any research breakthroughs regarding new medical uses for the plant.

» **Aromatic Qualities** explores the uses of scented herbs and spices, both for maintaining spiritual balance in the home and as part of aromatherapy—employing essential oils to remedy physical or emotional ills.

» **History and Lore** covers folktales, legends, unusual historical usages, or interesting facts.

» **Nutrition,** which is a separate heading in the Classic Culinary Herbs chapter, reveals the beneficial vitamins and minerals that are found in many herbs. Where applicable, this information is also included in the text of other entries.

Sidebars

The sidebars featured on each entry spread cover one of the following six topics:

» **In the Kitchen** showcases recipes or tips for the preparation of special dishes or even gift items.

» **In the Garden** offers tips on growing companion plants, keeping away pests, and other information about cultivating herbs and spices.

» **For Your Health** contains information on the health benefits of the entry and can also include helpful hints for turning herbs and spices into remedies you can make at home.

» **Make It Yourself** supplies readers with guidelines for creating gifts, crafts, or beauty products out of herbs and spices.

» **Cultural Connections** gives a glimpse of how seasonings have affected other cultures or been affected by historical happenings.

» **Curiosities** discusses unusual facts or bizarre traditions that involve the featured plant.

"Focus On" Features

There are also informational Focus On features scattered throughout the book.

These spreads furnish an in-depth look at a specific topic and can relate to cooking, gardening, medicine or health, or aromatic or cosmetic uses.

Grower's Guide

This handy reference chart at the back of the book (pages 296–303) features a photo of the plant, its Latin name, and a brief guide to planting, nurturing and harvesting most of the herbs, spices, and seasonings mentioned here. USDA hardiness zone restrictions are often included.

Usage Icons

Although the plants featured in *Herbs & Spices* have been placed into certain themed chapters, all of them have multiple uses—many culinary herbs, for instance, are also used medicinally, and a sweet spice may well be an aromatic. In the upper right-hand margin of each of the main entries you will therefore see five small icons: crossed kitchen utensils, a mortar and pestle, a perfume atomizer, a bee, and a seedling with leaves, which will show you the plant's multiple uses. If any of the top three icons is highlighted, it means that the plant may be culinary, medicinal, or aromatic. The fourth icon indicates that the plant is attractive to bees—something that is important to many gardeners who intentionally grow bee-specific flowers. If the fifth icon is highlighted, the plant is included in the Grower's Guide at the back of the book.

 Used in **cooking** (crossed utensils)

 Used in **medicine** (mortar and pestle)

 Used as an **aromatic** (perfume atomizer)

 Attracts bees (bee)

 Featured in **Grower's Guide**

USAGE ICONS
See above for key.

HERB/SPICE NAMES
The best known common name and the scientific name (genus and species)

TEXT HEADINGS
Each entry is broken down into main categories of discussion. See list opposite for individual headings.

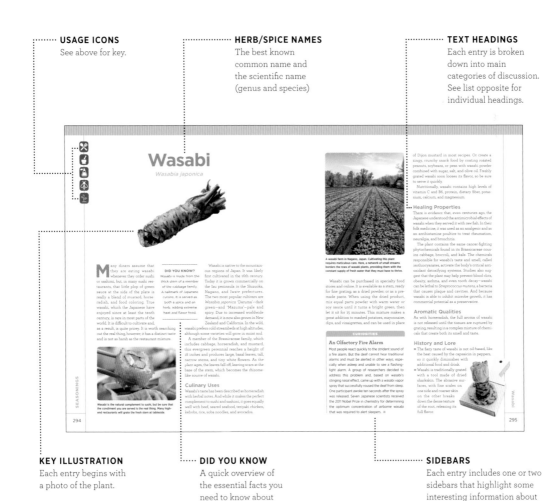

KEY ILLUSTRATION
Each entry begins with a photo of the plant.

DID YOU KNOW
A quick overview of the essential facts you need to know about the featured plant.

SIDEBARS
Each entry includes one or two sidebars that highlight some interesting information about the plant. See list opposite for individual sidebar headings.

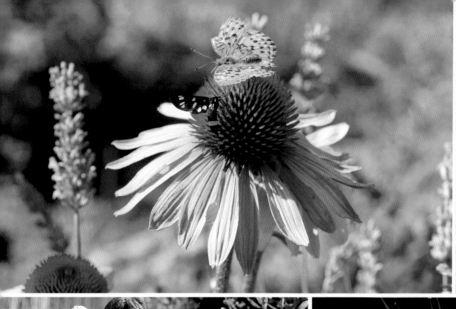
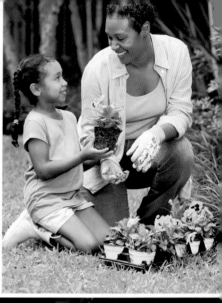
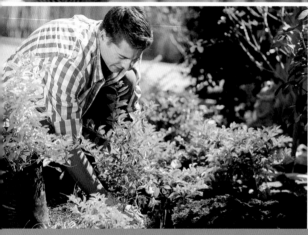
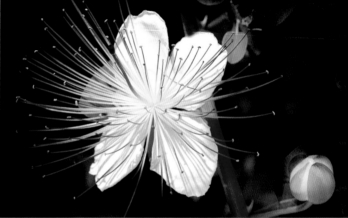

PART ONE
HERBS

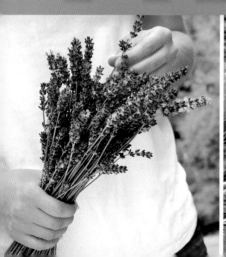
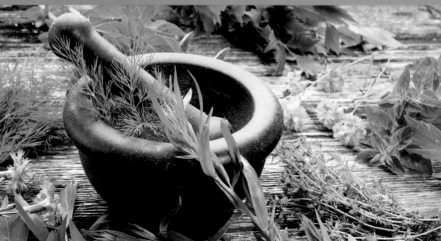

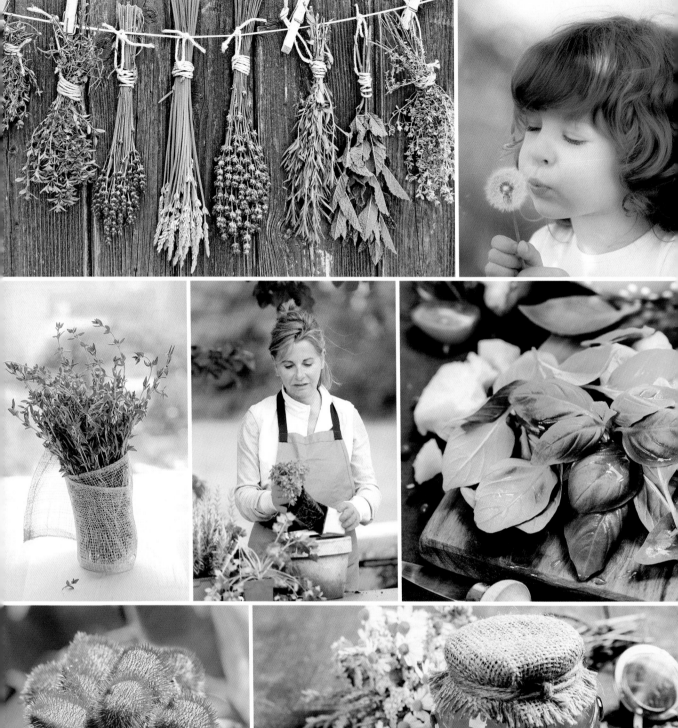
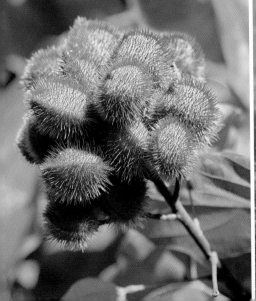
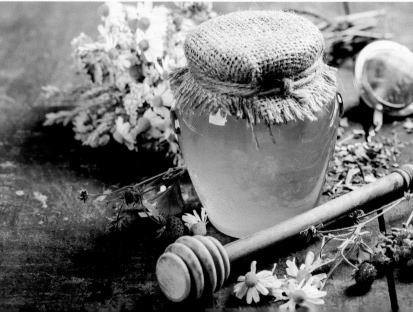

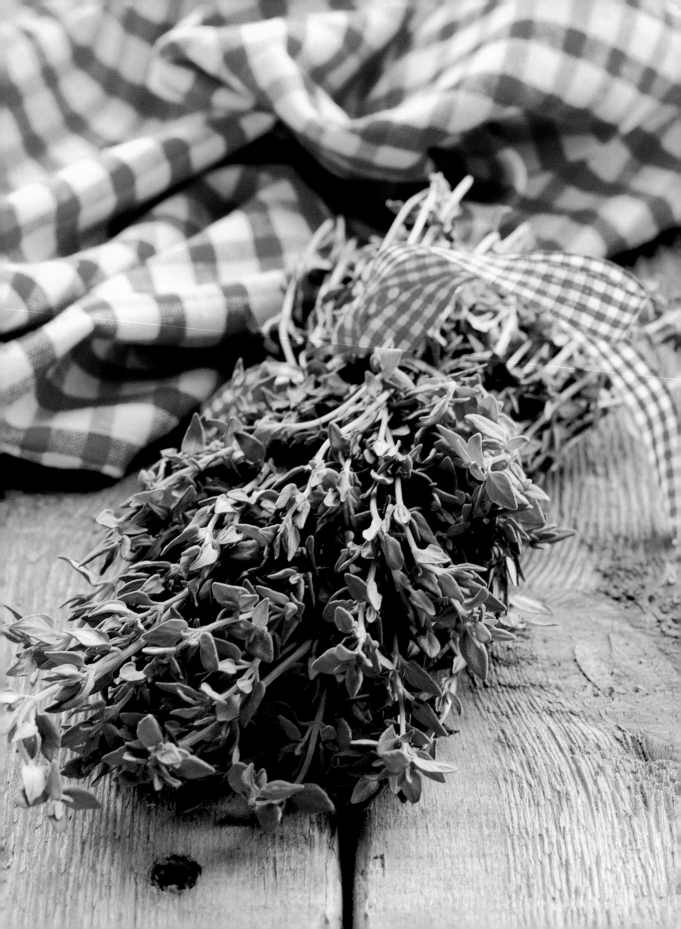

CLASSIC CULINARY HERBS

Opposite: **Thyme**

Herbs in
the Kitchen

ENHANCING THE FLAVOR OF FOOD
AND DEFINING INTERNATIONAL CUISINE

Forty years ago, American tourists traveling abroad would often be astonished at how rich and complex the cuisine tasted compared to the bland, "meat and potatoes" meals that they consumed back in the States. Much of this unfamiliar flavor could be attributed to the widespread use of herbs in foreign kitchens.

Happily, since that time, various culinary trends have swept this country—Asian food, Mediterranean or French cuisine, Mexican cookery, or the vegetarian lifestyle. The result? Savvy American cooks now know their way around the world's most flavorful herbs.

A LONG HISTORY OF TASTE

Herbs, either freshly picked or dried and powdered, have been used to enhance foods since the earliest days of human civilization. Charred fenugreek seeds have been carbon dated to 4000 B.C., and the seeds of various herbs show up in the tombs of the Egyptian kings. Ancient Greeks and Romans, no slouches when it came to

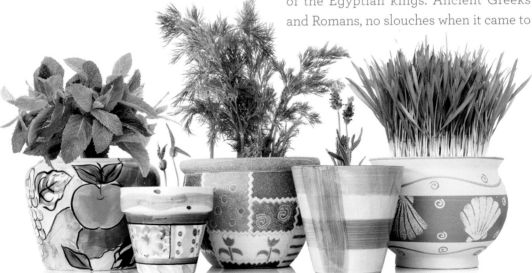

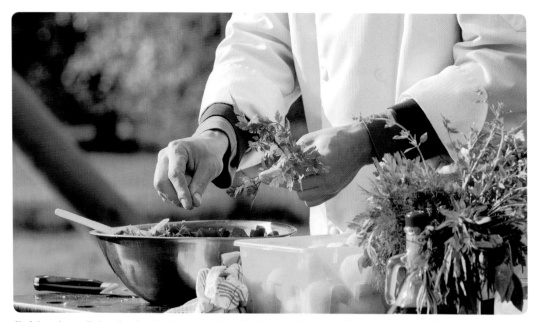

Chefs have long relied on the planet's abundant variety of herbaceous plants to add flavor and color to their culinary creations.

indulging themselves, regularly used the pungent local Mediterranean herbs when preparing feasts and banquets. It was the latter's armies that spread their indigenous herbs, such as chervil and fennel, to other countries during their campaigns to conquer Europe and the Middle East.

DEFINING FLAVORS

As the different nations of the world began to evolve and establish an identity, herbs helped distinguish their respective cuisines— the robust flavors of Italy or Greece in basil, bay leaf, and oregano; the aromatic rosemary and thyme of the Middle East; the tart citrus flavors of lemongrass or tamarind found in Asian food; or the slightly soapy taste of cilantro, that hallmark of Mexican cooking.

There were even early herbal fads—as when in the 1600s, European farming manuals insisted that chefs and cooks use new herbs and forego the older, traditional ones. Formerly popular herbs like cilantro fell out of fashion for centuries.

Doubtless, new and exotic cuisines will come into favor and new food fads will arise, but whatever the peregrinations of human taste, culinary herbs will always play a key part in the most delectable dishes.

> **"The first gatherings of the garden in May of salads, radishes and herbs made me feel like a mother about her baby—how could anything so beautiful be mine."**
>
> *—Alice B. Toklas*

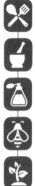

Basil

Ocimum basilicum

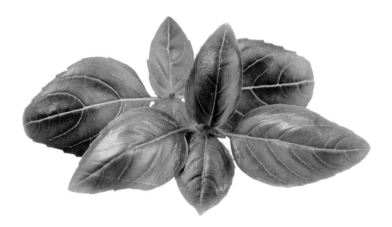

Basil, or sweet basil, is a member of the widespread mint family. Its slightly anise taste can be both pungent and sweet. It is originally native to India, where it has been cultivated for more than five thousand years—and remains a symbol of hospitality. Although most basil is considered a semi-hardy annual, in some tropical zones the herb can become perennial.

Culinary Uses

The French sometimes call it *l'herbe royale*, and for many chefs, basil still reigns as the king of herbs. According to the *Oxford English Dictionary*, basil might even have served as an unguent or medicinal bath for royalty.

DID YOU KNOW?

Basil is a leafy annual that yields a rich harvest of highly fragrant leaves. This classic culinary herb pairs well with tomatoes both in the kitchen and in the garden.

Although it is familiar as a dried herb, fresh leafy basil has become increasingly popular as an additive to soups or casseroles and as a salad ingredient. It can be blended with Parmesan cheese, olive oil, garlic, and pine nuts to make pesto sauce. When preparing hot dishes, fresh basil is typically added near the end—otherwise it loses much of its flavor. There are more than 60 kinds of basil, and some popular Mediterranean cultivars of the plant include 'Genovese', 'Purple Ruffles', 'Mammoth', 'African Blue', 'Lemon', 'Cinnamon', and 'Globe'.

Basil is a favorite in many Asian countries, including Indonesia, Vietnam, Cambodia, and Laos. It is added to Chinese and Taiwanese soups, and the Taiwanese also deep fry chicken with basil leaves. Thai cooks steep Thai basil in cream or milk as a flavoring for ice cream or chocolate delicacies. When the seeds are soaked in water, they become gelatinous and can be used in Asian drinks and desserts such as *feluda* and sherbet.

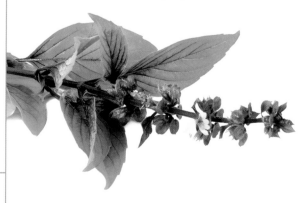

Smaller than sweet basil, Thai basil *(O. basilicum* var. *thyrsiflora)* is a striking plant with purple stems and purple-veined lance-shaped leaves surrounding delicate mauve flowers. Thai basil also has a stronger flavor than sweet basil, with subtle hints of licorice.

Opening the Gates of Heaven

In many early cultures, basil was thought to ensure a safe journey into the afterlife. The Greeks and Egyptians wrote of the herb "opening the gates of heaven" to those who had died. Later, Europeans would wrap the hands of the departed around a clump of basil, while in India the herb was placed in the mouths of the dying to guarantee their entry into the presence of God. ■

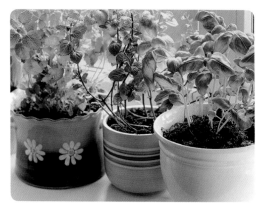

Basil adapts readily to both kitchen gardens and kitchen windowsills, where it will repel flies and mosquitoes.

Fresh basil should be wrapped in a damp paper towel and stored in the refrigerator. It can also be frozen in ice-cube trays for later use in recipes; this ensures a supply of fresh basil—always preferable to dry basil—during colder months. Organic basil is best for drying; irradiated plants can lose vitamin C and carotene.

Nutritional Value

Basil offers healthy doses of vitamin K (which aids in blood clotting) and vitamin A. It also contains manganese and magnesium.

Healing Properties

Traditional healers consider basil useful for treating coughs and bronchitis and for fighting depression. In India, it is used as a treatment for stress, asthma, and diabetes. Recent scientific studies have also found that the herb's flavonoids and volatile oils contain certain compounds that may offer significant antioxidant, antiviral, and antimicrobial benefits, and even have the potential to treat cancer.

History and Lore

» Basil takes its name from the Greek word *basilikon,* or "kingly," because it was so prized in the Mediterranean during the Middle Ages for its strong flavor and pungent aroma. Judges and other dignitaries would carry posies of basil to ward off unpleasant odors.

» Basil is associated with the Feast of the Cross, which commemorates St. Helena, mother of Holy Roman emperor St. Constantine, finding the True Cross with basil growing at its base. Stalks of basil are still used to sprinkle holy water by priests of the Greek Orthodox Church.

» Astrologers consider basil the essential oil of Scorpio, under the planetary rule of Pluto.

» In Portugal and Italy, the herb was once considered a symbol of love; a young Italian man would present his beloved with a pot of dwarf basil, along with a poem and a pom-pom, on the feast days of St. John and St. Anthony.

Classic Pesto

Use fresh basil leaves from the garden to create this simple but delicious classic pasta sauce.

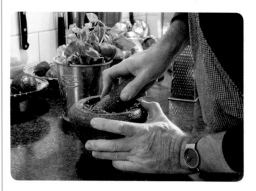

Ingredients
- 3 cups fresh basil leaves
- ½ cup olive oil
- ¼ cup pine nuts
- 4 garlic cloves
- ¾ cup freshly grated Parmesan cheese

Directions
Combine basil, garlic, Parmesan cheese, olive oil, and nuts with a mortar and pestle or in a food processor or blender. Blend to a smooth paste. Serve with your favorite pasta. ■

Basil

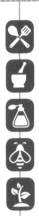

Bay Leaf

Laurus nobilis

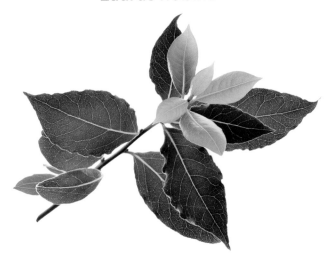

ay leaf can be used either fresh or dry to add flavor to soups, stews, braises, and sauces. It is harvested from the *Laurus nobilis,* or bay laurel tree, a conical evergreen that can reach 30 feet in height. The bay laurel is believed to have originated in Asia Minor, but it soon spread to most of the Mediterranean and some parts of Asia. The star-shaped flowers are yellow or greenish white and appear in clusters in the early spring; each flower produces a single, greenish purple seed berry. The elliptical, dark green leaves measure three to four inches and are thick and leathery.

Culinary Uses

Bay leaf has been a favored herb since the days of the ancient Greeks. In addition to Mediterranean cuisine, bay leaves feature in American as well as French cooking, where the leaves are part of a flavorsome bundle called a bouquet garni. Thai cuisine places them in

DID YOU KNOW?

Bay leaf comes from the bay laurel tree, an aromatic evergreen tree or large shrub with green, glossy leaves, native to the Mediterranean region.

its Arab-influenced dishes such as massaman curry. Dried leaves are added to the Filipino dish, adobo, and bay laurel leaves (as opposed to Indian bay leaves) are often found in Indian and Pakistani classics like rice biryani and as an ingredient in the spice mixture garam masala.

When fresh, the leaf's flavor is less aromatic; when dried for several weeks, the taste is sharp, bitter, and slightly floral, resembling thyme and oregano. Several other species of bay are also used in cooking. West Indian bay leaf (*Pimenta racemosa*) is used to produce the hair dressing cologne called bay rum. (A separate species, the mountain laurel of the United States, *Kalmia latifolia,* has poisonous leaves and should not be confused with the bay laurel.)

Bay leaves can irritate the digestive tract, so they should be removed from any dish before plating. If they are crushed before cooking, to impart richer flavor, the leaf fragments can be placed in a muslin bag for easy removal. Ground bay leaves do not need to be removed, but because their taste is far stronger, they need to be added sparingly.

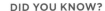

Dried and ground bay leaves are a kitchen herb staple.

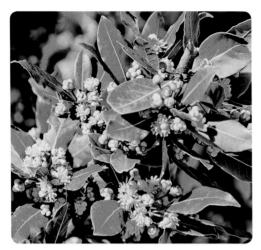

In spring, small yellow-green flowers cluster between the thick, glossy leaves of the bay laurel. In the home, the fresh leaves will help discourage pests, including flies, roaches, meal moths, silverfish, ants, and mice.

Nutritional Value

Bay leaves are a key source of the powerful antioxidant and immunity booster vitamin C, providing 77.5 percent of RDA (recommended dietary allowances) per 100 grams. They are also rich in folic acid, important in DNA synthesis, and vitamin A, an antioxidant necessary for healthy sight, maintaining mucus membranes, and clear skin. They contain the B-complex vitamins niacin, pyridoxine, pantothenic acid, and riboflavin, which contribute to enzyme synthesis, metabolic regulation, and nervous system function.

Their mineral content includes potassium (which helps control heart rate), calcium (bone strength), iron (red blood cell production), manganese, copper, selenium, zinc, and magnesium.

Healing Properties

In ancient times, the bay leaf was revered for its medicinal qualities—infusions were believed to relieve stomach ulcers and flatulence, as well as stimulate the appetite.

In traditional medicine, the leaves were known for their antiseptic and anti-inflammatory qualities. The components in the essential oil have been used as a liniment to treat arthritis, muscle aches, bruising and swelling, as well as to reduce flu and bronchitis symptoms, and treat dandruff. In spite of some unsubstantiated medicinal claims, treatment with bay leaves has been proven to reduce headaches and help the body process insulin, resulting in lowered blood sugar.

History and Lore

» In Europe and Britain, young girls once placed a posy of bay leaves under their pillows on the night before St. Valentine's Day so that they would have dreams of their future husbands.
» Entomologists use bay leaves in killing jars. The crushed, fresh leaves, when placed under a sheet of paper, emit toxic vapors—possibly cyanide—that slowly kill insects and leave the specimens pliant and easy to mount.

CULTURAL CONNECTIONS

Hail the Conquering Hero

According to Roman mythology, after Eros struck both the god Apollo and the nymph Daphne with golden arrows, Daphne fled from Apollo and was turned into a laurel tree. The despairing Apollo chose the leaves of her "noble laurel" to honor the athlete winners of his Pythian Games. The ancient Romans then presented circlets or crowns made of laurel leaves to military victors, athletic champions, and esteemed poets to signify they were special in the eyes of the gods. Examples of laurel wreaths can be seen on Roman statuary, pottery, and mosaics. This time-honored ritual of recognition gave rise to the expression "Resting on your laurels," or, in other words, relying on past glories rather than pursuing new achievements. ■

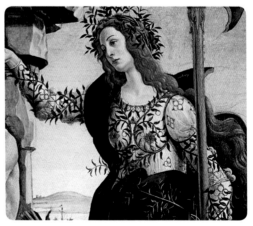

A detail from Botticelli's *Pallas and the Centaur* shows the goddess Athena draped in laurel. To the Greeks and Romans, the bay laurel symbolized wisdom, protection, and triumph.

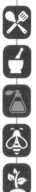

Borage

Borago officinalis

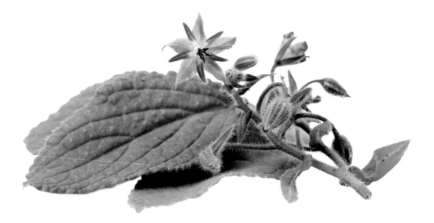

Also known as starflower, borage is an annual herb that had its origins in the Mediterranean, around Aleppo. This kitchen garden regular has naturalized over the years and is now found growing wild in many areas of the world. Borage is also grown commercially for its valuable seed oil.

The borage plant reaches a height of two to three feet, with stems and leaves covered with white, prickly hair. The leaves alternate and are deep green, wrinkled, and oval. The star-shaped flowers, which form floral

DID YOU KNOW?

Borage, an easy-growing annual, adds color to the garden with vivid star-shaped true-blue flowers. Its cucumber-flavored leaves make it a useful kitchen herb, too.

displays, are most often blue with distinctive black anthers—called the "beauty spot" by plant lovers. Pink flowers sometimes occur and there is a white variety. Many flowers bloom simultaneously, indicating that the plant has a high degree of intra-plant pollination. Borage spreads easily and in temperate zones will bloom from June to September. In milder climates, it may bloom all year.

In the Mediterranean, the name is spelled with two r's, so it is possible the name came from the Italian *borra* or the French *bourra,* meaning "hair" or "wool"—referring to the plant's hairy stems and leaves. Both words have their root in the Latin *burra,* which means "flock of wool."

Culinary Uses

Borage can be utilized either as a fresh vegetable—it tastes of cucumber and is often used in salads or as a garnish—or as a dried herb. The flowers, which contain a nontoxic pyrrolizidine alkaloid called thesinine, have a delightful honey-like taste and are used to decorate desserts, making them one of the few truly blue foods.

Borage is used as a vegetable in the cuisine of Crete and in Germany in soups and green sauce. In the Spanish regions of Navarre and Aragon, it

Prized for the blue of its mature flowers, a young borage blossom is still equally lovely in pink.

Crystallized Borage Flowers

Nothing makes a warm-weather dessert more appealing than the addition of delicate candied flowers. Pick borage blossoms on a dry, sunny morning, when the flowers are open wide.

Ingredients
- 1 handful of borage blossoms
- 1 egg white
- ¼ cup superfine granulated sugar

Directions
Lightly beat the egg white. Pour into a shallow bowl. Place superfine sugar into a slightly deeper bowl. Use tweezers to dip a blossom into the egg white and then the sugar. Use a paintbrush to get sugar into the folds of the flower. Shake off excess sugar, and then place blossoms on a fine wire rack to dry overnight. ■

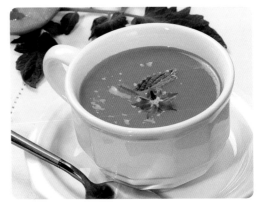

Borage works well as a garnish for savory dishes, such as tomato soup, adding cool contrast to the warm red-orange.

is boiled and served with garlic, and, in the northern Italian region of Liguria, it is traditionally used as a filling for ravioli and pansotti.

Borage is also the traditional garnish for that lawn party favorite Pimm's Cup cocktail, although it is often replaced by a cucumber peel or a sprig of mint. It is one of the botanical flavorings in Gilpin's Westmoreland Extra Dry Gin, and it is still used in Poland to pickle gherkins.

Nutritional Value
Borage contains the minerals potassium and calcium. It also contains nitrate of potash.

Healing Properties
Herbalists have used borage to treat everything from colic, cramps, and diarrhea to asthma and bronchitis, to cardiovascular and urinary disorders. Naturopathic healers use the herb for regulating hormones and metabolism, and for remedying symptoms of menopause, such as hot flashes.

In Iran, the plant is made into a tea for treating colds, flu, rheumatoid arthritis, and inflammation of the kidneys. The tea is also believed to bring more oxygen to the heart, which makes it a healthy choice for those suffering from heart conditions.

History and Lore
» The name *borage* may come from the Celtic term *barrach,* which means "man of courage."
» John Gerard, a 16th-century botanist, says that Roman naturalist Pliny called the herb *Euphrosinum* because it "maketh a man merry and joyfull." Pliny also claimed that borage was the "nepenthe" mentioned in Homer's *Odyssey,* which brought about total forgetfulness.
» In the early 17th century, English philosopher and scientist Francis Bacon wrote that borage "hath an excellent spirit to repress the fuliginous vapour of dusky melancholie."
» Nicholas Culpeper, a noted 17th-century English botanist, commented that the herb was beneficial for treating putrid fevers, venomous snakebite, jaundice, consumption, sore throat, and rheumatism.

The Babysitter Plant

Borage has a special quality that makes it a desirable addition to the vegetable garden—it is an ideal companion plant for promoting, protecting, or "nursing" legumes, squash, spinach, brassicas, and strawberries. When planted beside tomatoes, borage confuses the exploratory search of the mother moths of the destructive tomato hornworm (*Manduca quinquemaculata*), looking for a spot to lay their eggs. Reports that borage also improves the growth and taste of tomatoes have not been verified. ■

A tomato hornworm caterpillar

Borage

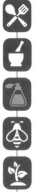

Capers

Capparis spinosa

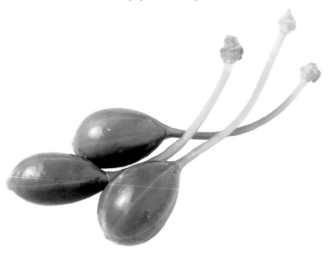

The caper bush, also called the Flinders rose, produces edible flower buds, which are used as a garnish, and edible fruit called the caper berry. Both buds and fruit are served pickled. Other parts of the plant are also used in medicinal applications.

This deciduous bush has round, fleshy leaves and bears large pinkish white flowers with a sweet scent. The blooms bear four sepals, four petals, numerous long, spidery violet stamens, and one protruding stigma.

The plant is widespread, and can be found in the Mediterranean region, Egypt and other parts of North Africa, on the island of Madagascar, in Central Asia, and throughout the Himalayas and the Pacific islands. Some botanists believe the bush originated in the tropics and later became naturalized along the more temperate Mediterranean rim.

Pickled caper buds

> **DID YOU KNOW?**
> The sweet-scented caper bush yields buds and berries that have become a staple of Mediterranean cuisine.

Culinary Uses

The buds of the caper flower have a piquant, salty, savory flavor after pickling. They have been used to garnish pasta sauces, meat, fish, salads, soups, and pizza. They are also used in the preparation of antipasto and fish or venison tartare. The young berries are added to sauces and salads. It is primarily Europeans who consume both forms of the garnish, with capers being essential parts of Italian and Cypriot cuisine.

Nutritional Value

Modern medicine hails capers for their low caloric content (only 23 calories per 100 grams), and their beneficial combination of phytonutrients, antioxidants, and vitamins, which include A, K, niacin, and riboflavin. They also contain the minerals calcium, iron, and copper. Unfortunately, bottled and prepared capers do have a high sodium content due to the pickling or brining process, which adds sea salt.

Healing Properties

Ancient Greeks and Romans found capers beneficial as a tonic, an analgesic, an expectorant, a diuretic, and a vasoconstrictor. Decoctions of the root bark have been used to treat dropsy,

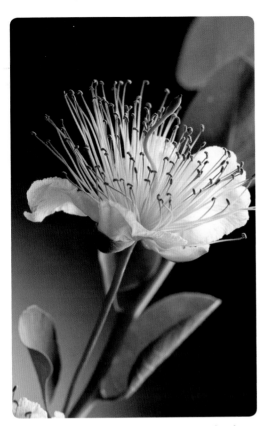

The caper flower opens at dawn, attracting a quantity of pollinators, and closes in the late afternoon.

arthritis, and anemia. As a poultice made of bruised leaves, they were used to ease gout. Ayurvedic physicians prescribe capers to improve liver function.

As well as increasing the appetite, capers can help soothe digestive complaints and curb flatulence. They contain the flavonoid compound rutin, which strengthens capillaries and helps prevent the clumping of platelets in the blood vessels.

History and Lore

» The name *caper* possibly comes from the Latin *capparis* borrowed from the Greek *kapparis,* a word thought to have Asian origins. The name might also have been taken from the island of Cyprus, where capers grow in profusion.

» People in Biblical times believed the caper berry acted as an aphrodisiac. In fact, the Hebrew word for "caper berry" is closely related to the Hebrew root word indicating "desire."

» Capers are 85 percent water. They contain mustard oil glycosides that are similar to those found in several spices in the cabbage family.

» Caper buds are sold by size. The smaller buds—nonpareils and surfines—taste better and so are more valuable than the larger ones—capucines, capotes, and grusas.

Tenacious Capers

The caper bush developed a group of survival mechanisms—reducing the impact of radiation, high temperatures, and drought—making it well suited to Mediterranean climates, and, as a result, its cultivation in certain at-risk areas might help to maintain delicate semiarid ecosystems. Capers are now produced commercially in Morocco, the southeastern region of Spain, Turkey, and the Italian islands of Pantelleria and Salina.

Capers not only tolerate dry conditions, they require long hours of intense sunlight. Crops need to be available for picking over a period of at least three months for cultivation to be profitable. The bush can withstand high temperatures, but it is at risk from frost. It is, however, not picky about soil quality. Bushes can be found growing on bare rock cliffs in Malta, in sand dunes in Pakistan, and in the coastal dunes of Australia. In the foothills of the Himalayas, they are found in both silty clay

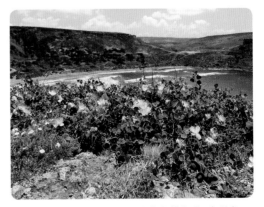

Capers grow on the cliffs above Ghajn Tuffieha Bay in Malta.

and gravelly surface soil with little organic matter. Caper bushes can even be found sprouting from the limestone Wailing Wall of the Temple Mount in Jerusalem. Their tenacity and affinity for stone structures make them threats to the preservation of ancient monuments. ■

Capers

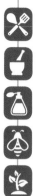

Chervil

Anthriscus cerefolium

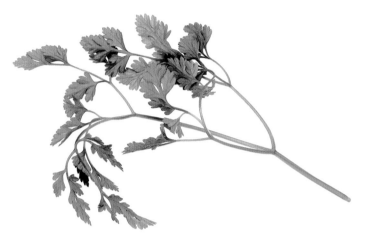

This classic garden herb has been an intrinsic part of French cuisine for centuries. Chervil possesses a delicate flavor with licorice undertones that makes it especially good in soups and salads, where its mild notes are not likely to be overwhelmed by more robust ingredients.

Chervil, a member of the widespread Apiaceae family (also known as Umbelliferae) that includes celery, carrot, and parsley, most likely originated in the Caucasus region and was spread through Europe by the Romans during their military campaigns. The leaves of this hardy annual plant

---

DID YOU KNOW?

A member of the parsley family, chervil is a delicate annual herb suitable for salads and cooking.

---

are lacelike and curly, reminiscent of carrot greens, and its inflorescence forms petite white umbels. The plant, typically 18 inches in height and 12 inches across, adapts well to indoor container gardening because it prefers growing in semi-shade.

Culinary Uses

One of the fines herbes—the favored herb mixture of traditional French cooking—chervil is also used in other types of cuisine. The frilly, pale-green leaves are part of the Provençal-based mesclun salad mix—along with arugula, lettuce, and endive—that became popular with urban gourmets in the 1990s.

Fresh chervil is perfect for accompanying lighter fare: salmon or trout, new potatoes, baby carrots, asparagus, or baby greens. It is delicious as an herbal butter or blended with goat cheese. Chervil is also ideal for seasoning omelets and frittatas, adding its own distinct flavor. When preparing hot dishes, chervil should be added at the very end to maintain its character.

Fresh chervil will keep for a week in the refrigerator inside a sealed plastic bag. Be aware that at the greengrocers it is known by several other names—cicely, sweet cicely, gourmet's parsley, French parsley, and, in France, *cerfeuil*.

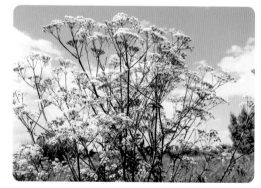

Chervil in bloom shows off its airy clusters of petite flowers, the defining characteristic of its Apiaceae family lineage.

Appearances Can Be Deceiving

One reason that chervil has not caught on with American gardeners, as other European herbs have, might be that it resembles the invasive British weed cow parsley *(Anthriscus sylvestris)*, to which it is related. Chervil also resembles the poisonous hemlock plant (the infamous cause of death for Greek philosopher Socrates) so it should never be picked in the wild—or anywhere that it is not clearly identifiable. ■

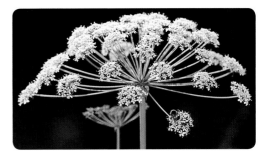

Cow parsley is an invasive chervil look-alike.

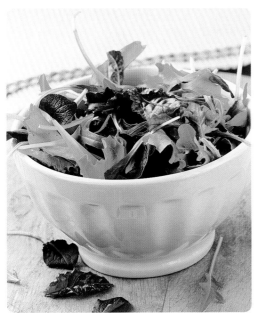

Chervil is a delicate herb, making it a mild counterpoint to more spicy greens, such as arugula, in mesclun salad mixes.

Nutritional Value

Chervil is a rich source of minerals—including calcium, potassium, phosphorus, selenium, manganese, and magnesium—and vitamins A, C, and D. The older leaves, which turn purple, offer fewer beneficial nutrients, so always try to purchase pale green sprigs.

Healing Properties

Chervil was popular with the ancient Romans (the name, from the Greek, translated as "the herb of rejoicing"), who used it to season food but also valued it for its "blood-purifying" and diuretic qualities. Roman naturalist Pliny considered the herb an aphrodisiac and a tonic for older men.

Although 17th-century botanist and herbalist Nicholas Culpeper wrote of chervil, "It doth much please and warm old and cold stomach," it had relatively limited medicinal value to the healers of that time. Perhaps they simply felt it was too mild to be effective against disease.

Chervil is now known to be an excellent source of antioxidants, which stabilize cell membranes and reduce the inflammation that causes headaches, peptic ulcers, and sinusitis. Modern-day herbalists recommend chervil tea for use as an eyewash, to relieve menstrual cramps, and as a spring tonic to rejuvenate both body and spirit. It is also used to treat coughs, flatulence, high blood pressure, depression, and digestive ailments. The fresh leaves can be applied directly to wounds, bites, and burns, and a warm chervil poultice can be used to relieve arthritis and painful, swollen joints.

History and Lore

» The ancients considered this spring herb the symbol of new life, and it has been used to celebrate the Easter calendar. In parts of Europe, chervil soup is served on Holy Thursday.

» The herb was traditionally believed to stop bad dreams or nightmares.

» Ninon de Lenclos, a 17th-century French courtesan, supposedly boiled chervil in water and then washed her face with it twice daily to prevent wrinkles.

» Chervil was sometimes called myrrhis because the scent of its volatile oil was similar to that of the aromatic resin myrrh.

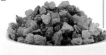

The aroma of chervil is reminiscent of myrrh.

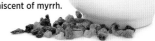

Chervil

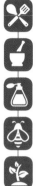

Chives

Allium schoenoprasum

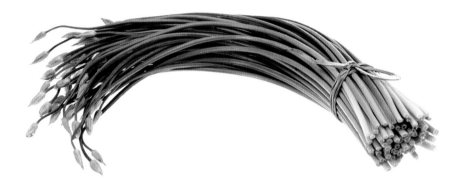

A component of the fines herbes mixture of France, chives are also popular in the cuisine of many other nations. They are the smallest of the edible onion species and are native to Europe, Asia, and North America. Chives were actively cultivated in the Middle Ages starting in the fifth century, but they have been used in food preparation for more than five thousand years.

The species name comes from the Greek *skhoinos*, "sedge" or "rush," and *prason,* for "leek." The English name derives from the French word *cive,* taken from the Latin word *cepa,* or "onion."

Chives, like all alliums, grow from bulbs, in this case, in tight clumps that reach a height of 18 inches. The hollow, tubular stems, or scapes, are soft until just before the flowers bloom. The leaves are short, almost an afterthought, and the pale purple or pink flowers are globular, with six star-like petals. The plant blooms

DID YOU KNOW?

Chives are a perennial herb, part of the onion family, with pale purple globe-shaped flowers. The delicate-tasting, hollow stems are used to flavor seafood, eggs, soups, and salads. Chives also have powerful anti-inflammatory and antibiotic properties.

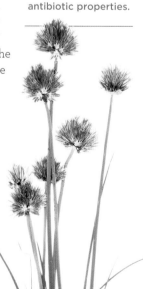

from April to May in warmer climates and in June in cooler regions. The dried blossoms are often used in flower arrangements.

Harvest by cutting stems with a scissor two inches above the soil; chives will quickly produce new, even more tender shoots.

Culinary Uses

With their delicate, zesty flavor, chopped chives make a good accompaniment to mild dishes such as omelets, potatoes, and fish. They are perfect for sprinkling over deviled eggs or baked potatoes with sour cream. Chives can be used either fresh, or dried and crushed. In addition to being a staple of French cuisine, chives are served with quark cheese by the Poles, while Swedish cooks use them to flavor pancakes, soups, sandwiches, and a sauce known as *graddfil,* which is served with herring at midsummer festivals.

The lovely round blossoms of chives are a cheerful pinkish lavender. Dried chive flowers retain their color and make pretty additions to decorative bouquets.

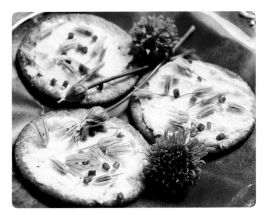

Chopped chives liven up mild cheese spreads, such as cream cheese, while adding a nutritious boost to an afternoon snack. You can also sprinkle on some of the flower petals.

Chives are available year-round in stores and will keep in the refrigerator for up to a week in a sealed bag. Or chop up and screen dry to preserve their flavor. If a gardener ends up with a bumper crop, chives can be frozen for later use.

Nutritional Value

Chives contain vitamins A, B6, C, E, and K, folic acid, and dietary fiber. They also contain the minerals calcium, copper, iron, magnesium, selenium, phosphorus, potassium, and zinc.

Healing Properties

Chives share with their cousin garlic (*Allium sativum*) the same amazing medicinal properties, but in a slightly less potent form. Their use by healers as an aid to the circulatory system is due to the presence of a number of organosulfur compounds.

Chives have proven antibiotic properties—natural antibacterial and antiviral agents in the herb interact with its vitamin C to attack microbes, making them an excellent defense against colds and flu. The flavonoids present in the herb can aid in the regulation of blood pressure, and its sulfides can help to lower blood lipids—both factors in heart health.

The herb's anti-inflammatory properties can lower the risk of rheumatoid arthritis, and its high levels of antioxidant vitamin E boost the immune system. Chives have even been used to inhibit the growth of tumors in cases of esophageal, stomach, prostate, and gastrointestinal tract cancer.

History and Lore

» Chives are the only species of allium to occur naturally in both the Old and New Worlds.

» Ancient Romans used chives to ease the pain of sunburn and sore throats.

» The sulfur compounds in chives repel many insect pests, yet their blossoms attract bees, making them doubly valuable to gardeners.

» These herbs were once used by Romanian gypsies for fortune-telling.

» During the Middle Ages, chives were hung in bunches around village homes to ward off evil—similar to the garlic festoons used to discourage vampires.

IN THE KITCHEN

Chives, Scallions, or Green Onions?

Some home cooks are just not sure how to distinguish chives, scallions, and green onions. Many grocery stores label any long, skinny green-leafed plants with a conspicuous white bottom as either scallions or green onions. It turns out they are exactly the same plant, *Allium fistulosum,* also called the Japanese bunching onion and the Welsh onion. To complicate matters further, regular cooking onions, *A. cepa,* may be sold as scallions if harvested young, before the bulbs fully form. The flavor of scallions is strong compared with chives, though not as robust as *A. cepa.* Chives have finer stems, less white at the base, and are classified as herbs; they offer a more refined flavor. ■

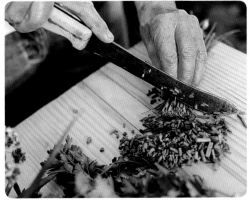

To achieve crisp cuts of chives, scallions, or green onions, hold the herbs in a tight bunch, keeping the stems taut so that you can chop quickly and cleanly without crushing the herbs.

MINGLED FLAVORS

Blend your own herbs to create classic culinary mixtures.

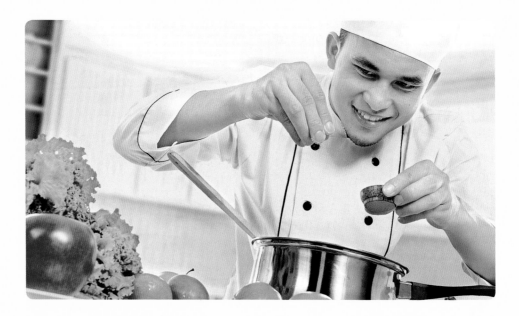

One of the most delightful aspects of cooking with herbs is the way their flavors blend—bitter with sweet, pungent with minty, or delicate with earthy—but are rarely obscured. Home chefs should try experimenting with various herbal combinations: surprisingly complex flavors are often the result. Three famous blends are bouquet garni, fines herbes, and herbes de Provence.

In France, that bastion of haute—and herbal—cuisine, these three different traditional blends have evolved over the centuries, each one adding a distinct character to the dishes they complement.

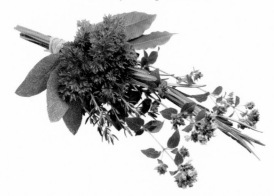

Bouquet Garni

Unlike fines herbes or herbes de Provence, which are consumed with the dish, the bouquet garni—French for "garnished bouquet"—is used as a flavoring to enhance soups, stews, or stocks and then discarded. Bay leaf and thyme are almost always included, and other favorites are parsley, basil, salad burnet, chervil, rosemary, peppercorns, savory, and tarragon. Vegetables are also often added to the bundle, most often carrots, celery, celeriac, leeks, onions, and parsley root.

To create a bouquet garni, gather a number of basil, parsley, and rosemary sprigs, as well as several bay leaves. Add a small celery stalk and carrot. Bundle the ingredients all together inside a coffee filter or a piece of cheesecloth, and then tie with butcher's twine. Some cooks favor wrapping the herbs inside leek leaves and tying them with string, while others use a mesh bag or sachet for the ingredients. Your bouquet can be used to season chicken stock, fish stock, or to make a flavorful poaching liquid called court-bouillon.

Fines Herbes

Fines herbes are a mainstay of French cuisine—refined but flavorful. The term *fines herbes* describes the kind of delicate herbs that make up this culinary mixture: parsley, chives, tarragon, and chervil. Marjoram, cress, cicely, or lemon balm may also be included. Ideally, the herbs should be fresh for optimum taste and chopped fine just before use. Fines herbes are especially effective when preparing lighter fare, such as roasted or baked fish, omelets, potato dishes, soups, and vinaigrettes.

Make Your Own Herbes de Provence

This robust mixture of dried summer herbs includes thyme, marjoram, savory, and other pungent herbs. Its most telling note is the inclusion of lavender, one of Provence's most famous crops. This blend is best used when preparing hearty dishes such as meat, poultry, casseroles, and winter soups. Just choose a selection from the dried herbs shown below. ■

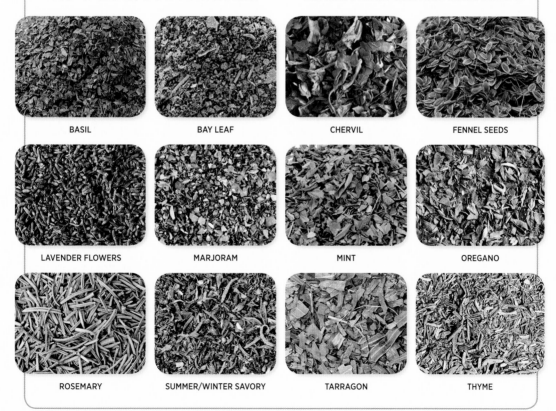

BASIL   BAY LEAF   CHERVIL   FENNEL SEEDS

LAVENDER FLOWERS   MARJORAM   MINT   OREGANO

ROSEMARY   SUMMER/WINTER SAVORY   TARRAGON   THYME

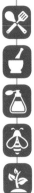

Cilantro

Coriandrum sativum

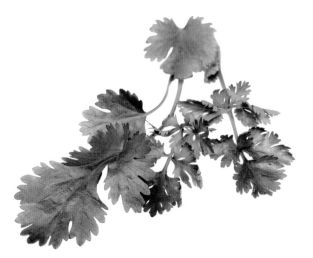

Cilantro originates from the same plant as the spice coriander (the seeds), but cilantro (the lacy green leaves) has recently become a kitchen favorite for use in Mexican and Asian cooking and for imparting its sweet, earthy flavor to salads and seafood.

The plant grows to a height of one or two feet and bears small white, pink, or pale lavender flowers that form umbels. It is native to the Mediterranean and Asia Minor, where it has been flavoring food for more than five thousand years. The Egyptians cultivated it, and it was popular with both the Greeks and Romans. European cooks seasoned with it throughout most of the Middle Ages. But, by 1600, many medieval dishes began to fall from favor after the publication of French and English farming books that encouraged cooks to try newer, less familiar herbs and forego the old ones.

Cilantro again became popular when modern home cooks began to dabble in exotic cuisines, many of which rely on this flavorsome herb.

DID YOU KNOW?
This staple of Mexican and Asian cooking is the lacy green leaf of the coriander plant. The leaves contain many beneficial substances, including antioxidants, phyto-nutrients, and significant amounts of vitamin K.

It is easy to grow in the garden, and it can be harvested continuously during the spring and fall. Leaves should be trimmed off near the ground, but never more than one third of the plant should be taken at a time.

Culinary Uses

Closely associated with Mexican dishes, cilantro is also used extensively in the cuisine of the Middle East, the Mediterranean, India, China, Southeast Asia, Latin America, and Africa. It can be added to hot dishes or served as a garnish; its taste blends especially well with avocado, chicken, fish, lamb, lentils, shellfish, and yogurt. It's also great in chili or curry, as a meat marinade, and as an alternative to basil in pesto.

Because fresh cilantro resembles flat-leaf parsley, always check for that distinctive aroma. Wash at home by swishing in water to remove any residual grit, and then pat dry. Store it in the refrigerator with the cut ends

Cilantro flowers are surrounded by the delicate fernlike upper leaves of the plant. The herb's broad-lobed lower leaves (shown above) resemble those of Italian parsley.

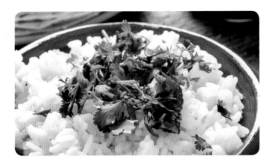

Cilantro is a staple herb of traditional Mexican cuisine, lending its flavor to dishes like Cilantro and Lime Rice.

placed in a jar of fresh water and a loose plastic bag over the top. The leaves can be frozen in an airtight container or with a small amount of water or stock in an ice-cube tray.

Nutritional Value

Cilantro's leaves furnish dietary fiber—necessary for reducing low-density lipoprotein (LDL), the "bad" cholesterol—as well as the minerals iron, copper, manganese, magnesium, potassium, and calcium. The herb provides significant amounts of vitamins A and C, and especially K—believed to limit neuronal damage in the brains of Alzheimer's patients. It also contains folic acid, niacin, riboflavin, and beta-carotene. Its beneficial phytonutrient profile is as impressive as high-calorie foods like nuts, cereal, or meats.

CURIOSITIES

Scent-sational . . . or Not?

This herb's distinctive scent was not always appreciated—the name "coriander" was derived from the Greek word *koris,* or "bedbug," because many people thought the plant smelled like bug-infested linens. In modern times, noted TV chef Julia Child was not a fan; she said if she ever found it on her plate she would "pick it off if I saw it and throw it on the floor." Others find the citrus-sage odor pleasing, similar to hand soap or body lotion. The scent is actually a combination of several modified fragments of fat molecules called aldehydes. Not surprisingly, these same aldehydes are found in soaps, lotions . . . and some insects. Researchers have discovered a way to reduce the scent—crushed cilantro leaves soon lose their strong odor and can be consumed without the buggy or soapy associations. ■

Healing Properties

The early Greek physician Hippocrates used cilantro as an aromatic stimulant. Traditional healers have found it effective in numerous applications—as an analgesic, antispasmodic, aphrodisiac, flatulence reducer, digestive aid, antifungal, deodorant, and stimulant.

Modern medical researchers have discovered that cilantro leaves and stem tips are rich in antioxidant polyphenolic flavonoids, while the leaves and seeds (coriander) are a source of many essential volatile oils.

History and Lore

» Cilantro is mentioned in the Ebers Papyrus, an Egyptian medical papyrus of herbal knowledge dating from 1552 B.C.; the herb is listed as one of the plants that grew in the Hanging Gardens of Babylon.

» In *Arabian Nights,* the herb is referred to as an aphrodisiac.

» British colonists brought *Coriandrum sativum* to Massachusetts in 1670, and it may have been one of the earliest cultivated herbs in North America. After the plant appeared in South America, the leaves rather than the seeds became most desirable.

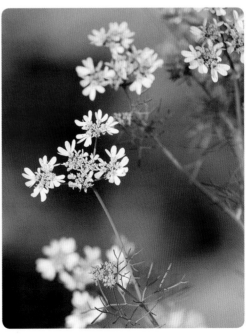

The airy cilantro plant in bloom. The flowers, which appear in umbels, can be white, a range of pinks, or pale lavender.

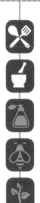
Curry Leaf

Murraya koenigii

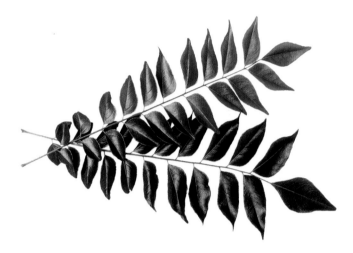

Curry, the perennially popular spicy dish of India and Southeast Asia, is flavored with a variety of seasonings, but the leaf of the curry tree is the foundation for a really authentic curry. The use of this leaf in Indian cooking goes back millennia.

The tropical or subtropical curry tree is native to India and Sri Lanka, where it typically grows from 12 to 20 feet high. It bears small-to-medium pinnate leaves that release a scent that is similar to tangerines or nutty with a hint of lemon. The small, fragrant white flowers produce shiny black berries. An attractive garden addition, curry trees can be found in many homes throughout the Asian tropics. Their range extends almost everywhere on the subcontinent except the higher reaches of the Himalayas.

DID YOU KNOW?

This traditional addition to curry recipes is also used in many other Asian dishes from India and Sri Lanka to Indonesia and Cambodia. The leaf is a valued part of alternative Indian medicine for treating stomach and blood disorders.

The modern Indian name for the leaves, *meethi neem,* translates to "sweet neem leaves"—as opposed to regular neem leaves, which are bitter. In Indonesia, the leaves are called *fogli di cari.*

There is also a European curry plant, *Helichrysum italicum,* that has an aroma similar to the curry leaf, but its young leaves and shoots are most often used in Mediterranean stews to flavor meat rather than in masala to flavor curry or other Asian dishes. The blossoms of this curry plant produce an oil with anti-inflammatory, antifungal, and astringent properties that is soothing to burns and chapped skin.

Culinary Uses

The leaves of the curry tree are prized in southern and west-coast Indian and Sri Lankan cuisine. During the first stage of curry preparation, fresh curry leaves are fried with chopped onions to form an aromatic base. Cambodian Khmer crush the leaves and add them to a sour soup called *maju krueng.*

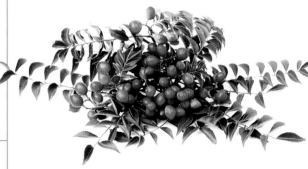

As it ripens, the yellow-green fruit of the curry leaf tree turns to bright red and then darkens to deep purplish black. Although the fruit is edible, the seeds are poisonous.

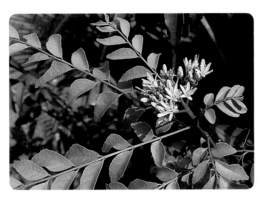

In late spring to summer, small white flowers appear on the curry leaf tree. Like the leaves, the blooms are fragrant.

Fresh curry leaves should be used up quickly; storing or freezing them causes a loss of taste, aroma, and even their medicinal value. Even though curry leaf is available dried, the taste and aroma do not compare to fresh.

Nutritional Value

Curry leaves contain calcium, phosphorus, iron, nicotinic acid, and vitamins A and C. They are also a source of antioxidants and alkaloids.

Healing Properties

Throughout India and much of Asia, curry leaves are a valuable healing herb used for treating piles, skin problems, and blood disorders, and to lower fevers. In Ayurvedic and other traditional medicines, they are used to treat stomach disorders. Pregnant women with morning sickness are advised to mix curry leaf juice with lime juice and sugar for a stomach-soothing tonic. Because the leaves are a rich source of iron, a meal of curry leaf paste over fish or meat is recommended for anyone who has undergone an operation or suffered blood loss.

As a "grandmother's cure" for dry hair or split ends, mix curry leaves with heated coconut oil for a scalp massage that leaves hair gleaming. For relief from constipation, a soak a handful in hot water, leave for a few hours, and then drink with a spoonful of honey.

Modern healers use curry leaf to treat diabetes because it can control blood glucose levels. It is also used to control high cholesterol—the antioxidants in curry leaves can reduce low-density lipoprotein (LDL), or bad cholesterol while increasing levels of high-density lipoprotein (HDL), or good cholesterol. In addition, curry leaf can protect the gastrointestinal tract. Regularly consuming this herb can also protect the liver and other organs from free radicals.

History and Lore

» The Latin name of the curry tree honors 18th-century German botanist Johann König, who worked as a naturalist for the Nawab of Arcot in southern India and recorded descriptions of many plants used in Indian medicine.
» If the leaves of *tulasi* (holy basil, *Ocimum tenuiflorum*) are not available for the religious rituals performed by Hindus, Buddhists, Jains, and Sikhs to honor a deity, curry leaves may be used instead.

IN THE KITCHEN

Deconstructing Curry Powder

The English term *curry* is given to a host of popular, pungent meat, fish, or vegetable dishes prepared in many parts of Asia. Curries can either be "wet," featuring a sauce or gravy, or "dry," where the spicy mixture coats the other ingredients. Commercial curry powder includes only a few of the ingredients that are found in traditional curry mixtures, which, depending on country of origin, might contain curry leaves, tamarind, coriander, turmeric, ginger, garlic, chili, pepper, mustard seeds, cumin, anise, fenugreek, fennel, poppy seeds, cinnamon, cloves, cardamom, and rosewater. ■

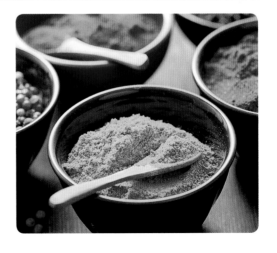

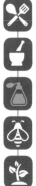

Dandelion

Taraxacum officinale

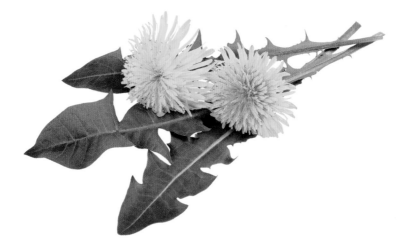

This familiar lawn-invading weed not only makes a tasty salad ingredient if harvested early, nutritionists also recognize it as a prime source of valuable vitamins and minerals, and medical researchers believe it could be a powerful disease-fighting agent.

Dandelions thrive in most temperate regions, as likely to spring up in lush grassy fields as in littered waste grounds. The plant grows prolifically in spring and early summer, but it can bloom and disperse its seeds throughout the growing season.

Dandelion's genus name comes from the Greek words *taraxos*, meaning "disorder," and *akos*, meaning "remedy," indicating that the ancients already understood the healing powers of this humble plant.

The English name is derived from the French *dent de lion*, or "teeth of the lion," which is likely a reference to the jagged-edged leaves (although some varieties have rounded lobes, and some have no indents at all). It is also possible the name refers not to the leaves, but to the flower's color, as in the yellow teeth of the heraldic lion, or to the white, toothlike shade of the root's interior.

A deep, brown taproot leads to a single, purplish stalk topped by a bright yellow bloom of star-shaped florets. When the blooms fade, the head closes up inside its bracts—looking like the nose of a pig or "swine's snout." When all the petals have fallen away, the seeds mature. Prompted by sun and wind, the head reopens, revealing the ball of white fluff that children love. After the plumed seeds, or pappus, have dispersed, the top of the stem appears white, surrounded by drooping bracts. During the Middle Ages, this similarity to a monk's tonsure led to the nickname "priest's crown."

The cheerful yellow flower heads of dandelions mature into fluffy round seed heads. When the seeds are released, the wind can send them drifting up to several hundred yards.

Dandelion Syrup

Make this tasty alternative to maple syrup.

Ingredients
- 4 handfuls of dandelion blossoms
- 1 quart water
- 2 pounds granulated sugar (approximate)
- 2 lemons sliced

Directions

Bring dandelions and water to a boil in medium pan; remove from heat and let sit for 24 hours. Strain and weigh; return to pan and add equal amount of sugar. Add lemon juice, and bring to a boil, them simmer until thick and syrupy. Transfer to sterilized jars while hot. ■

Culinary Uses

Country folk know that young dandelion greens made excellent additions to summer meals, especially if blanched. The leaves can be torn—never cut—into pieces and served in a salad or made into delicate sandwiches with butter and salt. In Wales, the mature root is chopped and added to salads. The young greens can also be boiled and served as a vegetable; if the result is too bitter, spinach can be added.

Nutritional Value

Over the years, so many claims have been made for this plant's astonishing powers that it began to be regarded as a cure-all. The reality is not far off—a 1984 U.S.D.A. bulletin, "Composition of Foods," ranked dandelions among the top-four green vegetables in nutritional value. In addition to offering vitamin B, calcium, potassium, and fiber, they are the richest source of beta-carotene of all green vegetables, and the third-best source for vitamin A, after cod-liver oil and beef liver. Impressive credentials for a plant most homeowners spend money trying to eradicate.

Healing Properties

Arab physicians first wrote about the healing powers of dandelions in the 10th and 11th centuries, calling the plant wild endive. Dandelions were also mentioned in 13th-century Welsh medical literature. Traditional healers used the

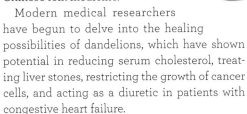

Dandelion salad makes a healthy meal.

root, fresh and dried, as well as the young leaves, while Indian healers cultivated dandelions for treating liver complaints. The plant is still one of the top-six herbs of Chinese folk medicine.

Modern medical researchers have begun to delve into the healing possibilities of dandelions, which have shown potential in reducing serum cholesterol, treating liver stones, restricting the growth of cancer cells, and acting as a diuretic in patients with congestive heart failure.

History and Lore

» Dandelions can predict bad weather. In bright sunlight, the yellow heads are wide open, but if rain threatens, they close up tight.

» At least 93 different types of insects have been identified feeding from the plants' bountiful supply of nectar.

The Beekeeper's Friend

Beekeepers in particular appreciate this plant, because, as one of spring's first arrivals, dandelions furnish bees with nectar and pollen before most other spring plants have bloomed and after fruit trees have stopped flowering. Sufficient dandelions bloom in the fall to nourish bees well into that season, delaying the time when beekeepers have to feed the colony supplemental food. ■

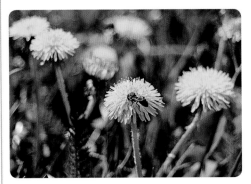

Dandelions are crucial to the survival of the disappearing honeybee, offering pollen and nectar in early spring, when other sources of nutrition are scarce.

Dandelion

Dill

Anethum graveolens

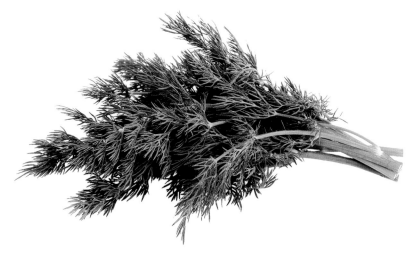

Feathery dill is known for its delicate flavor, as well as its equally delicate presence in the garden. But it is much more than a tasty ornamental. This ancient plant—a rarity that produces both an herb and a spice—was documented as a powerful healing agent as far back as the Bible and in early Egyptian writings. The Romans called it *aneth,* made a tonic from its oil, and considered it a sign of wealth.

Dill, a member of the Apiaceae family, typically reaches two feet in height. The soft, spindly leaves, known as the herb dill weed, have a grassy flavor. Dill seed, the light brown fruit of the tiny yellow flowers, is an aromatic spice with a sweet citrus flavor and bitter undertones. Dill seeds, more intense than dill weed, are similar in appearance and taste to caraway seeds, and are a signature taste profile of the cuisine of Scandinavia and Germany.

DID YOU KNOW?
Grown for the culinary uses of both its leaves and seeds, dill is also a flowering ornamental that attracts beneficial insects to your kitchen garden.

Native to the Mediterranean and western Asia, the plant's name comes from the old Norse *dylla,* meaning "to lull." This reflects dill's effectiveness at calming gastric distress—the Vikings used it to treat infant colic—and treating insomnia.

Culinary Uses

Today, dill is found in the cuisines of Northern and Central Europe, North America, North Africa, the Russian Federation, and the Indian subcontinent. It is typically used to flavor vegetables, potato salad, sauerkraut, German pork roast, cabbage dishes, stews, soups, apple pie, chutney, and breads. In the Middle East, dill seeds perk up cold dishes like *fattosh,* and they are also found in Vietnamese, Thai, and Laotian coconut milk-based fish curries. Iranians use dill in rice dishes, and in Indian Gujarat cuisine it is traditionally given to new mothers.

Dill seed and dill weed are often used together in potato dishes, pickling brine, salad dressings, vinegars, and sauces. The seeds can be rubbed into meats before broiling, while dill weed adds a boost to sweet-fleshed fish, such as salmon and trout, and egg salad and other egg dishes.

Nutritionally, both dill weed and dill seed are good sources of calcium, important for reducing

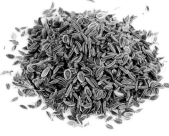

The airy upper leaves of *Anethum graveolens* (above) are used as a the culinary herb dill weed, while the plant's seeds are sold as a savory spice.

Dill and Cucumber Salad

This creamy luncheon side dish tastes best after being refrigerated for at least two hours after preparation. The recipe serves six.

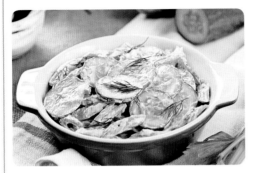

Ingredients
- 5 large cucumbers, sliced and seeded
- 2 teaspoons salt
- ¼ cup fine chopped dill
- 1½ cups sour cream
- ¼ cup apple cider vinegar
- 1½ teaspoons granulated sugar

Directions
Toss cucumbers with 2 teaspoons salt, let drain for an hour or two. Prepare sauce by combining sugar, vinegar, dill, and sour cream, and then spoon over vegetables. Season with salt and pepper, and serve with dill garnish. ■

bone loss after menopause. Dill also offers beneficial levels of vitamin A, vitamin C, dietary fiber, iron, and magnesium.

Healing Properties

Dill has always been valued as a cure for indigestion. Charlemagne offered it to his banquet guests to ease any discomfort after rich, festive meals, and 12th-century Benedictine abbess Hildegard of Bingen, often credited as the first herbalist and naturopath of the Middle Ages, mentioned it in her two treatises on medicine and natural history, *Physica* and *Causae et Curae*.

Dill is known to support the endocrine, immune, and circulatory systems. Its chemical compounds, including monoterpenes and flavonoids, provide antioxidant, disease-preventing, and health-promoting properties. The plant's volatile oils are capable of neutralizing certain types of cancer-causing agents, such as the benzopyrenes in the smoke from cigarettes and charcoal grills. These oils, like garlic, also prevent bacterial overgrowth. Diabetes researchers at the University of Cairo have investigated dill's ability to lower glucose levels and normalize insulin levels (due to the presence of eugenol) and to support pancreatic function.

Aromatic Qualities

Dill's essential oil has a spicy, fresh, invigorating aroma, and in aromatherapy it is used to treat digestive ailments, liver deficiencies, bronchial problems, and headaches. Dill diffused with chamomile is extremely calming to the nervous system. The essential oil also combines well with nutmeg and the citrus oils lemon, orange, grapefruit. The oil can be applied topically to the abdomen and the bottom of feet, or taken as a supplement in food or rice milk.

History and Lore

» First-century Romans believed dill was good luck. They made wreaths and garlands out of the plant, while gladiators rubbed their skin with the herb before combat.

» According to folklore, dill has the power to keep witches away.

» In the United States, dill is indelibly linked with pickles, which Americans consume nine pounds of each year.

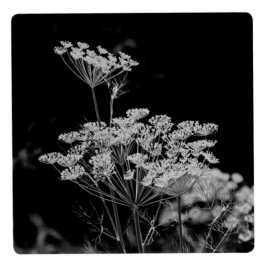

Yellow dill flowers are typical of the Apiaceae family, with large, rounded, compound umbels atop stiff, hollow stems.

Dill

Fennel

Foeniculum vulgare

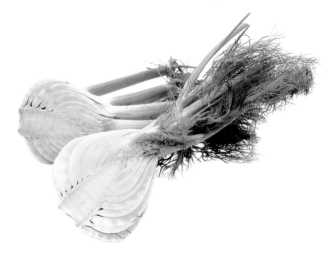

ennel is a versatile plant; in fact, all parts of the plant are edible, from the white or pale green bulb to the multiple stalks to the airy green leaves to the seeds (fruit), which develop from its bright yellow flowers.

The genus name comes from the Latin *foeniculum,* or "little hay." In the Middle Ages, the common name evolved to *fanculum,* and was then popularized as "fenkel" or "finule." Fennel is today considered the only member of the genus. A native of the Mediterranean, this perennial plant was utilized by the ancient Greeks and was spread throughout Europe by invading Roman armies. It now also grows in India, Asia, Australia, and South America, and it has become naturalized in North America.

A member of the vast Apiaceae family, it grows best in dry soil near seacoasts or on riverbanks. In the garden, it is a striking plant, with many sturdy sleek green stems rising four feet

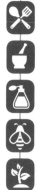

A fennel flower goes to seed.

DID YOU KNOW?
A crunchy, sweet-tasting staple of Italian cooking, fennel is classified as both an herb and a spice.

or more; narrow, threadlike leaves; and sunny yellow flowers that form large, flat umbels that bloom in July and August. As Longfellow wrote: "Above the lower plants it towers; The Fennel with its yellow flowers."

Culinary Uses

The Romans enjoyed fennel as a vegetable; fennel seed and fennel shoots were mentioned in records of Spanish agriculture dating from A.D. 961; and it was a documented part of Anglo-Saxon cookery—and medicine—before the Norman Conquest.

The fresh seeds, identified by their green color, have a pleasant taste reminiscent of anise and are used to flavor cake, pastries, bread, soups, stews, pickles, fish, and sauerkraut. Italian cooks use the seeds to flavor sausage and the stems in soup or salad. The dill-like leaves can be added to seafood dishes or soups, while the crisp bulbs are typically served as a vegetable, either sautéed, braised, stewed, grilled, or raw. In France, it is one of the three main ingredients of absinthe, and it is an important spice in regional Indian cookery, as well as in Pakistan, Afghanistan, and Iran. In India and Pakistan, the roasted seeds are often chewed as a post-meal breath freshener. In China, it is an essential component of five-spice powders.

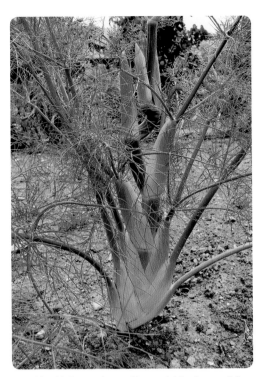

Fennel is a kitchen garden workhorse, yielding leaves, stalks, seeds, and bulbs that are all edible.

Nutritional Value

Fennel seeds are a rich source of dietary fiber. They also contain the minerals copper, iron, calcium, potassium, manganese, and magnesium, and the A, B-complex, C, and E vitamins.

Healing Properties

This herb has been used in alternative medicine to prevent gas, gout, cramps, heartburn, cystitis, colic, and spasms. It is sometimes used to flavor natural toothpaste.

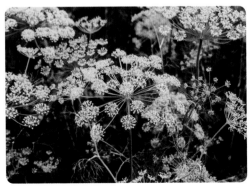

The flower head of fennel consists of umbels with 20 to 50 tiny yellow flowers extending from single stalks called pedicels.

The Origins of the Marathon

The plains of Marathon, where the outnumbered Athenians defeated the invading Persian army in 490 B.C., was so named because fennel, called *marathon* in Greek, grew there in great profusion. At the end of the critical battle, the Athenians sent messenger Pheidippides back to their city with the news. He ran a distance of approximately 26 miles and died after reporting the victory. ■

In 1657, botanist William Coles commented in *Adam in Eden, or Nature's Paradise* that drinks or broths made from the leaves and roots caused the stout patient to become gaunt and lank. This might explain the ancient Greek name for the herb, *marathon,* from *maraino,* "to grow thin."

Fennel has been found by modern researchers to contain beneficial volatile essential oil compounds such as anethole, limonene, anisic aldehyde, pinene, myrcene, fenchone, chavicol, and cineol. These account for the herb's digestive, antioxidant, carminative, and antiflatulent properties. The seeds also contain flavonoid antioxidants such as kaempferol and quercetin, which help the body remove harmful free radicals.

History and Lore

» The Puritans called fennel the "meeting" seed because they often chewed it during long church services. Similarly, many poor Catholics ate fennel seeds to ward off hunger on fast days.

» Medieval villagers hung fennel, along with St. John's wort and other herbs, over their doors on Midsummer's Eve to protect their homes from witchcraft and other evils.

» In the Middle Ages, it was believed that serpents or snakes sharpened their eyesight by rubbing against the plant: "Whaune the adder is hurt in eye, Ye red fenel is hys prey."

» Modern Roman bakers place fennel under their bread while baking to add flavor to the loaves.

» Fennel gives off ozone, and, in its powered form, it is said to repel fleas from stables and kennels.

Fennel

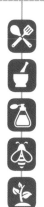

Fenugreek

Trigonella foenum-graecum

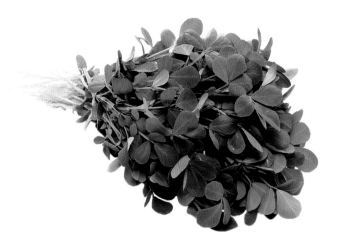

Fenugreek, an annual plant in the legume family Fabaceae, has long been used as a flavoring agent and an herbal supplement. Charred remains of the seeds have been carbon dated to 4000 B.C., while desiccated seeds were found in the tomb of Tutankhamun. The first written record of the herb was on an Egyptian papyrus dating from 1500 B.C.

The fenugreek plant reaches a height of two feet, and features small, light green, cloverlike leaves and long yellow seedpods. The yellow

DID YOU KNOW?

Fenugreek is a versatile plant whose fresh leaves, sprouts, and dried leaves and seeds are, respectively, an herb, a vegetable, and a spice.

or white flowers grow singly or in pairs. It is grown commercially as a semi-arid crop, most notably in Afghanistan, Pakistan, Argentina, Egypt, France, Spain, Turkey, and Morocco. India is the main commercial producer worldwide (with 80 percent grown in Rajasthan). Not surprisingly, fenugreek seeds are a mainstay of Indian cuisine.

Culinary Uses

The seeds, whole or powdered, are used in India for pickling and to make vegetable dishes, daals, and spice mixtures such as *panch phoron* and *sambar*. The leaves are sometimes used in curries, while the sprouts are mixed into salads. In Persian cuisine, the leaves are used to make *ghormeh sabzi,* an herb stew that is often called the Iranian national dish. Yemenite Jews believe that fenugreek is the Talmudic herb rubia; they use it to prepare a curry-like sauce called *hilbeh* that is eaten on the first and second night of Rosh Hashanah , the Jewish New Year.

Nutritional Value

Fenugreek leaves and seeds are rich in fiber and contain thiamin, folic acid, riboflavin, niacin, and vitamins A, B6, C, E, and K. They supply

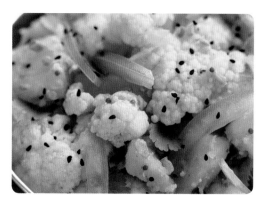

Dried fenugreek leaves are a key ingredient in *aloo gobi,* a cauliflower and potato dish that is found on many Indian restaurant menus in the United States.

Nutritional Value

Hibiscus packs a powerful nutritional punch. Hibiscus tea, for example, contains 31 percent of the daily requirement of vitamin C, a hefty 85 percent of thiamin, and 48 percent of the daily iron requirement.

Healing Properties

Natural healers have used hibiscus for many centuries; in ancient Indian scriptures, *Hibiscus rosa-sinensis* was recommended for treating numerous ailments. It offers a wealth of medicinal possibilities to herbalists, who use all parts of the plant. It is known to be a laxative, diuretic, antibacterial, and antiscorbutic (prevents scurvy) due to its high levels of vitamin C. This also makes it a good choice for treating colds and the flu. Hibiscus tea, sometimes called sour tea for its tart taste, is full of antioxidants that protect the liver, stimulate appetite, reduce fevers, ease coughs, and help repair chapped or irritated skin.

Recently, scientists studying metabolic syndrome, the name given to group of risk factors for heart disease—including high blood sugar, high triglycerides, high blood pressure, and large waistline—have proposed that the antioxidant and anti-inflammatory polyphenols in hibiscus might be useful in treating or even preventing

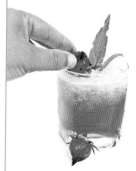
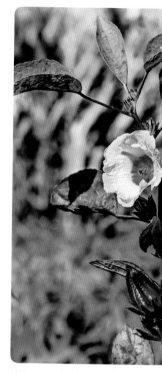

Sitting on reddish stems, the yellow or [...] *Hibiscus sabdariffa* feature a deep-red [...] At the end of the day, the blooms will f[...]

this condition. Studies have s[...] *dariffa* can lower blood pressure[...] ACE inhibitor (angiotensin-cc[...] inhibitor), something the Iran[...] to have known for decades, w[...] glasses of sour tea. Other resea[...] the plant's antioxidants might [...] tain cancers. After a 2009 study[...] tions that consuming hibiscus t[...] help diabetes patients manag[...] lowering their LDL (low-densi[...] "bad cholesterol") and raising [...] density lipoprotein or "good ch[...]

History and Lore

» The genus name comes from t[...] which was what they called th[...]
» This is a plant of many names. [...] cus, roselle, and Jamaican sor[...] Indian sorrel, red sorrel, *ma[...] cabitutu, rosa de Jamaica,* an[...]
» *H. sabdariffa* is often cultiva[...] fiber, which can be used as a [...] fashion durable rope.

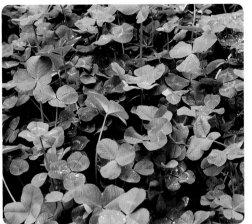

Fenugreek, with its cloverlike leaves, is a fast growing plant.

copper, calcium, potassium, iron, selenium, zinc, manganese, and magnesium. The seeds also contain the alkaloid trigonelline, the amino acids l-tryptophan and lysine, as well as large amounts of the natural detergent saponin.

Healing Properties

In traditional medicine, especially among the Chinese and Indians, fenugreek seeds were used as an aid for gastritis or constipation (the mucilage the seeds release creates a soothing coating on the digestive organs), to treat high blood pressure and high cholesterol, as an aphrodisiac, to induce labor, to stimulate the production of milk in new mothers, and to treat kidney ailments, beriberi, mouth ulcers, cellulite, cancer, and diabetes. Applied in a poultice, powdered seeds were used to treat swelling, muscle aches, wounds, and eczema.

Fenugreek is a potent source of alkaloids and estrogens. Early research indicates that the plant slows the

Fenugreek leaves, pods, and seeds

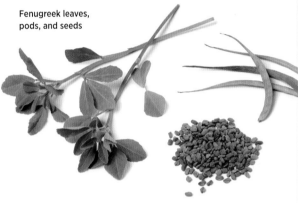

absorption of sugars in the stomach and can lower serum glucose levels (fenugreek contains an amino acid called 4-hydroxyisoleucine, which appears to increase the body's production of insulin when blood sugar levels are high). This data is not yet definitive, however. There is also some evidence that fenugreek can help restore healthy levels of cholesterol, and it may also reduce the amount of calcium oxalate in the kidneys, a contributing factor to the formation of kidney stones.

The seeds are rich in diogenin, a substance that mimics estrogen and may have anti-cancer properties.

History and Lore

» Cato the Elder listed fenugreek with clover and vetch as crops grown to feed cattle.
» The herb's sweet, maple-like flavor allows it to mask the taste of other medications. Sotolon is the chemical responsible for that distinctive sweet smell.
» Fenugreek is also known as Greek hay seed and bird's foot.

Hibiscus

Hibiscus sabdariffa

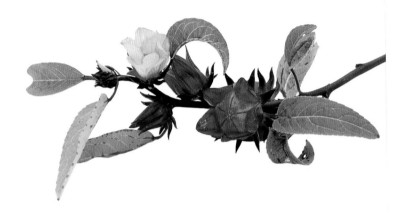

Although it is believed to have originated in Egypt, the hibiscus is now found in many parts of the world, including India, Africa, Sudan, Jamaica, China, Philippines, Mexico, and the United States. There are more than two hundred species, including hybrids. The culinary species of hibiscus, also known as the roselle, bears striking yellow or buff flowers with rose or maroon eyes. The flowers turn pink as they wither at the end of the day. After blooming, the flower sepals enlarge, becoming fleshy and crisp but juicy, with a cranberry-like flavor.

The plant flourishes in tropical or warm-temperate gardens; it is popular with landscapers, and is a major attractant to butterflies, bees, hummingbirds, and other pollinators.

DID YOU KNOW?

Plant lovers know the hibiscus, a member of the Malvaceae, or mallow family, as a bushy annual that produces large, graceful, trumpet-shaped flowers in vibrant colors.

Culinary Us[...]

Hibiscus flowers [...] known as the s[...] herbal tea, which [...] and cold, but the [...] also edible and o[...] can cooking. The [...] made into a delici[...] be blended into s[...] make granita or [...] vinaigrette, or mi[...] fruit vodka for a "Jamaican [...] jam or jelly is especially good [...] on a cracker or crostini.

The plant is often called Jam[...] in Mexico and the Caribbean [...] sepals are boiled down into a re[...] *agua de flor de Jamaica,* whi[...] and sold commercially. In Jama[...] *Hibiscus sabdariffa* are used t[...] red drink called sorrel. Despite [...] hibiscus is not related to *Rume[...]* is also commonly known as sor[...]

In Egypt, parts of the flower [...] *karkadé,* a popular drink serve[...] China, the seeds are used to pro[...] oil. They can also be dried and g[...] as a coffee substitute. The plant's [...] an aperitif in the Philippines.

In Jamaica and other parts of the Caribbean, the ruby-colored sorrel drink made from *Hibiscus sabdariffa* is considered an integral part of Christmas celebrations.

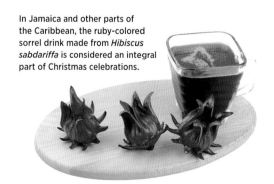

Hops

Humulus lupulus

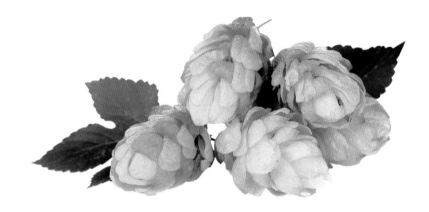

Hops, the female flowers (also known as seed cones or strobiles) of the hop plant, are used to stabilize beer as well as lend it a tangy flavor. This vigorous climbing perennial, which can reach 20 feet in length, is typically trained to grow up strings or trellises. The plant was most likely first cultivated in Germany—there is mention of a hops garden in the eighth-century will of Pepin III, the father of Charlemagne, but there is no indication of hops being used to flavor beer until at least the ninth century.

DID YOU KNOW?

For centuries, the ripened seed cones of the female hop plant *(Humulus lupulus)* have been used to brew beer, one of the world's oldest beverages.

Today, hops are grown worldwide in any moist, temperate climate. Key production centers are the Hallertau in Germany, the Yakima Valley in Washington, the Willamette Valley in Oregon, Canyon County in Idaho, and Kent in the United Kingdom.

Culinary Uses

Beer is an alcoholic malt beverage—created by the fermentation of starch into sugar—that possibly dates back to 9500 B.C. Some time around the tenth century, hops were added to the basic recipe of malted grain, brewer's yeast, and water. Hops furnish a needed bitter counterpoint to the sweet taste of the malt, and they also supply an antibacterial effect that favors brewer's yeast over other less-desirable microorganisms formed during the fermenting process. Early brewers who used gruit, an herbal mixture, to flavor their beer, switched to hops when they realized it reduced spoilage. In the Middle Ages, when untreated water was not safe to drink, weak or "small" beer was the thirst quencher of choice, even for children. Most villages boasted their own hop garden, barley field, and a small brewery or two.

Modern beer production is a billion-dollar industry, and many varieties of hops are grown

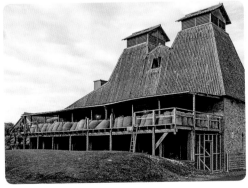

A functioning hop house in Kent, England. Also known as an oast house or hop kiln, this type of building was designed for drying hops as part of the beer and ale brewing process.

commercially, allowing brewers to create different styles of beer. Microbreweries that specialized in artisanal beers sprang up in many cities near the end of the 20th century, while home-brewing also became popular.

Nutritional Value

Hops contain antiseptic and pain-relieving essential oils, as well as the antioxidant vitamins E, C, and B6. The phytoestrogens hops supply to the body mimic estrogen and support bone and heart health.

Healing Properties

Traditional healers use hops to treat insomnia—sometimes in conjunction with valerian or melatonin, as well as to combat anxiety. Hops are also used to relieve gastric distress, and the plant's estrogenic effects may ease menstrual cramps.

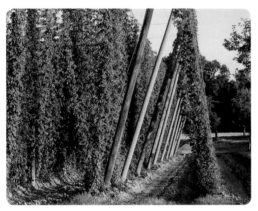

Hop vines need a strong support; tall poles or a sturdy trellis and heavy twine will encourage the growing vines. Healthy hop plants can grow as much as a foot in one day.

Drink to Your Health!

Raising a glass was not always a healthy bet; water once often carried deadly pathogens, such as cholera and typhoid. These days, most of us take a plentiful supply of clean drinking water piped directly to our homes for granted, but before the days of public sanitation, the thirst quencher of choice was beer. Water could easily make one sick, so even children partook of this hop-based beverage in the form of small beer. It contained very little alcohol, but there was enough to kill most water-borne pathogens, and the boiling that takes place during the brewing process further ensured a safe quaff. ■

Modern research shows that hops are a significant source of antioxidants, on a par with red wine. They contain organic compounds believed to fight, or even prevent, osteoporosis, and they can also reduce levels of calcium and so halt the formation of kidney stones. You can take hops as a supplement, or simply imbibe it in a cup of tea or glass of beer. On the other hand, an excess of hops consumption might result in gastric distress, irregular menstruation, and loss of libido in men.

History and Lore

» The species name, *lupulus,* means "small wolf" in Latin and refers to the plant's aggressive habit of smothering other growth.
» Hop farmers in southern England sometimes issued their own coins to pay harvesters; some featured beautiful images of hops.

A Family Affair: Society and Harvesting Hops

The harvesting of hops before the days of agricultural mechanization was so labor intensive that, in addition to migrant workers, entire families would be recruited from the larger cities to bring in the crop. In spite of the hard work, this arrangement offered poor urban families a chance to experience healthful country life and live in "hopper's huts" for the duration of the harvest.

At the turn of the 20th century, German-American entrepreneur Emil Clemons Horst owned vast acres of hops farms in the American West, which required extensive labor camps to maintain them. When the conditions at these camps became "unspeakably" bad, both his American and Japanese workers went on strike. In 1913, the Wheatland Hop Riot broke out at Horst's Durst Ranch, resulting in four deaths. This conflict, one of the first farm labor confrontations in California, was blamed on the radical Industrial Workers of the World (IWW). In 1909, Horst invented a mechanical hops separator that revolutionized harvesting—and soon did away with the culture of the "hopper hut" workers. ■

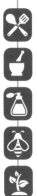

Lemongrass

Cymbopogon citratus, C. flexuosus

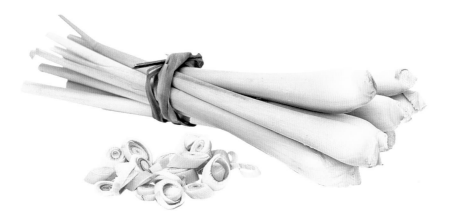

Originating in India and tropical Asia, this tall, perennial grass now boasts as many as 45 species and can be found in most warm-temperate or tropical regions of the Old World and Oceania.

West Indian lemongrass (*Cymbopogon citratus*) furnishes a pleasing citrus flavor to Southeast Asian teas, soups, marinades, and curries, as well as to Jamaican dishes. In the United States, where

DID YOU KNOW?

The subtle citrus taste and aroma of lemongrass has made this Southeast Asian native a welcome addition to gardens and kitchens everywhere.

the herb has become a favorite of home cooks, the chief commercial sources are California and Florida. A related species, Indian lemongrass (*C. flexuosus*), is used as a fragrance in soaps and cosmetics.

Lemongrass rarely flowers, but it is an attractive, willowy addition to the garden, growing in dense clumps from a bulbous base to a height of about three feet. When harvesting for cooking, look for fresh green blades.

Culinary Uses

Lemongrass's entire stalk—the stems and leaf buds—can be finely sliced and added to recipes, although some cooks prefer to discard the grass after cooking. Whether used fresh or dried and powdered, lemongrass adds a zesty note to poultry, fish, and seafood dishes. It blends especially well with cilantro, garlic, and chilies. The herb can end up tasting pungent, however, so it should be added in small amounts.

Tom yum, one of Thailand's favorite soups, is made from fresh lemongrass, kaffir lime leaves, galangal, lime juice, fish sauce, and crushed chili peppers, often with the addition of prawns, fish, poultry, or mushrooms. Lemongrass is also delicious brewed into tea, either hot or iced.

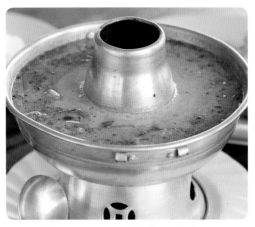

Made with lemongrass, *tom yum* is a hot and spicy soup enjoyed in Thailand and also in Laos. Variations of this soup include additional meats such as prawns or chicken.

Fresh lemongrass can be found in Asian or Mexican markets all year long. It will keep in a plastic bag for several weeks; frozen, it will last up to six months. Dried lemongrass needs to be soaked in water to reconstitute it prior to use.

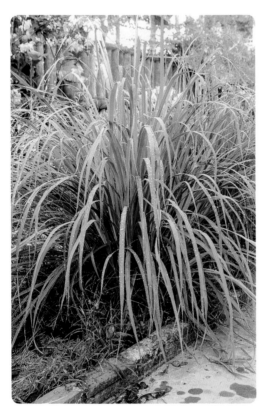

Its fragrant swordlike leaves make lemongrass an attention-grabbing garden plant. Although its essential oil repels many insects, honeybees are attracted to it.

CURIOSITIES

Versatile Citronella Oil

Two species related to lemongrass, called citronella grass (*Cymbopogon nardus* and *C. winterianus),* contain essential oils that repel insects, most notably, mosquitoes. The oils are used commercially in insect-repelling soaps, sprays, and candles. When grown in gardens, these plants will also discourage white flies and other garden invaders.

Conservators at museums in India that collect ancient manuscripts also use citronella oil as a preservative for their fragile palm leaf books. The essential oil makes the leaves supple, while keeping them dry enough to prevent humidity from destroying the text. ■

IN THE KITCHEN

Lemongrass-Infused Olive Oil

This herb-infused oil is delicious as a bread dip, salad dressing, or marinade.

Ingredients
- ⅓ cup olive oil
- fresh rosemary twig
- fresh lemongrass blades
- fresh thyme twig
- 1 clove of garlic
- salt
- red and black peppercorns

Directions
Combine all ingredients in a glass container; let sit for a week. Shake vigorously, and serve. ■

Nutritional Value

Lemongrass is an excellent source of folic acid, as well as vitamin B5, vitamin B6, and vitamin B1 (thiamin). The herb contains significant amounts of potassium, zinc, calcium, iron, manganese, copper, and magnesium.

Healing Properties

Traditional healers have used lemongrass to treat digestive tract spasms, stomach pain, high blood pressure, convulsions, vomiting, coughing, sore throat, joint aches, fever, colds, and exhaustion. The herb also possesses mild astringent properties and is used to kill germs. The essential oil can be placed directly on the skin to treat headaches, stomachaches, and muscle pain.

Lemongrass's main chemical component is an antimicrobial and antifungal aldehyde called citral, the active ingredient in lemon peel, which has been shown to ease spasms and relieve pain.

History and Lore

» Lemongrass oil is an effective lure to help recapture honeybees that have swarmed away from the hive.
» If you like the taste of lemon *and* cream in your tea, add lemongrass—it won't curdle cream.
» International names include: *citronnelle* in France; *zitronengras* in Germany; *erba di limone* in Italy; and *bhustrina, sera* in India.

Lemongrass

49

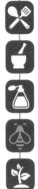

Licorice

Glycyrrhiza glabra

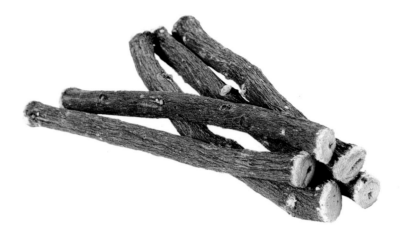

This distinctive flavor—used in candy whips and "allsorts" mixtures—is familiar to most people since childhood. Licorice flavoring is processed from the root of the licorice plant, a tall, perennial legume with purple or lavender flowers that grows in southern Europe and parts of Asia. Traditional healers as far back as ancient Egypt and Syria used it to treat a wide range of ailments, and vast stores of the root were found in

DID YOU KNOW?
The fibrous root of the licorice plant produces the distinctive flavoring often found in candy and other sweets. It is also used medicinally.

Tutankhamun's tomb. The name—often spelled "liquorice"—comes from the Old French *licoresse*, which in turn came from the Greek *glukurrhiza*, which means "sweet root."

Culinary Uses

In more modern times, licorice was first combined with sugar and used to flavor cakes (round candies) in Pontefract, Yorkshire, where there is still an annual licorice festival. Today, most licorice-flavored sweets have the taste augmented by aniseed oil, and the amount of actual licorice is low, except in the Netherlands, the "licorice drop capital," where supplemental anise flavorings are rarely used. The Dutch do, however, mix licorice with mint, menthol, or laurel. The distinctive flavor of licorice comes from a sweet-tasting compound called anethole, an aromatic, unsaturated ether also found in other anise-flavored plants. Even though their flavors are similar, licorice is not botanically related to anise, star anise, or fennel.

Licorice in its natural form is popular in southern Italy and Spain, where the root is dug up, cleansed, and chewed as a mouth freshener. The Chinese use it as a culinary spice and add it to savory dishes. It is also enjoyed around the world

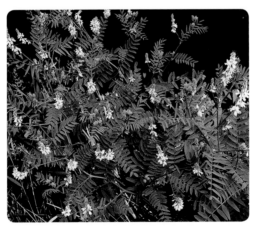

A licorice plant. Licorice has a long history of use in Western herbal medicine, and it has often been employed to disguise the unpleasant taste of other medications.

as a soothing, stomach-calming tea, and a beverage called *mai sus,* brewed from the sweet root, is popular in the Middle East.

Nutritional Value

Licorice root contains healthful amino acids, amines, and flavonoids, as well as beta-carotene, vitamin C. It also contains the minerals calcium, iron, magnesium, manganese, selenium, phosphorus, potassium, silicon, and zinc.

Healing Properties

Herbal healers recommend licorice for treating asthma, athlete's foot, baldness, body odor, bursitis, colds and flu, tooth decay, gout, fatigue, depression, Lyme disease, liver problems, shingles, prostate enlargement, yeast infections, and arthritis. In Chinese herbal medicine, it is considered a "balancing" or "stabilizing" agent. As such, it is added to many herbal formulas, including those for treating ulcers, canker sores, and cold sores, for soothing coughs, and for reducing inflammation.

Modern researchers have documented many of the effects of this "wonder herb," and they concur that licorice does relieve ulcers, not by reducing stomach acid, but by enabling the digestive mucosal tissues to protect themselves from stomach acid. The botanical increases the action of mucus-secreting cells, thus prolonging the life of surface cells in the intestines.

Research has also discovered that the saponin found in licorice, glyzcyrrhizic acid (or glycyrrhizin), extends the time that inflammation-reducing cortisol circulates through the body. Licorice has been used to treat inflammation of

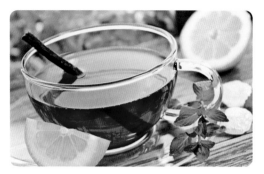
Licorice makes a healthful, soothing, and appetizing tea.

the lungs, bowels, and skin, and it may also play a key role in boosting immunity by raising levels of interferon, a chemical that fights off viruses. Moderate doses of licorice, 100 milligrams a day, can also counteract LDL (low-density lipoprotein, often called the "bad cholesterol") and prevent plaque from forming and clogging arteries.

The glycyrrhizin in licorice can mimic the hormone aldosterone, which causes water retention and raises blood pressure, so consumption should be monitored. A licorice product made without glycyrrhizin is called deglycyrrhizinated licorice, or DGL.

History and Lore

» The glycyrrhizin in licorice is 30 to 60 times sweeter than sugar.
» The ancient Greeks learned of the health benefits of licorice from the Scythians in the third century B.C.
» Alexander the Great supplied his troops with sticks of licorice root to ease their thirst and increase their vigor prior to battle.

The Tobacco Connection

Even though natural healers laud licorice as a versatile herbal remedy, an estimated 90 percent of licorice extract is added to tobacco products. Licorice, which blends easily with the other natural and artificial flavorings used in tobacco, can be found in cigarettes, moist snuff, chewing tobacco, and pipe tobacco. Licorice cuts down on harshness, and also makes it easier to inhale by creating bronchodilators that open up the lungs. Some people claim licorice candy help them quit cigarettes by satisfying some part of their craving. ■

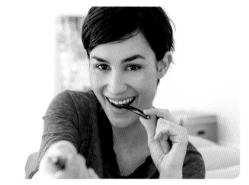
Have a bite of licorice instead of lighting up.

Licorice

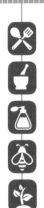

Lovage

Levisticum officinale

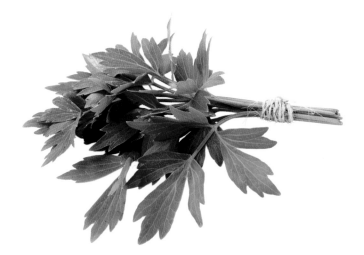

It may not be as popular as other traditional herbs, but lovage is a versatile garden plant—the leaves can be used as an herb, the root as a vegetable, and the seeds as a spice.

It is most likely native to Europe, the Middle East, and central Asia, although some botanists believe that the plant was spread and naturalized throughout Europe by the Romans. However it spread, though, lovage has a long history as a taste enhancer, an aromatic, and an herbal remedy.

It is a strapping, spreading plant that can grow as tall as four feet if given good soil, sun, and sufficient water. An erect perennial, this member of the carrot family features a basal rosette of finely cut leaves with additional leaves on the stem. Both its stem and leaves are a bright, shiny green, like an oversized version of Italian parsley, and the tiny yellow-green flowers form graceful umbels.

The plant's name comes from love-ache, *(ache* being the medieval name for parsley), and was derived from the old French *levesche.*

Culinary Uses

Lovage leaves smell of lime when crushed, although their taste is more like a blend of celery

DID YOU KNOW?

The attractive foliage of lovage, along with its pleasing scent, make it a welcome addition to the backyard garden. It is also used commercially as a fragrance in cosmetics, lotions, and soaps.

and parsley. They are most often used in salads or to season soups, especially in Romania, where lovage flavors the local broth. In Mediterranean countries, the chopped leaves are added to tomato sauce.

Lovage's clean, crisp taste works well with egg and potato dishes, rice, cream soups, and cucumbers. It can also be used wherever celery is recommended—in stews, casseroles, and stuffing. Tender, delicate young leaves are best for cooking, but both leaves and stems can be dried and stored for winter use.

The root is often grated or sliced before serving. The brown seeds are similar in taste to fennel, celery, or caraway seeds and may be substituted for them.

Nutritional Value

Lovage is rich in vitamin C and the B-complex vitamins. It is also high in the antioxidant quercetin.

Healing Properties

This herb could be found growing in many village or monastery physic gardens during the Middle Ages; it was used for treating stomach complaints and urinary tract ailments, to prevent kidney stones, as an antiseptic, and to relieve gout, boils, and migraines. Earlier, the Greeks chewed it to improve digestion and relieve gas.

The plant is unusually high in quercetin (third behind green tea and capers), an antioxidant flavonoid. Ongoing medical research indicates that quercetin acts as bronchodilator when prescribed for asthma, has a remarkably high inhibitory effect on hepatitis C virus replication, and can reduce inflammation in the urinary tract. A 2010 study at the University of Mainz in Germany observed that essential oil of lovage inhibited the growth of squamous carcinoma cells of the head and neck. Other chemical compounds in the essential oils may prove to destroy viruses or lower bad cholesterol.

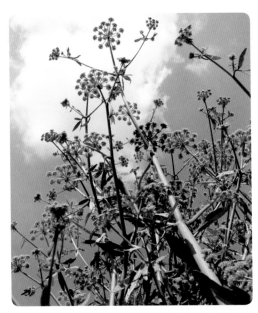

This tall, erect plant makes a statement in the garden and will prove a favorite of bees. In the spring, the larvae of the black swallowtail butterfly may nibble the leaves.

History and Lore

» Dr. Samuel Johnson recommended the herb for rheumatism.

» Colonial Americans brought the herb from England and drank it as a tea to cure aches and pains.

» In England, the nonalcoholic lovage cordial becomes a warming winter drink when mixed with brandy.

» As the name may suggest, this herb was used in love potions or worn in a sachet when visiting the love object.

Light and Tasty Lovage Soup

This creamy soup, seasoned with lovage, is perfect for a spring or summer luncheon.

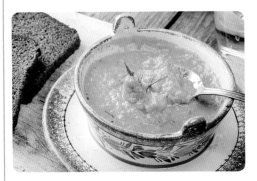

Ingredients

- 2 tablespoons butter
- 1 bunch chives, white and light-green parts chopped
- 1 medium yellow onion, peeled and chopped
- 2 quarts chicken stock
- 3 medium potatoes, peeled and chopped
- 1 bunch (1 ounce) lovage leaves, chopped fine
- heavy cream, to taste

Directions

Melt butter in stockpot over medium-high heat until it froths; reduce heat to medium, and stir in onions. Sauté until fragrant, about five minutes. Pour in chicken stock, and stir in chopped potatoes. Simmer covered, about 30 minutes, until potatoes are tender. Stir in lovage and simmer, covered, five or six minutes. Remove from heat and blend well with immersion blender. Season with sea salt and freshly ground pepper. Stir in heavy cream and serve. Serves six to eight. ■

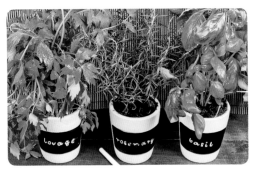

Lovage can be planted in pots for a kitchen garden.

Lovage

53

KITCHEN GARDENS

Add flavorful and attractive herbs to your landscape.

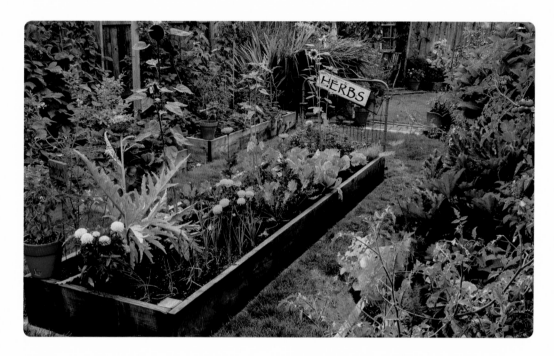

Herbs are not only delicious and beneficial, many of them—with their wide variety of leaves and striking flowers—also make wonderful visual additions to the garden. They can be grown in a casual kitchen garden, offering the option of fresh flavors just outside the back door, or can be used to define a more structured parterre. Ornamental herbs taste just as good as the ones grown for the table, so don't feel bad if you pluck a few leaves as you stroll the formal paths.

Kitchen Gardens

From the time humans began to culti-vate crops, they understood the wisdom of keeping a garden with certain essen-tials—fruits, vegetables, and herbs—near their main dwellings. This gave rise to the potager, or kitchen garden, a space dedicated to supplying fresh produce on a daily basis, an idea that modern gar-deners and cooks have readily adopted.

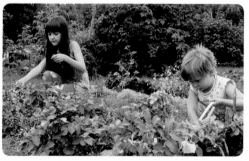

Anyone who has walked a few yards from the house to pick zucchini or carrots, collect a handful of basil, or fill a basket of strawberries understands the joys of a kitchen garden.

Parterres: Displaying Herbs in a Formal Setting

Parterres are symmetrical formal gardens laid out on a level surface, with crisp edges and gravel walkways. They were first created during the French Renaissance by landscapers who arranged elegant, geometric gardens for their noble patrons, and who based them on earlier knot gardens. The parterre reached its height at the palace of Versailles, where the elaborate patterns were best viewed from above.

As envisioned by 16th-century landscaper Claude Mollet, the parterre consisted of interlaces made of herbs, their centers filled with sand or flowers. The parterre fell out of favor by the 18th century, when more naturalistic British landscaping became the rage.

Small home parterres are relatively easy to create. Simply block out your cultivation areas on a cleared, level space with landscaping paint and a yardstick or string, edge them with flexible plastic, and fill in with herbs. Use pea gravel or crushed rock for smooth, weed-free walkways. Woody herbs, especially, make superior edging plants for parterres because they can be clipped and shaped. Low, spreading, flowering herbs, such as sage, are effective as center plantings. ■

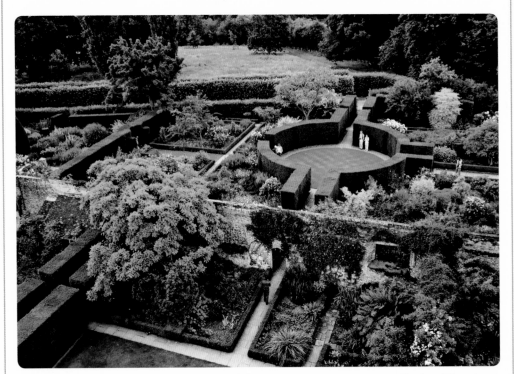

The garden as Sissinghurst Castle in England allows luxurious plantings to spill from the structured borders of the parterres.

Herbs do especially well in a kitchen garden and attract beneficial insects. Locate your garden away from overhanging trees for better sun exposure, and augment with well-drained soil (easy to accomplish using raised beds). A few small trees, perennial shrubs, or evergreens will add interest before the growing season begins and after the annuals have died back. And don't forget to plant protective companion herbs, such as borage, next to their corresponding vegetables—tomatoes and cabbage.

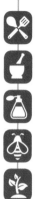

Marjoram

Origanum majorana

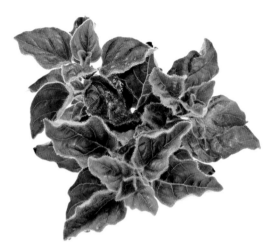

Marjoram, also known as sweet marjoram, is a favored herb in the kitchen and a powerful curative in the herbal pharmacopoeia. Most likely originating in Northern Africa and Arabia, this member of the mint family is now cultivated in gardens around the world—although it also grows wild in grassy areas.

A perennial herb, and a member of the Lamiaceae, marjoram can be cold sensitive. It has a downy stem and oval, opposite leaves of a soft gray-green. The tiny white or pink flowers emerge from knot-shaped buds, leading some gardeners to call the herb "knot marjoram." In a 2013 study, scientists found that the flowers of marjoram, along with those of lavender and borage, were among the ones most attractive to honeybees.

DID YOU KNOW?

A low-growing plant, marjoram thrives in an outdoor garden or in a kitchen window. It also makes a pretty summer ground cover or edging.

Culinary Uses

With its piney-citrus notes, marjoram is one of the main components of Mediterranean cuisine. Its taste is similar to oregano, but marjoram has a milder flavor profile than its cousin. It can be used fresh, dried, or powdered in soups, sauces, egg and meat dishes, and salad dressings. It enhances the flavor of vegetables like cauliflower, spinach, peas, and tomatoes, and it also blends well with other herbs—when combined with thyme, tarragon, bay leaf, and parsley it forms the bouquet garni used in classic French cuisine. This herb is familiar to most Americans as a key flavoring of turkey stuffing, pizza sauce, and Italian sausage links.

When shopping for fresh marjoram, choose gray-green leaves, and avoid yellow leaves. At home, rinse well under water to remove dust and pesticides, and store in the refrigerator. To make your own dried marjoram from any leftover leaves, dry the stem tips on a cookie sheet in a 150-degree oven for three hours. Dried marjoram is always a good option—delivering almost as much flavor as the fresh leaves.

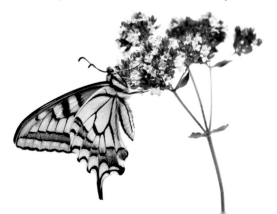

A common yellow swallowtail *(Papilio machaon)* butterfly visits a marjoram flower. The plant will attract butterflies, bees, and other pollinators during its summer bloom.

Stress-Buster Tea

Perhaps the easiest way to enjoy the health benefits of this herb is in a simple tea, which can soothe an anxious or upset stomach. Add a teaspoon of ground marjoram to a cup of cold water, and let it sit over night. Add a spoonful of honey or a dash of lemon juice before drinking it hot or iced. ■

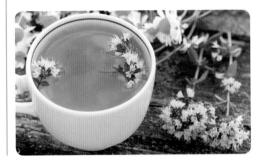

Nutritional Value

This herb contains substantial levels of vitamins A and C, and is an important source of vitamin K, which promotes bone health and limits neuronal damage in the brain. Marjoram also supplies high amounts of iron, as well as calcium, potassium, copper, zinc, manganese, and magnesium.

Healing Properties

In the past, marjoram has been used by healers to relieve digestive complaints such as nervous stomach, loss of appetite, gas, cramps, diarrhea and constipation. With its antiseptic, antiviral, and antifungal benefits, it has been effective against staph infections, typhoid, malaria, flu,

Marjoram has a spicy citrus scent—similar to oregano—that appeals to both men and women. It is sometimes used commercially in skin creams, shaving gels, bath soaps, and body lotions.

colds, mumps, and measles, and it has improved heart health by lowering bad cholesterol, lowering blood pressure, and improving circulation by dilating the arteries. Its anti-inflammatory properties make it useful for treating asthma, sinus headaches and migraines, fever, and body aches. It even offers psychological benefits: it relieves insomnia, reduces anxiety, and calms emotions and may be useful in treating clinical depression.

With all the restorative claims made for marjoram, it's not surprising that medical researchers are studying its healing potential. The plant contains high levels of antioxidants and notable phytonutrients, and its many chemical compounds have anti-inflammatory and anti-bacterial properties. It also contains zea-xanthin, a dietary carotenoid that can protect the eyes from macular degeneration. The eugenol found in the herb acts as an anti-inflammatory, making marjoram useful for treating rheumatoid arthritis, osteoarthritis, and irritable bowel syndrome.

History and Lore

» Wreaths and garlands of marjoram, the herb of "marital bliss"—and a favorite of Aphrodite—were worn at ancient Greek weddings.

» During the Middle Ages, mourners planted marjoram on graves to ensure the happiness of the departed loved ones.

Companion Planting

Many plants have natural substances in their roots, leaves, flowers, and other parts that can either repel or attract insects. Experienced gardeners find that they can discourage harmful pests, without losing beneficial allies, by carefully plotting out which plants should share a garden. Marjoram makes an excellent addition to a vegetable garden. It is particularly useful for repelling harmful cabbage moths, so plant it between rows of brassicas for this purpose. It's also a good companion to asparagus and basil. ■

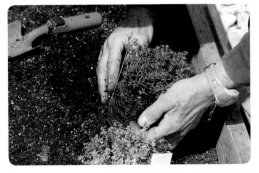

If you choose its neighbors wisely, marjoram can keep garden pests away from cabbage and other brassicas.

Marjoram

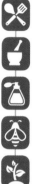

Oregano

Origanum vulgare

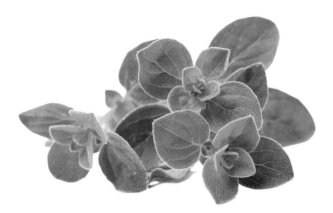

Oregano is the herbal heavy hitter—a kitchen must-have with a long history and one of the most identifiable tastes and fragrances in the world. The plant, whose name derives from the Greek *oros ganos*, or "mountain joy," was originally native to northern Europe but soon spread to many parts of the world. Even though it has been cultivated in France since the Middle Ages, few American were familiar with the herb until after World War II, when G.I.s returned from Italy praising the pungent sprigs.

Mature oregano forms a small shrub with many branches, grayish green oval leaves, and purple, pink, or white flowers. A perennial in warmer climates, it grows so well, it even makes an attractive ground cover.

DID YOU KNOW?

A true culinary classic, oregano is a hardy perennial with delicate flowers that enliven an herb garden and leaves that add a zesty tang to savory dishes.

Culinary Uses

Oregano is most often thought of as an Italian or Mediterranean herb, but its woody balsamic flavor works with a variety of cuisines, including Asian and South American. It is the heart of a savory vinaigrette and the soul of a proper tomato sauce. Its signature taste enhances vegetable dishes, such as sautéed mushrooms, kick-starts omelets, and puts the finishing touch on garlic bread.

When using fresh oregano, look for supple, bright green leaves and firm stems; avoid dark spots or yellowing. Wash thoroughly, and then store in the refrigerator in a damp paper towel. If you grow your own oregano, be sure to dry some and store it. Drying the herb actually helps concentrate the oil, resulting in a stronger flavor than fresh leaves. If store-bought dried oregano has been shelved too long, however, it may have lost much of its strength.

Nutritional Value

Oregano contains impressive amounts of vitamin K, which the body requires to modify certain proteins that aid in the coagulation of blood. The herb is also a good source of dietary fiber and the vital minerals manganese, iron, and calcium.

Oregano is sold as both a fresh and a dried herb. Although the fresh leaves are preferable, dried oregano is a useful pantry staple. Stored in a cool, dark, and dry place, it can last up to six months.

Soothing Oil of Oregano

This pungent oil can be used as a body rub for muscle aches or sinus pain or a few drops can be mixed with water to treat colds and sore throat.

Ingredients
- ½ cup oregano leaves, washed
- ½ cup olive or grape-seed oil
- glass container

Directions

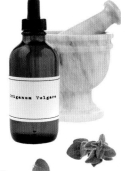

Place leaves in plastic bag, cover with cloth, and pound with a mallet or pestle. Then heat olive oil in a pan until warm. Do not boil. Add olive oil to leaves in bag and work through. Place mixture in glass jar or bottle and store in a cool, dry place for two weeks. Strain before use. (Note: Do not use if pregnant.) ▪

Medicinal Properties

For thousands of years, healers have relied on oregano to treat respiratory tract and gastrointestinal disorders, menstrual cramps, and urinary tract problems. It has also been applied topically for various skin conditions, and drunk as tea to settle the stomach and relax the nerves.

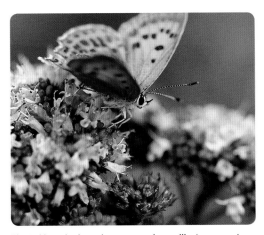

Planted in an herb garden, oregano is a pollinator magnet, bringing honeybees and butterflies, such as this scarce copper (*Lycaena virgaureae*), to your backyard.

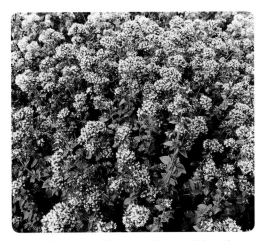

Oregano flowers range from near white to pinkish purple.

Modern research has discovered that the plant's volatile oils, including thymol and carvacrol, inhibit the growth of bacteria such as *Pseudomonas aeruginosa* and *Staphylococcus aureus*. In Mexican studies, the herb has proven more effective against the intestinal amoeba *Giardia lamblia* than prescription medications. The phytonutrients found in oregano act as antioxidants, preventing damage to cell structures.

History and Lore

» Oregano was once used to relieve the "sour humors" that plagued elderly farmers.

» It is thought to be an effective treatment for scorpion and spider bites.

» The woodsy flavor of *Origanum vulgare* is closely approximated in other species, such as *O. syriacum, O. heracleoticum, O. x majoricum, O. majorana, O. onites, Lippia graveolens, L. palmeri, Coleus anboinicus,* and *Thymus nummularius.*

A Greek Favorite

Although oregano is indelibly linked with Italy in the minds of many cooks, it was the Greeks who first used it—and considered it a symbol of joy and happiness. To the ancient Greeks the herb possessed special powers. They believed that a tortoise bitten by a poisonous snake could eat oregano to counteract the toxins, that cattle grazing on fields of oregano produced tastier meat, and that chewing the leaves was a cure for seasickness. ▪

Oregano

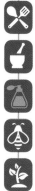

Parsley

Petroselinum crispum, P. neapolitanum crispum

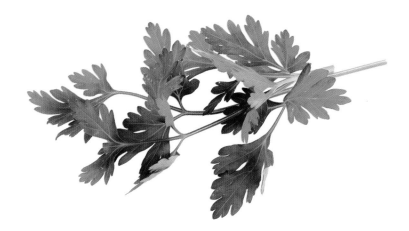

Sadly, parsley is the herb most likely to be thrown away. It is so often used as a garnish at the edge of a dinner plate that no one thinks to actually eat it. The Romans knew better: they chewed parsley at the end of a meal to freshen their breath. Serving it as a garnish is only one of the many uses for parsley, which can lend its delicately bitter flavor to many dishes.

A popular garden plant that originated in the Mediterranean more than two thousand years ago, parsley was a healing agent before it became a culinary herb. By the 18th century, it had become established in the kitchen. Thomas Jefferson included both curly- and flat-leaf parsley in his vegetable gardens at Monticello.

This self-seeding biennial features bright green frilled leaves and tiny yellowish flowers. It is an umbellifer, related to dill and celery—not surprising,

DID YOU KNOW?
This bright-green herb has many more uses than just its traditional role as a plate garnish. Try one of its many varieties as a main ingredient in a salad or sauce.

because its name comes from the Greek term for "rock celery."

Culinary Uses

In spite of its reputation as a "toss away" herb, parsley serves a very important function in cooking—it actually heightens the taste of other ingredients. Think of adding it to dishes for the same reason that you add lemon juice, to brighten a recipe. Parsley can be used in soups—where it lessens the need for salt—sauces, marinades, and salads. The leaves can be chopped fine and sprinkled over egg or seafood dishes, or shredded for use in casseroles or stews. For light-colored recipes, use only the stems; this will add taste but eliminate any green color.

Curly-leaf parsley makes a pretty garnish, but most cooks prefer the Italian flat-leaf varieties because they have better flavor and are easier to work with. Wash fresh parsley by swishing it in a bowl of water, and then gently pat dry.

Nutritional Value

Parsley, like many leafy green plants, is highly nutritious. It is impressively rich in iron, calcium, and vitamin K, as well as vitamins A, B12, C, and folic acid, which is important to cardiac health.

Curly-leaf parsley *(Petroselinum crispum)* makes a pretty garnish or potted plant, but most cooks prefer the taste of Italian parsley *(P. crispum neapolitanum).*

CLASSIC CULINARY HERBS

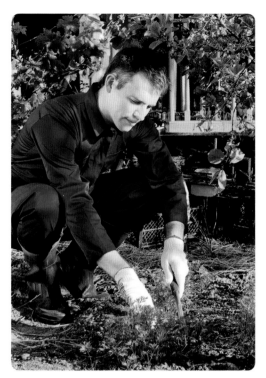

Both the flat-leaf and curly species of parsley work as seasonal edging plants that provide a crisp backdrop for brightly colored annuals, such as pansies or petunias.

Healing Properties

Parsley has been valued for its healing attributes since the ancient Greeks. Pliny recommended it for ailing fish, while medieval folklore maintained that the herb cured baldness. For centuries, a parsley infusion in bath water was considered both soothing and cleansing. Parsley was also reported to aid digestion, act as a diuretic, and bring on and relieve a woman's monthly courses. Conversely, it was believed to be harmful to small birds, injurious to the sight, and, when wet, cause glass to become brittle.

Modern science has discovered that parsley's benefits far outweigh its negatives, yet it contains oxalates that can form crystals in body fluids and should be avoided by anyone with kidney or gall bladder issues. Chemically, parsley contains two components that offer unique health benefits—volatile oils, such as myristicin, which inhibits the formation of tumors in animals, and flavonoid antioxidants that protect cell structure. The herb's antioxidant properties make it effective against joint pain, while its essential oils qualify it as a chemoprotective food.

History and Lore

» Parsley was used by the ancient Greeks to make funeral wreaths and to adorn tombs. This led to the saying "He is in need of parsley," meaning the person was near death.

» Charlemagne, who enjoyed cheese flavored with parsley, grew it on his estates in France.

» The herb was once believed to repel head lice and attract rabbits; today it is known to keep bugs and slugs away from the garden.

» Slow to germinate, parsley was said to "go to the Devil and back nine times" before sprouting.

IN THE KITCHEN

Chimichurri

When there is too much parsley left over after you've added a few diced leaves to a baked potato, try this popular Argentinean sauce, which is similar to pesto.

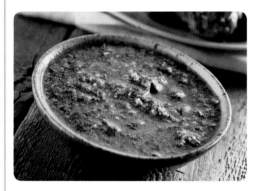

Ingredients
- 1 cup fresh flat-leaf parsley, stems trimmed
- 2 tablespoons fresh oregano leaves (or 2 teaspoons dried oregano)
- 3–4 garlic cloves
- ½ cup olive oil
- 2 tablespoons wine vinegar
- 1 teaspoon sea salt
- ¼ teaspoon ground black pepper
- ¼ teaspoon red pepper flakes

Directions
Finely chop parsley, oregano, and garlic (or pulse several times in food processor). Place in bowl, and mix in olive oil, vinegar, salt, pepper, and pepper flakes. Serve heated over pasta, or use it as a marinade for meat, poultry, and fish or as a sauce for grilled beef. Serves four. ■

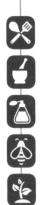

Peppermint

Mentha x piperita

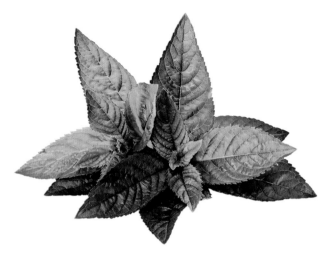

CLASSIC CULINARY HERBS

Since ancient times, this distinctive-smelling herb has been valued for its cool, prickly effect on the palate, its fruity aroma, and its medicinal benefits. A native of Europe, peppermint can now be found in most regions of the world, including Asia and North America, where the majority of commercial peppermint is produced.

It is easy to grow and makes a graceful addition to a border or herb garden. Mature plants reach 18 to 24 inches in height and produce toothed green leaves, with lavender-colored blossoms following in late summer. Leaves should be picked frequently to encourage tender new growth.

Culinary Uses

Peppermint is best known as a flavoring for candy, gum, lozenges, and ice cream. In the kitchen, young peppermint leaves add zest to salads and can be included in soups and sauces. Peppermint also

Peppermint flowers produce an abundance of nectar, which honeybees and other nectar harvesters love.

DID YOU KNOW?

This hybrid mint has much to offer. It is a classic component of many confections and teas, and it has strong aromatic and medicinal qualities. It will also attract bees to your kitchen garden.

makes one of the most popular herbal teas. Fresh leaves can be crushed and mixed into whipped cream—especially good with chocolate mousse—added to sorbet, or sprinkled over tomatoes. Dried leaves can be added to sweet beverages or cocktails and to desserts like meringues, cookies, or cakes. Simple, refreshing mint water is made by adding a cup of bruised leaves to a gallon of water. Chill, then strain, and serve over ice.

Whenever possible, use fresh peppermint when preparing dishes. It can be found year round in grocery stores. Wash thoroughly, pat dry, and store in the refrigerator in a zip pouch.

Nutritional Value

Peppermint is high in essential oils, vitamin A, beta-carotene, vitamins C and E, important B-complex vitamins like folates, riboflavin, and pyridoxine (B6), and vitamin K, as well as in dietary fiber. It is also an important source of potassium, calcium, iron, manganese, and magnesium.

Healing Properties

For millennia, traditional healers turned to peppermint: the medically sophisticated Egyptians cultivated it for use as a digestive aid and

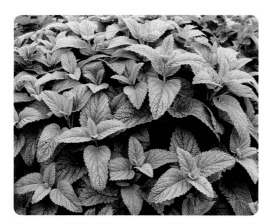

The peppermint plant *(Mentha x piperita)* is a natural hybrid, a cross between water mint *(M. aquatica)* and spearmint *(M. spicata)*. Because it is a hybrid, peppermint is usually sterile, producing no seeds and reproducing vegetatively.

stomach soother, as did the Greeks and Romans. It was also used throughout the Middle Ages as a treatment for the common cold, sinus infections, and menstrual disorders.

Many of the medical claims for peppermint have been born out by research and trials. Studies indicate that the chemical compounds found in peppermint can help relax intestinal walls and sphincter smooth muscles, making it an effective tool in treating irritable bowel syndrome and other colon-related conditions. Peppermint is often used to treat colds and flu; the menthol it contains eases congestion and helps sufferers to breathe more easily. Medicinal peppermint can be either taken as a tea or applied to the skin in the form of an oil.

Many members of the mint family, including peppermint, contain an organic compound called menthol, which binds with the cold receptors in the skin, mouth, and throat and makes them extra sensitive. This accounts for the pleasant cooling sensation mint provides when it is inhaled, eaten, or smoothed onto the skin. Menthol also has anesthetic properties, which make it useful for easing sore throats.

History and Lore

» Ancient Romans wore wreaths of peppermint leaves on their heads.
» During the Middle Ages, mint was believed to cure hiccups and counteract sea serpent stings.
» American colonists enjoyed peppermint tea because it was not taxed by the British.

CULTURAL CONNECTIONS

A Multitude of Mints

Around the world, there are more than seven thousand species and 236 genera of mints. They all belong to the family Lamiaceae, also called deadnettles. The original family name was Labiateae, so called for flower petals that fuse into an upper and lower lip, but botanists prefer the former designation. Mints are identifiable by their square stems and simple, opposite leaves. Most are aromatic, and many are edible—the family includes classic herbs like basil, rosemary, sage, and lavender. Popular mint varieties and hybrids include chocolate mint, fruit-flavored mints (such as lemon, lime, banana, and pineapple), tiny Corsican mint, and Bowles mint, which is popular in England.

The history of mint goes back to the Egyptians and the ancient Greeks, who bruised the leaves to make an after-bath lotion. During the Middle Ages, mint was used to purify drinking water gone stale during long sea voyages. Some cultures believed it could ward off the "evil eye," while others used it to produce aggression. ∎

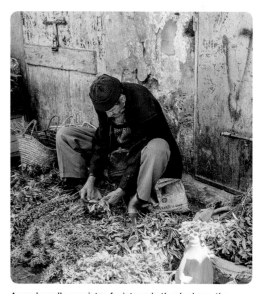

A vendor sells a variety of mints and other herbs on the streets of Rabat, Morocco. Mint is sold in large quantities for making the national drink of mint tea, which is made from mint leaves, gunpowder tea, and sugar. It is served all day long, and, taking great pride in their tea-making skills, Moroccan hosts offer it as a sign of hospitality and friendship.

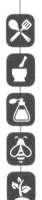

Rosemary
Rosmarinus officinalis

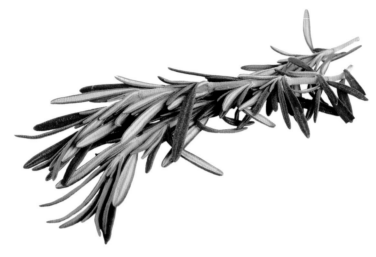

A member of the vast mint family, rosemary has a long and venerable history as a culinary herb, a medicinal plant, and an aromatic garden favorite. Native to the Mediterranean, it is now naturalized in many temperate regions of Europe and America. It dates back to ancient Egypt, where it was placed on a coffin or tombstone for remembrance, a custom that continued into the Middle Ages. It also gets a recommendation in one of the earliest known herbals printed in England.

Originally a coastal plant, rosemary's Latin genus name, *Rosmarinus,* means "dew of the sea." The bush grows to a height of three to five feet and spreads outward on straight stems. Its flat, pine-like needles are deep green on the top, silvery white on the underside, and the delicate flowers can be white, pink, blue, or purple.

Culinary Uses
Often thought of as an accompaniment to roast lamb, rosemary's pungent scent and complex flavor can augment the taste of red meats, pork, chicken,

DID YOU KNOW?
This fragrant evergreen member of the mint family has many culinary and medical uses. It is also valued as a decorative addition to container and herb gardens.

salmon, and tuna steak. Plus, it stands up to longer cooking times, unlike more delicate herbs. It gives a boost to omelets and frittatas, as well as potato and vegetable dishes and tomato sauce. It blends well with other Mediterranean herbs and is often included in the mix for herbes de Provence and bouquet garni.

You can remove the leaves from the stem if a recipe calls for them alone—rosemary leaves pureed with olive oil makes a memorable dipping sauce—or add entire sprigs to soups, casseroles, stews, and meat dishes, and then remove before serving. Sprigs can also be added to vinegar or used to flavor oil and butter.

If possible, opt for fresh rosemary, which is far superior to the dried version. Organic rosemary is even better; it is not likely to have been irradiated, a process that can decrease the valuable phytonutrient content of the herb. Rinse it under cool water, and pat dry.

Rosemary oil is used commercially to make hand soaps and perfumes. At home, it can enhance the scent of bath oil, a wreath, or a sachet. Just infuse rosemary in water and coconut oil, and use when needed.

Scarborough Fair Butter

Serving herb butter is a simple way to make a meal special. This version combines the classic quartet of parsley, sage, rosemary, and thyme.

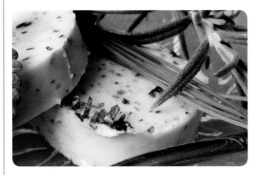

Ingredients
- ½ cup butter, softened
- 2 teaspoons minced fresh rosemary
- 1 teaspoon minced fresh parsley
- ½ teaspoon minced fresh sage
- ½ teaspoon minced fresh thyme
- ½ teaspoon lemon zest

Directions
Using a blender, food processor, or mixer, cream the butter and blend in the herbs. Mix in the lemon zest. Lay out flat a sheet of plastic wrap, and spoon the mixed butter onto it. Roll into a log shape, and place in the freezer to chill for half an hour. Serve on bread, meats, or vegetables. ■

Nutritional Value

Rosemary contains vitamin A, in the form of carotenoid phytonutrients, and vitamin B6. It also contains the minerals iron, calcium, copper, and magnesium.

Healing Properties

Traditional healers used rosemary to improve memory, ease muscle pain, settle a sour stomach, relieve anxiety, aid impotence, banish nightmares, boost the immune system, and cure hair loss. Healthful teas and liquid extracts were made from both fresh and dried leaves.

During the 18th century, the herb served a more macabre purpose—it was used to dress dead bodies. French botanist Jacques-Christophe Valmont de Bomare reported that when coffins were occasionally opened for legal reasons, the rosemary branches in the hands of the deceased would have kept growing until they covered the corpse.

It turns out rosemary really *is* brain food—according to research published in *Therapeutic Advances in Psychopharmacology,* rosemary oil can improve the cognitive performance of the brain and keep the organ from aging. Its essential oil can block histamines, the chemicals that cause asthma and allergies. The plant also contains salicylic acid, the forerunner of aspirin, explaining its traditional use as a pain reliever; and the powerful anti-inflammatory antioxidant, rosmarinic acid.

History and Lore

» In ancient Greece, students braided rosemary sprigs into their hair to improve memory before taking exams.

» Rosemary oil was first extracted in the 14th century and was used to make Queen of Hungary water, a popular cosmetic of the time, and which supposedly cured the queen of paralysis.

» Wise women wash with the herb to retain their youthful looks (rosemary is full of antioxidants that slow down the aging process). It also treats dry scalp and promotes hair growth.

» Australians and New Zealanders wear rosemary on Anzac Day, their national day of remembrance, as a mark of respect for the servicepeople who never returned from war.

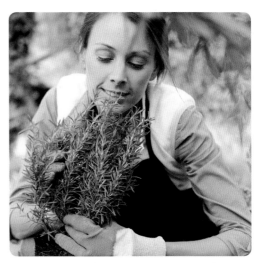

This small drought-tolerant evergreen shrub gives off the essence of warm hillsides, brisk surf, and fresh pine greenery. Its scent also acts as an effective bug repellent.

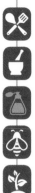

Safflower

Carthamus tinctorius

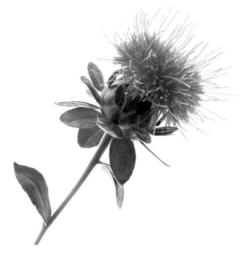

The safflower, an annual plant with bright, thistle-like flowers, is a member of the Asteraceae, or daisy, family and is related to the sunflower. Also called American or bastard saffron, safflower originally grew in the arid Middle East but can now be found in Europe and North America, where it is commercially cultivated for its seed oil. For centuries, Chinese and European herbalists have used the seeds medicinally to treat a variety of ailments.

The safflower plant reaches a height of two to four feet and has a single, smooth, upright stem with shiny, ragged-edged, oval leaves. It produces

striking flowers, ranging from yellow to dark red, that make jaunty additions to the home garden. Seeds typically occur in August, surrounded by a downy globe.

Safflower is one of history's oldest crops, and its richly hued flowers have been used for millennia as a coloring agent in cosmetics and fabric dye. Egyptian textile samples have been dated back to the 12th dynasty (1991–1778 B.C.), while safflower garlands were found in the tomb of Tutankhamun (circa 1323 B.C.). Today, the plant is not only a valuable source of seed oil, but it also supplies livestock meal and bird feed.

Culinary Uses

Both the flowers and the seeds of the safflower plant produce an oil. Safflower seeds can be pressed into two types of oil: one that is high in monounsaturated fatty acids (oleic acid), and another that has high concentrations of polyunsaturated fatty acids (linoleic acid). Either type is very low in saturated fatty acids compared to other cooking oils, and even though its other health benefits are still debated by scientists and researchers, safflower oil remains a high-quality product.

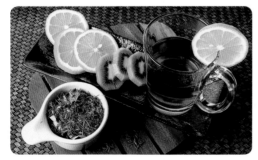

Safflower petals can be used as a cheaper substitute for saffron, which is made from the stigmas of *Crocus sativus*. The petals can also be brewed into a deep orange tea.

DILL

(Anethum graveolens)

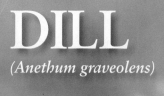

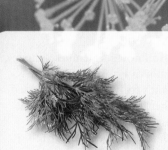

Like cilantro, the dill plant provides an herb, dill weed (the feathery leaves), and a spice, dill seed. This ancient plant goes back at least to Biblical times, when it was used as both a seasoning and a tonic for gastric relief. With its delicate, grassy flavor, it is found today in European, North American, North African, East Asian, and Indian cuisine. Dill weed is used in stews, soups, roasted pork or cabbage dishes, breads, and chutneys. The seeds are used for pickling, vinegars, and salad dressings, or can be rubbed into meat or fish prior to grilling. Dill is a good source of calcium, dietary fiber, and vitamins A and C.

This aromatic annual can be grown indoors from seeds sown ¼ inch deep in well-drained, compost-rich soil. Transplant the healthiest seedlings to their own eight-inch pots, and place them in a sunny window—or hang a fluorescent light at least eight inches above the plants. For a continuous supply of dill, seed plants at staggered intervals. The compact cultivar Fernleaf is ideal for growing indoors.

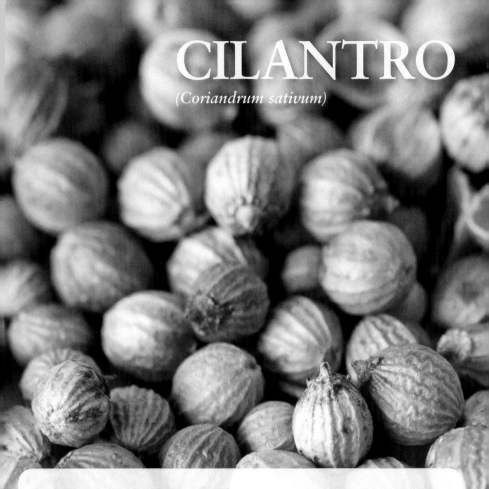

CILANTRO

(Coriandrum sativum)

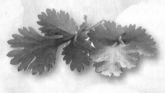

Cilantro, also known as Chinese parsley, is native to Southern Europe and North Africa. The plant's frilly leaves can be used as an herb, either fresh or dried, while the seeds can be used as a spice, known as coriander. With its slightly soapy taste—a blend of parsley, sage, and citrus—cilantro is a mainstay of Mexican cooking and is also found in many Asian dishes. Coriander has a milder flavor and is used in Asian, Indian, Middle Eastern, Tex-Mex, Latin American, and Scandinavian cooking. The plant supplies significant amounts of dietary fiber and vitamins A, C, and K.

This annual is best started from seeds planted ¼ inch deep in rich, well-drained soil. Although cilantro grows quickly, once picked, the stems will not regenerate. Therefore, it's best to stagger your harvest by cultivating three pots at different stages—seeded, intermediate growth, and ready to trim. If the plant is left to flower, the herb will rapidly lose it's flavor, but the coriander seeds can still be used whole or ground.

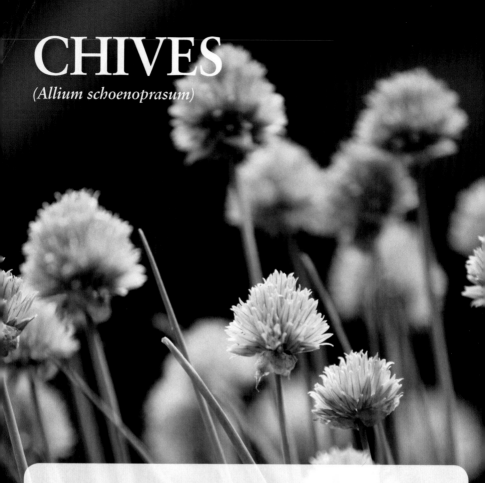

CHIVES
(Allium schoenoprasum)

Chives, the smallest of the edible alliums, are native to Europe, Asia, and North America, accounting for their popularity in many cultures. With their sweet, mild, onion flavor, they are especially good in light dishes such as omelets, cream soups, potatoes, sauces, and savory pancakes. Use the leaves of the classic cultivar Grolau, or garlic chives *(A. tuberosum)* for a mild garlic taste. Chives contain vitamins A, B6, C, E, and K, and dietary fiber, as well as calcium, iron, copper, and magnesium.

It is best to begin growing chives indoors in the fall. Begin by transplanting a clump of garden chives to a clay pot and leaving it outside until the leaves die back. Then place it in your coolest indoor spot—a basement or attached garage—for a week or so, before moving it to your brightest window to stimulate growth. Rotate the pot if the plants are "reaching" toward the light, and keep it on or near a wet pebble tray for humidity. To harvest chives, cut off small bunches at soil level.

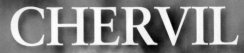

CHERVIL
(Anthriscus cerefolium)

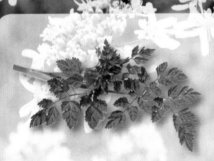

Also known as French parsley, this mainstay of Gallic cooking can be identified by its delicate, slightly licorice taste. Chervil often accompanies lighter fare, such as soups, baby vegetables, sauces, egg and fish dishes, and goat cheese, and can also be found in the Provençal salad mix called mesclun. When cooking with this herb, it's best to add it at the very end of preparation. Chervil supplies high levels of calcium, potassium, phosphorus, selenium, manganese, and magnesium, as well as vitamins A, C, and D.

Chervil can be grown indoors from seeds in the late summer. It can handle low light, but requires cooler temperatures, between 65°F and 70°F, to do well. To harvest fresh chervil for cooking, snip off the outer leaves and stems, or gather a handful of sprigs and cut them off an inch or two above the soil line.

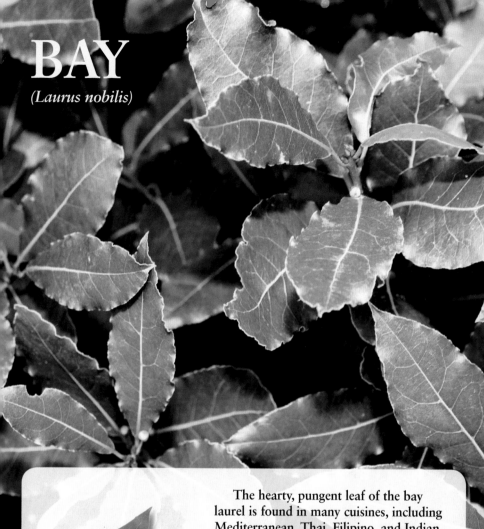

BAY

(Laurus nobilis)

The hearty, pungent leaf of the bay laurel is found in many cuisines, including Mediterranean, Thai, Filipino, and Indian. In French cooking, it is an intrinsic part of the savory herb bundle called a bouquet garni. The leathery leaves can be used either fresh or dried, and are typically removed from a dish before plating, as they are difficult to digest.

The leaves of the bay laurel contain the powerful antioxidant vitamin C and are also rich in folic acid, vitamin A, and B-complex vitamins. Traditionally, bay has been considered an appetite stimulant. The perennial bay laurel tree does well in indoor containers all year long. It grows slowly, but will eventually form a small bush that can easily be trimmed into topiary. The easiest course is to purchase a young 1- to 2-foot plant. Place the pot in an east- or west-facing window, and make sure not to crowd the plant. These small trees need good air circulation to remain healthy.

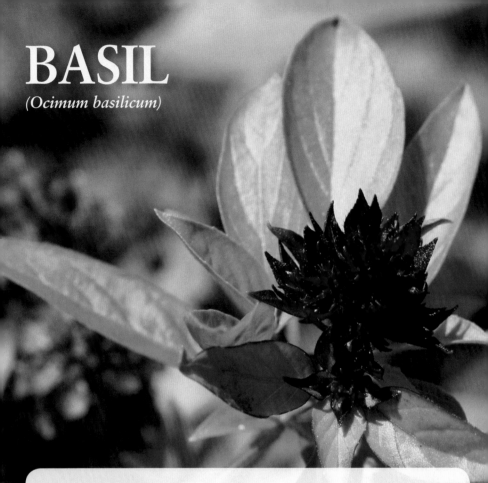

BASIL
(Ocimum basilicum)

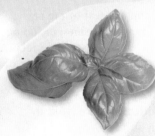

Hardy, aromatic basil is known as the "king of herbs." With its pungent sweetness, it takes a starring role in Mediterranean dishes, including red sauces, pesto, soups, stews, and salads. It is also a favorite in Asian cookery. A member of the mint family, basil is high in vitamins A and K, and its volatile oils furnish antioxidant, antiviral, and antimicrobial benefits.

Start growing basil from seeds and place the pots in a south-facing window, as it prefers lots of sun and warmth. It can be grown outdoors during the summer in temperate climates, but will also do fine indoors all year—just prune the tips back to keep those tender leaves coming. Try Genovese for classic taste, Lemon for citrus notes, Spicy Globe for its compact size, or Siam Queen for its spicy flavor. Fresh basil can be used in hot dishes as well as salads. Store in the refrigerator in a damp paper towel, or dry the herb by hanging clumps inside a brown paper bag until brittle.

Introduction

Herbs are among the most versatile plants—whether culti-vated indoors or out, they provide attractive foliage, welcoming scents, and signature flavors for cooking. Many are easy to grow inside the home with only basic maintenance, and some also have medicinal value as teas or infusions. In temperate regions, creating a windowsill garden allows your herbs to grow in spite of the harsh elements and offer their bounty during even the chilliest months.

When planning your garden, be sure to include a variety of culinary herbs to choose from. Rosemary, thyme, and sage are considered warming herbs; dill and parsley are cooling. Chives add a mild onion tang; mint adds zest. Bay and oregano are woody; marjoram has subtle citrus notes; basil and chervil give off hints of anise. Bright, grassy cilantro is perfect in Mexican dishes. And once your garden is flourishing, don't be afraid to experiment by mixing and matching flavors.

Text by Nancy Hajeski

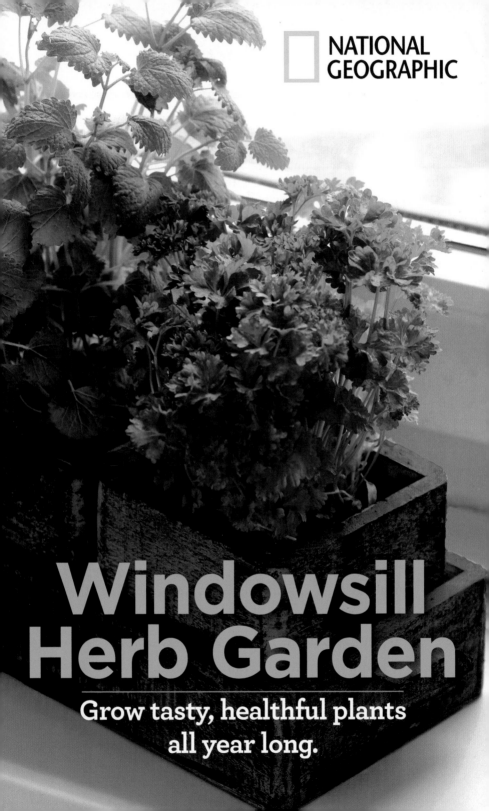

National Geographic

Windowsill
Herb Garden

Grow tasty, healthful plants
all year long.

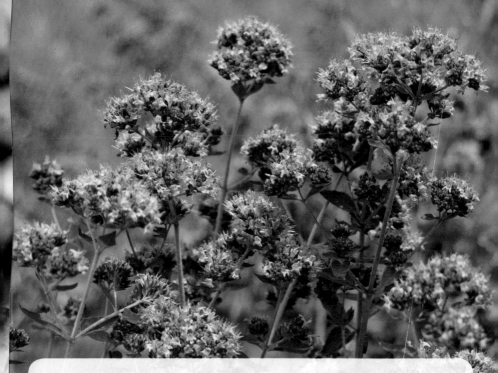

MARJORAM

(Origanum spp.)

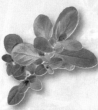

A cousin to oregano, marjoram has its own distinct pine/citrus flavor—delicate and sweet. This North African native soon spread to the Mediterranean and beyond, integrating into the cuisines of France, Italy, and North America, especially in vegetable, egg, and meat dishes, soups, sauces, salad dressings, and turkey stuffing. The herb supplies vitamins A and C and is an important source of vitamin K, which promotes bone and brain health.

Marjoram will live for years in a mild indoor climate, but a good source of sun and consistent watering are key. Seeds sown directly in potting soil can be slow to germinate, so employing cuttings or root division is more efficient. Pinch back plant tips before they bloom in late summer to keep the herb compact. Sweet marjoram *(O. majorana)* is popular for indoor cultivation. Italian marjoram *(O. x majoricum)* is another windowsill option that offers a delicious blend of sweet and spicy flavors. The tiny gray-green leaves of either cultivar can be harvested at all times.

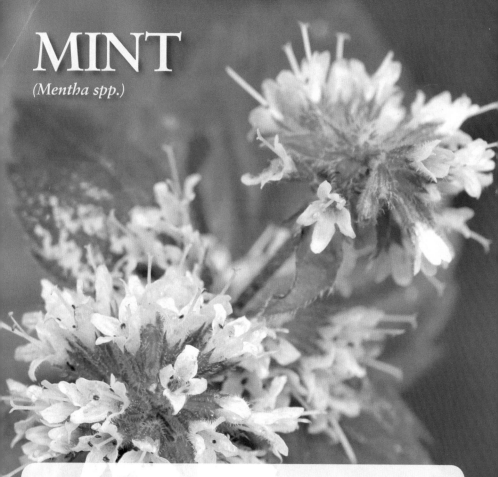

MINT
(Mentha spp.)

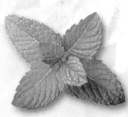

Hardy mint has been providing unique flavor to dishes for centuries. Peppermint, *(M. x piperita)* with its menthol bite, originated in Europe and is a popular flavoring for candy and gum. Spearmint *(M. spicata)* is native to Europe and Southwest Asia, and can now be found in Middle Eastern and North African cuisine. Mints supply vitamins A, C, and E, the B-complex vitamins, and potassium. From ancient times to modern day, mints have been used to ease digestive problems.

Spearmint and peppermint are two of the easiest herbs to grow indoors. Simply pot up plants in commercial soil or in a mix of peat, sand, and perlite, and place in a cool location with indirect light. English mint is a non-invasive spearmint cultivar with attractive, deep-green leaves that is great for cooking and making tea. Catnip, or catmint *(Nepeta Cataria)*, can keep your cats entertained all winter long, and also adapts easily to the windowsill.

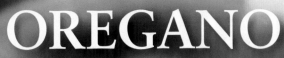

OREGANO
(Origanum vulgare spp. hirtum)

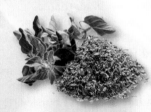

This Northern European native, with its woody, balsamic essence, provides one of the most distinctive tastes found in the modern kitchen. Although associated with Mediterranean cuisine, oregano also features in Asian and Latin American cookery. Fresh or dried, it can be used to flavor meat dishes, tomato sauce, vinaigrettes, sautéed vegetables and mushrooms, and garlic bread. It is a major source of vitamin K and also supplies dietary fiber, manganese, iron, and calcium.

This small, sun-loving perennial shrub will grow indoors from seeds or tip cuttings planted in loamy soil and placed in a south-facing window. Thin the healthiest seedlings to individual pots. One popular indoor cultivar is Kaliteri *(O. vulgare "Kaliteri")*, a Greek strain that is spicy but never bitter. Water plants only when soil feels dry to the touch and harvest leaves often to encourage new growth. Oregano remains productive for up to two years, but should be replaced when plants become woody.

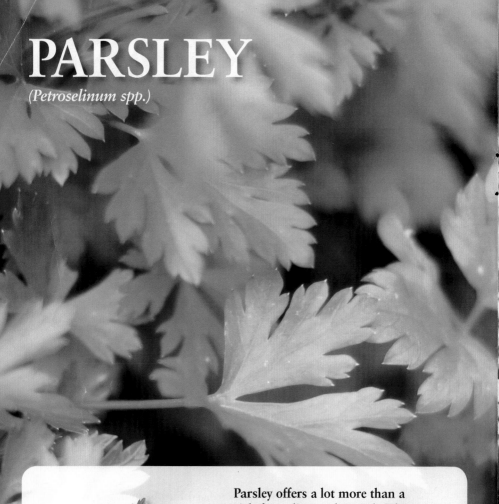

PARSLEY
(Petroselinum spp.)

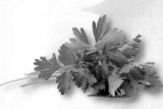

Parsley offers a lot more than a garnish for a dinner plate. It brightens the flavors of foods and other herbs, and lessens the need for salt. Originating in the Mediterranean more than 2,000 years ago, it is found today in cuisines around the globe, with Italian flat leaf parsley *(P. crispum* var. *neapolitanum)* providing more robust flavor than the curly-leaf variety *(P. crispum)*. The herb is rich in iron, calcium, and vitamin K, and also supplies vitamins A, B12, and C.

Both types of parsley grow well indoors. Start plants from seeds sown directly into a container of well-drained potting mix and covered with ¼ inch of soil, or dig up a clump from your garden at the end of the growing season. Parsley likes full sun in a south-facing window, but will tolerate eastern or western exposure. Trim only the outer leaves when harvesting to encourage new growth from the center. This will keep your plant productive for several months.

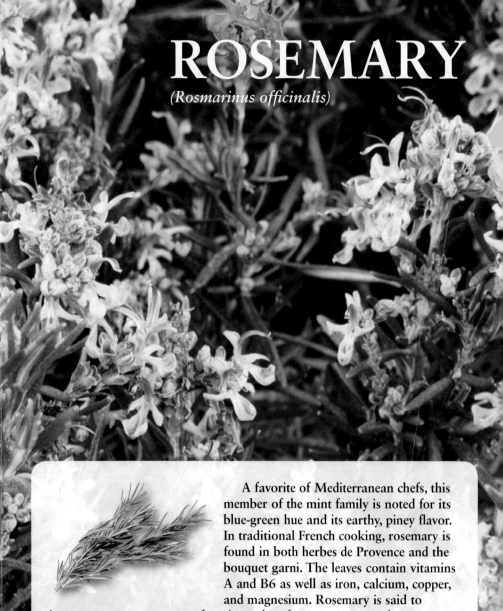

ROSEMARY

(Rosmarinus officinalis)

A favorite of Mediterranean chefs, this member of the mint family is noted for its blue-green hue and its earthy, piney flavor. In traditional French cooking, rosemary is found in both herbes de Provence and the bouquet garni. The leaves contain vitamins A and B6 as well as iron, calcium, copper, and magnesium. Rosemary is said to improve memory, ease muscle pain, and settle an upset stomach.

Perennial rosemary can be found in trailing forms, such as the creeping Blue Boy variety, or in compact upright forms like flavorful Taylor's Blue or Salem. To grow any variety indoors, start with a cutting of rosemary in a soil-less mixture, and keep it moist until it roots. Alternately, you could pot up some garden rosemary in September. Set the plant in the shade for several weeks to acclimate to less light, then place it inside in a cool spot with lots of southern or western light. Water sparingly, but keep the pot on a wet pebble tray to provide humidity.

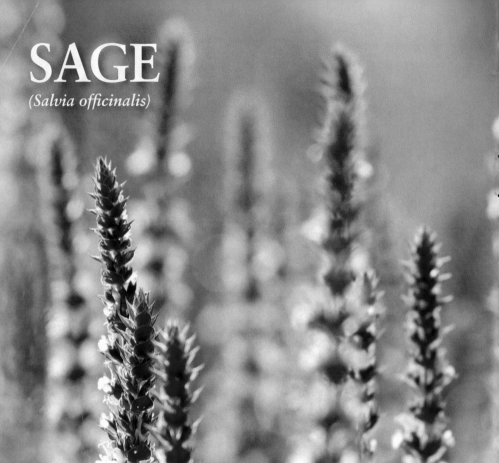

SAGE
(Salvia officinalis)

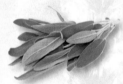

In addition to its culinary benefits, this ancient, gray-green herb was once used as a medicine—its scientific name comes from the Latin *salvare*, or "to save." Native to the limestone coasts of the Mediterranean, sage has a savory flavor and sweet, earthy aroma that makes it a perfect addition to soups, stews, casseroles, pork, duck, liver, and turkey stuffing. Nutritionally, the plant contains significant amounts of vitamin K as well as vitamin A, calcium, and iron.

The key to growing sage indoors is providing six to eight hours of light daily. For best results, consider supplemental fluorescent lighting. To start growing indoors, plant a tipcutting or two from an outdoor plant into a clay pot with well-drained soil. Fortunately, sage tolerates dry, indoor air and dryish soil—simply place a humidifying tray of wet gravel under the plant. Cultivars that do well in containers include 15-inch dwarf common sage (*S. officinalis* "*Minimus*"); flavorful dwarf garden sage (*S. officinalis* "*Compacta*"), which grows to 10 inches high; and nonflowering *Berggarten*, a small, vigorous, low-growing culinary variety.

THYME

(Thymus spp.)

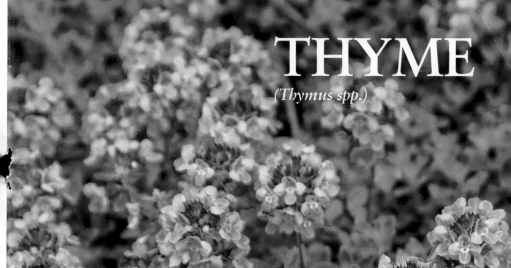

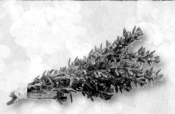

Common thyme, also called English or French thyme, is a popular Mediterranean herb that was spread throughout Europe by the Romans. Today, its delicate, aromatic leaves are used in the cuisine of many cultures to prepare egg, fish, and bean dishes, and sauces, soups, and stocks. Thyme is a traditional component of the French bouquet garni and is a rich source of vitamin C. It also supplies vitamin A, iron, manganese, copper, and dietary fiber.

Start growing thyme indoors by rooting a soft tip cutting or transplanting an outdoor specimen into a clay pot with well-drained soil. Thyme prefers full sun, but will manage with an east- or west-facing window. Repot each season if necessary to allow for growth. Lemon thyme *(T. x citriodorus)* and Narrow Leaf French thyme *(T. vulgaris)* are two tasty varieties, or try creeping Oregano thyme. Broadleaf thyme *(Plectranthus amboinicus* or *Coleus amboinicus)*, known as Spanish or Cuban thyme, is a windowsill champ with a spicy thyme-oregano flavor that reaches only 12 inches in height.

Discover the benefits of windowsill gardening
and enjoy the appearance, aroma, and flavors
of healthful herbs throughout the year.

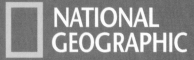

NATIONAL
GEOGRAPHIC

1145 17th Street N.W.
Washington, D.C. 20036-4688

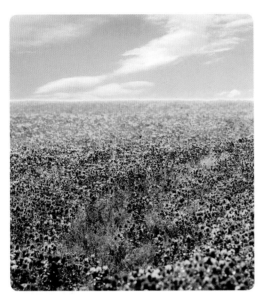

A field of commercially grown safflower. It is usually harvested for its oil, which is often used for cooking that demands high temperatures—to fry potato chips or French fries, for example.

The linoleic variety is a "cold" oil used primarily in salad oils and soft margarines. It is perishable and needs to be refrigerated. The oleic-rich oil is shelf stable and most often used for high-temperature cooking. It is also used in industry as a drying oil in the manufacture of paints, stains, and linoleum tiles—because it does not yellow over time, it is especially valuable for white or lighter-colored pigments.

The petals of the safflower have been used as a substitute for pricey saffron. They have a similar color and flavor and have also become popular in their own right. A tea can be made from the petals by soaking them in water.

Nutritional Value

Safflower oil contains more vitamin E than olive oil, as well as thiamin, folate, vitamin B6, pantothenic acid, niacin, and riboflavin. The seeds furnish substantial amounts of the minerals manganese, magnesium, and copper, as well as zinc, phosphorus, potassium, and iron.

Healing Properties

Traditional healers have used the plant to treat fevers, tumors, coughs, clotting conditions, pain, heart disease, and traumatic injuries. It has also been used to induce sweating, as a laxative, stimulant, antiperspirant, and expectorant. Over the years it has come to be associated with the treatment of painful menstrual periods and even with inducing abortions.

Although there is a belief among traditional healers that the plant's beneficial polyunsaturated fatty acids, including the linoleic and oleic acids found in the seed oil, might help prevent hardening of the arteries, lower bad cholesterol levels, and reduce the risk of heart disease, there is no conclusive evidence from clinical trials to support most of these claims. The N-(p-coumaroyl) serotonin found in the oil, however, is acknowledged to be a powerful antioxidant, and the seed extract has been shown in experiments to have a protective effect against estrogen-related osteoporosis.

History and Lore

» Safflower extracts were used to dye the wrappings of Egyptian mummies.
» Chinese herbalists used the plant to invigorate the blood and reduce pain.
» During the 19th century, the red dye produced from the safflower was known as carthamine. Today it is known as Natural Red 26. Both the red and yellow dyes were important to textile manufacturing before the advent of cheaper aniline dyes.

FOR YOUR HEALTH

The Beauty Factor

Safflower oil makes a useful addition to your daily beauty routine. When lightly rubbed onto the roots and scalp, the oil improves hair quality and will also give it a lustrous sheen. It can also be massaged into fingernails and cuticles. The oil is an effective moisturizer and is often added to bath and beauty products—it is non-comodegenic, which means it does not clog pores. When applied directly to facial skin, safflower oil will reduce the look of fine lines and wrinkles. It can also be massaged into elbows and heels for smooth arms and pretty, sandal-ready feet. It has even been used to treat eczema, soothing inflammation and redness. ■

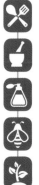

Sage

Salvia officinalis

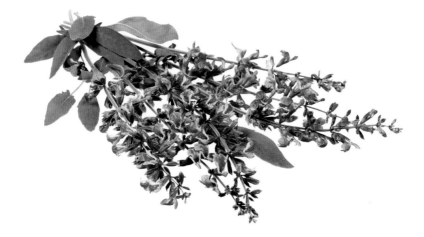

Sage is an ancient herb that has long been esteemed for its savory taste, its medicinal qualities, and its sweet, earthy aroma. For eons, sage has grown along the limestone coasts of the Mediterranean Sea, and some early cultures used it as a preservative for meat. In A.D. 812, Charlemagne ordered sage to be planted at the German imperial farms. In the 17th century, the Chinese so craved sage tea that they offered Dutch traders four pounds of valuable black tea leaves for one pound of sage. The plant eventually naturalized in England, France, and Germany.

Sage is a perennial evergreen shrub, a member of the ubiquitous mint family. It can reach a foot or more in height and is typically wider than it is tall. The lance-shaped leaves grow in pairs on the

DID YOU KNOW?

Sage, with its slightly peppery taste, has a long history of culinary use. Its essential oil has also been preeminent in the traditional pharmacopoeia. It also makes a striking garden plant, which will attract honeybees.

wiry stems; they are grayish green with a silvery bloom and prominent veins. The purple flowers are whorled, with lipped corollas, and bloom from June to August.

Culinary Uses

Most Americans recognize sage as the predominant flavor in Thanksgiving turkey stuffing. Its taste is less robust than some Mediterranean herbs, yet it works well in soups, stews, and casseroles, and with pork, duck, liver, seafood, and even burgers. When baking fish or chicken in parchment or tin foil, place fresh sage on top before putting it into the oven. You can also toss it into a salad with cucumber, bell peppers, and onions. Sage makes a wonderful addition to cornbread or muffins; serve either one with an herbed butter. Dried or powdered sage is stronger than fresh leaves, so use sparingly.

Some edible cultivars include 'Berggarten' (with large leaves), 'Purpurascens' (with purple leaves), and 'Tricolor' (with white-purple-and-green variegated leaves).

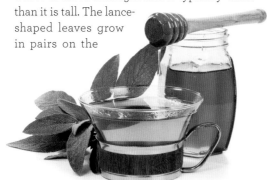

Bees love the scent of sage, either growing wild on a hillside or confined in a garden, and will cluster around the blooming plants collecting nectar. The rich, complex taste of sage honey makes it one of the most expensive varieties.

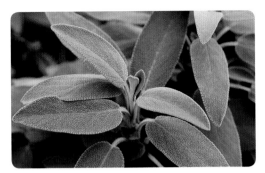
The aromatic leaves of sage have a pebble-like texture.

Nutritional Value

In addition to healthful flavonoids and volatile oils, sage contains significant amounts of vitamin K. It also contains a decent amount of vitamin A, calcium, iron, magnesium, and manganese.

Medicinal Properties

In the first century A.D., Roman physician Dioscorides described how a decoction of sage stopped wounds from bleeding and cleansed ulcers. Traditional herbalists believed it was useful for treating sprains, swelling, rheumatism, sore throats, coughs, and excessive menstrual bleeding, as well as to dry up mother's milk and to curb hot flashes. It was also used to sharpen the memory and strengthen the nervous system.

FOR YOUR HEALTH

Herb of Salvation

Sage was the cornerstone of the traditional herbal healer's pharmacopoeia. Its very name, *salvia,* came from the Latin *salvare,* or "to save"—giving an indication of just how important it was. One Latin maxim ran: *Cur moriatur homo cui salvia crescit in horto?* or "Why should a man die while sage grows in his garden?" There was also an English recommendation: "He that would live for aye, must eat sage in May." Sage was also thought to be the guardian of all other herbs.

John Gerard, a 16th-century herbalist, noted, "Sage is singularly good for the head and brain, it quickeneth the senses and memory, strengtheneth the sinews, restoreth health to those that have the palsy, and taketh away trembling of the members." Modern medical research bears out many of the early claims for this most honored herb. ■

Modern medical research has corroborated many of those early claims. Sage has been found to contain beneficial compounds like tannin, an astringent; phenolic acid, potent against staph infections and yeast; and, like sage's sister plant rosemary, rosmarinic acid, which is an anti-inflammatory. Sage is currently used to treat mouth and throat infections, tooth abscesses, excessive menstrual bleeding, and symptoms of menopause. Its perspiration-inhibiting effect makes it useful for treating night sweats in tuberculosis patients and excessive salivation in Parkinson's patients. Like rosemary, it can be used to enhance brain function and memory. Sage can be prescribed as a tea, an alcoholic tincture, a fresh tincture, an alcoholic fluid extract, a fresh juice, or a leaf.

History and Lore

» Some ancient cultures thought sage promoted strength and longevity. Early Arabs believed that the herb bestowed immortality.
» Ancient Romans took it to aid their digestion after consuming fatty meats.
» American Indians used a stalk of sage as a toothbrush and as a cure for bleeding gums. It is still used today—just make a sage powder and mix with sea salt to prevent gum disease,
» Americans in the early 1900s believed that an application of sage would remove warts.

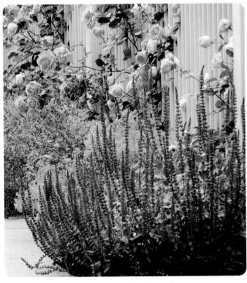
With its dramatic spikes of purplish blossoms, sage works as well in an ornamental garden as it does in a kitchen garden.

SHELF LIFE

Learn how to keep your herbs fresh tasting and flavorful.

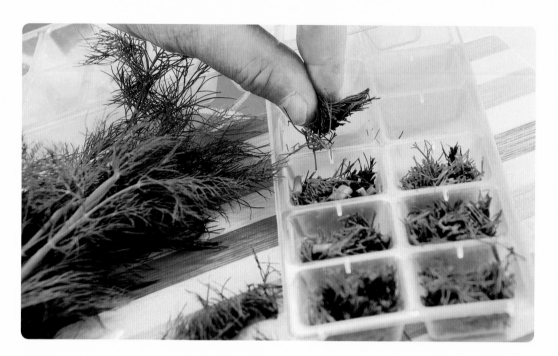

Anyone who shops for fresh herbs in a grocery or farmers' market knows that many of them can be pricey. So it's naturally upsetting when they go limp and soggy or turn yellow and wither within a few days. And dried herbs might be even worse—containers of herbs that cost a fortune just sit there in the spice rack for years . . . losing their potency and flavor. There are some tricks, however, that you can try to extend the shelf life of herbs, both fresh and dried.

Keeping Fresh Herbs Potent

Here are a few tips for maximizing the freshness and flavor of your fresh herbs:

» For high-moisture herbs, such as parsley and cilantro, cut off the excess stems, place the bundle in a glass or jar, and fill with water. Keep leaves above the water level, similar to a floral arrangement. Cover loosely with a plastic bag and store in the refrigerator. Change the water if it gets cloudy, and trim off any yellow or brown leaves. When ready for use, rinse the herbs well under cool water, shake off excess, and pat dry with paper towels. Basil can be stored in the same way, but on the countertop rather than in the refrigerator. Most herbs last two weeks or more using this method.

» For woody, low-moisture herbs such as bay, dill, rosemary, and thyme, as well as chives, wrap loosely in plastic, and place in a door compartment or any relatively warmer part of the refrigerator. Add a crumpled paper towel to absorb moisture. Do not cleanse until just before using: excess water might cause mold.

» To keep fresh herbs on hand, place them in ice cube trays with water or stock and freeze them to use later. Another way to freeze fresh herbs is to use olive oil or butter instead of water or stock. The fats will absorb the flavors of the herbs, making a tasty addition to many dishes.

Drying Herbs for Long-term Life
You have no way of knowing how long a container of dried herbs sat on the grocer's shelf before you brought it home. Yet, most food experts recommend discarding packaged herbs after a year or so—*Yes, we know there is a decade-old jar of cloves in your cupboard*—and that's money down the drain. The best way to ensure the flavor and health benefits of herbs is to grow them and dry them yourself. Here are some tips on drying:

» Harvest herbs right before the flowers bloom, in mid-morning, after the dew has dried from them. This when they are at peak flavor.

» To air-dry herbs, just gather the fresh-cut stems together, and tie them with a string. Punch holes in a paper bag, place the herbs upside down in the bag, and then gather the bag's edges together, and seal it with an elastic band. Hang the bag in a warm spot with good circulation. The stems will shrink over time, so check the string occasionally for tightness. Once the herbs are completely dry and brittle, crush them in a paper bag with a mallet or powder them in a food mill. Place herbs into airtight containers, label with the date, and store in a cool, dark spot—definitely not above the stove. Whole leaves will last longer than crushed ones.

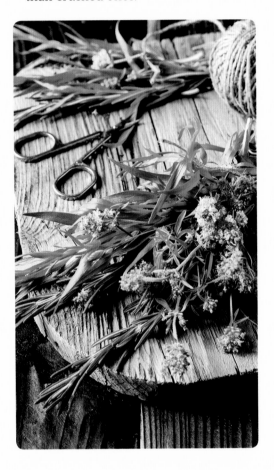

» Fresh herbs can also be quick dried without too much loss of flavor or oils. Chop up basil or parsley leaves or use whole sprigs of rosemary or thyme, spread on a cookie sheet in an open oven at low heat (less than 180 degrees) for about 15 minutes. Afterward, place in a zip bag and store in the refrigerator.

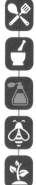

Salad Burnet

Sanguisorba minor

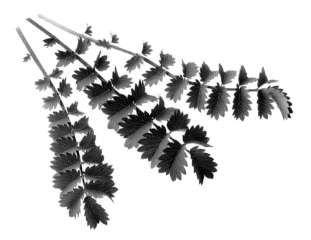

This attractive perennial herb, also called pimprenelle, is part of the rose family. Native to the dry grassy meadows of western, central, and southern Europe, northwest Africa, and southwest Asia, salad burnet is now naturalized in most of North America. Medicinally, the herb's use is documented as far back as the Han dynasty of China, around 200 B.C.

The plant has slender stems that can reach two feet in height; small, gray-green "pinked" leaves; and rosy or purple flowers that form on raspberry-shaped globes. Because it possesses both male and female flowers, salad burnet is able to self-pollinate. The name *burnet* comes from Middle English, derived from the Old French; *brunete,* or *burnete,* was a diminutive of brown, referring to the brown seed heads.

Culinary Uses

This herb possesses a light cucumber flavor, and continental cooks, especially, enjoy mixing it with other greens. In fact, an Italian proverb declares, *"L' insalata non è buona ne bella, ove non è la pimpinella"*—meaning, "a salad is neither good nor pretty without burnet." It can accompany rich meats, such as lamb

---

DID YOU KNOW?

As its name implies, this old-fashioned herb will add flavor to your salad, but its delicate leaves will lend a graceful touch to a container or windowsill garden

---

and rabbit, yet it is quite good with fish. It is a key ingredient, along with parsley, cress, chives, borage, and sorrel in Frankfurt green sauce. It can also be used to make vinegars, marinades, and herb butters, or as a garnish. Some cooks use salad burnet interchangeably with mint. The seeds can also be used in vinegar, marinades, or cheese dishes, or to make authentic French dressing.

A handful of finely chopped burnet leaves (scissors are recommended) can be combined with cream cheese, pepper, salt, and a little milk or cream, to create a tasty dip. They can be sprinkled into a Bloody Mary to replace the usual celery stick. Or freeze the leaves in fruit juice in an ice cube tray to decorate a party punch. Remember to use young, tender leaves in recipes, because they become increasingly bitter as they mature. Dried salad burnet has little flavor, so the best way to preserve it for out-of-season use is to strip off the leaves and freeze them.

Nutritional Value

Salad burnet is not as nutrient rich as some of its herbal cousins. It does contain vitamins A and C, and some of the B-complex vitamins, as well as the minerals iron and potassium.

The Soldier's Ally

The plant's genus, *Sanguisorba*, is taken from the Latin for "blood absorber" because it was reputed to stop bleeding. Nicholas Culpeper suggested the leaves "to staunch bleeding inward or outward," but the usage went back to early Chinese herbalists who made a poultice of the root. Many stories were spread of the herb's powers, and according to legend, King Chaba of Hungary cured the wounds of 15,000 of his soldiers by applying the juice of burnet. Revolutionary War soldiers dosed themselves with burnet tea before battle in the belief that, if wounded, the burnet would keep them from bleeding to death. The plant does exhibit astringent properties, so tales of its healing abilities are not that farfetched. ■

Healing Properties

Salad burnet has many of the same healing benefits as medicinal burnet (*Sanguisorba officinalis*). Early healers used the herb to ease indigestion, rheumatism, and gout, and even to treat the plague. English colonists brought salad burnet to America, and Thomas Jefferson himself mentioned his admiration for the plant. It was considered a restorative tonic for the "morning after"—pouring boiling water over the leaves was supposed to create "a cure for, or an alleviant of, drunkard's thirst." The herb was also used in tea and tisanes to relieve diarrhea.

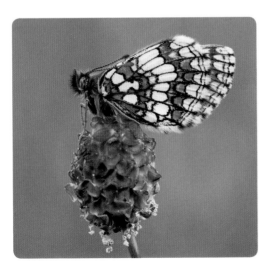

Pollinators, such as a Nickerl's fritillary butterfly *(Melitaea aurelia)* are attracted to the flowers of salad burnet.

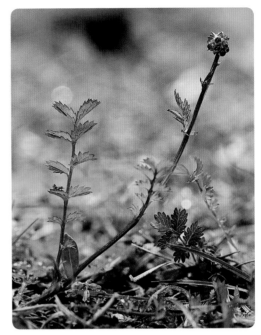

A young shoot of salad burnet. Cultivate it an herb garden, where it will produce fresh edible leaves all year round.

Recent studies by scientists in Spain have found that extracts of the herb displayed anti-HIV effects in vitro. In Germany, researchers concluded that *Sanguisorba* extracts considerably reduced blood sugar levels in laboratory mice. A study in Turkey indicated that the extracts prevented ulcers. The extracts are also believed, based on research from Iran and Canada, to have antifungal properties.

The plant contains several unique and beneficial organic compounds. Its glycosides, called sanguisorbines, lower bad cholesterol, improve bone health, and stimulate the immune system. Its flavonoids neutralize free radicals and have anti-cancer and anti-inflammatory effects.

History and Lore

» Salad burnet was said to "lighten the heart" and was often served in wine.
» Scientist-philosopher Sir Francis Bacon, in a 1625 essay on which herbs to plant in walkways, suggested salad burnet combined with thyme or water mint—"to perfume the air most delightfully, being trodden on and crushed."
» Tudor-era gardeners admired the plant's graceful fountain shape and often located it at the edge of knot gardens.

Salad Burnet

73

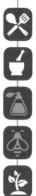

Sorrel

Rumex acetosa, R. scutatus

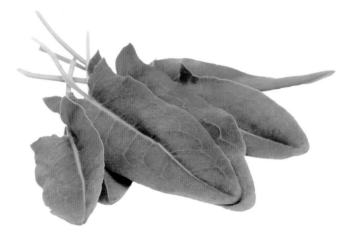

Two types of sorrel are grown for culinary use: citrus-flavored garden or common sorrel *(Rumex acetosa)* was once a popular English herb that could be found throughout Europe in both gardens and meadows. French sorrel *(R. scutatus),* which developed in Italy and France, has a milder lemon flavor. In the 16th century, succulent-leafed French sorrel increased in popularity until it replaced garden sorrel in the kitchen. Oddly, over time both species fell into disuse and ceased to be cultivated in home gardens.

A mature sorrel plant reaches two feet in height, with juicy stems and leaves and reddish green flowers that form whorled spikes, which often turn purple or rusty as they age.

Culinary Uses

Before it fell from favor, sorrel was a kitchen staple all over Europe. French chefs included it in ragouts, fricassees, and soups, and it is still the main ingredient of the favorite *soupe aux herbes.* The English country

---

DID YOU KNOW?

Genus *Rumex* contains about 200 species of common herbs. Called both sorrel and dock, many are nuisance weeds, but *R. acetosa* and *R. scutatus* make delightful additions to your herbal pantry.

---

folk would mash it into a pulp, and then mix it with vinegar and sugar to serve over cold meat, leading to "greensauce" becoming one of *R. scutatus*'s popular names. Scandinavians sometimes added it to bread, if flour was scarce—the leaves contain a little starch and mucilage—while Laplanders used it in place of rennet to curdle milk.

Contemporary cooks are rediscovering the tart herb, using tender young leaves to flavor salads, goat cheese, and eggs, and the older, more bitter leaves in stews, soups, and sauces. Alas, fresh sorrel must be used almost immediately after picking, so it is rarely found in markets. Yet, it is easy to grow from seeds, and it should become a part of every cook's herb garden.

Nutritional Value

Sorrel, rich in vitamin C, was valued for centuries for its ability to prevent scurvy, a condition brought on by lack of citric acid, which was once

Sorrel's tiny green flowers grow in terminal clusters and turn a rusty red as they age.

Sorrel Soup

This light summer soup is a French classic.

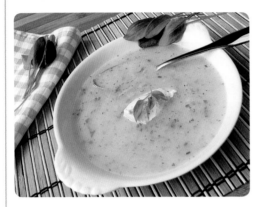

Ingredients

- 3 cups vegetable broth
- 2 tablespoons uncooked white rice
- 1 bunch sorrel, stemmed and rinsed
- ½ cup heavy cream
- salt and pepper to taste

Directions

In a large saucepan, bring broth to a boil over medium heat. Stir in rice, and continue to boil for about 8 minutes. Add the sorrel and a pinch of salt, and stir well. When the sorrel is mostly wilted, reduce heat to medium-low, cover and cook 10 minutes. Remove from heat, and puree in batches in a blender or food processor. Return to medium-low heat, and stir in cream, salt, and pepper. ■

especially rife among men who lived at sea for long stretches. It is also a key source of vitamins A and B9 and vital minerals such as potassium, magnesium, sodium, iron, and calcium.

Healing Properties

Nicholas Culpeper wrote of the herb: "Sorrel is prevalent in all hot diseases, to cool any inflammation and heat of blood in agues pestilential or choleric, or sickness or fainting, arising from heat, and to refresh the overspent spirits with the violence of furious or fiery fits of agues." He also recommended its use for thirst, to stimulate appetite, kill worms, aid the heart, cure scorpion bites, and open boils. At the turn of the 20th century, sheep sorrel (*R. acetosella*), a plant poisonous to livestock, was an ingredient in Essiac, an herbal mixture promoted as a cancer remedy.

Researchers have discovered that sorrel contains flavonoids, antioxidants, and anthocyanins that make it effective in treating or preventing a range of ailments including cancer, hypertension, diabetes, and heart disease. Sorrel also contains tannins, which reduce the production of mucous and help in the treatment of sinusitis and swelling of the nasal passages. Sorrel is an effective diuretic and has been used, along with conventional medicines, to treat bacterial infections.

Due to its high acidity, sorrel should be consumed sparingly by those who suffer from arthritis, kidney stones, or gout.

History and Lore

» The plant is sometimes called cuckoo's meate, from the old belief that the bird used the herb to clear its voice. In Scotland it is known as gowkemeat. *R. acetosa* is also known as spinach dock, sour dock, sour grabs, or sour grass. *R. scutatus* also goes by the names buckler-leaf sorrel, buckleaf sorrel, and shield-leaf sorrel.

» Noted diarist and gardener John Evelyn wrote that sorrel imparted "so grateful a quickness to the salad that it should never be left out."

» The sap of garden sorrel can be used as a laundry stain-remover.

The Salt of Sorrel

Binoxalate of potash (oxalic acid and potash), also known as the salt of sorrel, is a chemical compound in the plant that is responsible for both its acidic taste and its medicinal value. The salt is used to bleach straw and to remove ink stains from linen; in shops, it is sold as "essential salt of lemons." Perhaps the most unconventional application of the salt is by forgers—when they wish to make the ink in counterfeit documents appear old, they mix ordinary ink with muriatic acid and binoxalate of potash for a properly aged effect. ■

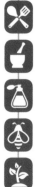

Spearmint

Mentha spicata

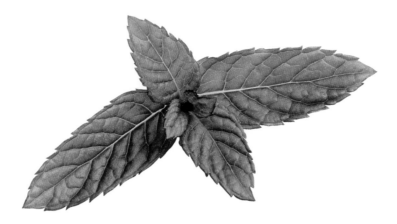

T**his herb possesses the most robust aroma in the mint family. Originating in Europe and southwest Asia, spearmint was extensively cultivated from early times onward, making its natural range hard to pinpoint. The first recorded use of the herb goes back to 400 B.C. in the Mediterranean region, where it was used as a breath freshener and to keep mice away from grain stores. The Romans used it as a medicinal herb and brought it north with them, where it became established in Britain. The plant is not native to America, but escapees from colonial gardens quickly naturalized it in the United States and Canada.

This branching perennial herb reaches two feet in height, can be hairless or hairy, and produces serrated, spear-shaped leaves, which are responsible for its name, and small, pinkish flowers that bloom on slender spikes.

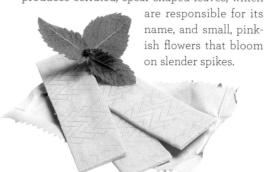

DID YOU KNOW?

Spearmint, with its crisply fragrant leaves, can be grown as a culinary or ornamental plant. It is also used to flavor toothpaste and confections, and is often added to shampoos, soaps, and cosmetics.

Culinary Uses

With only small amounts of menthol, spearmint leaves taste less intensely minty than its hybrid cousin peppermint's leaves. They can be used fresh or dried, or they can be preserved in salt, sugar, sugar syrup, alcohol, or oil. The leaves make a crisp addition to salads, a soothing tea, and a jaunty cocktail garnish. They have been used by Middle Eastern cultures as the basis of dipping sauces. The cultivar 'Nana', the nana mint of Morocco, is used to make Touareg tea, known for its mild but pungent aroma. As an herbal tea, spearmint has welcome stomach-soothing qualities. It is also used to flavor gum and candy mints.

When cooking with spearmint, for fullest flavor, wait until the end of preparation to add the herb. It is available year round in most markets; choose bright green bundles with a sharp scent. Wash thoroughly, pat dry, and store in the refrigerator. Spearmint can also be easily air-dried: just spread the leaves on a tray, place it outdoors in semi-shade for several hours, and then store the leaves in an airtight container.

In 1893, Wrigley Incorporated boosted spearmint's popularity in America by introducing it as a breath-freshening gum.

Piquant Mint Sauce

Mint sauces are refreshing staples of Middle Eastern and Indian cuisine. They are used as dipping sauces for bread, meat, or Indian samosas. This version uses spearmint as its base flavor. ■

Ingredients
- ¼ cup fresh spearmint
- 1 clove garlic
- 1 cup yogurt
- 1 tablespoon lime juice
- 2 tablespoons olive oil
- pinch of cumin or turmeric
- ½ teaspoon sea salt

Directions
Grind the spearmint, mash the garlic, and whisk together with the other ingredients until a smooth paste is formed. Refrigerate before serving. Serves four. ■

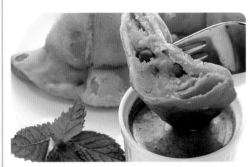

The coolness of yogurt and spearmint counteracts the hot sensation of biting into a samosa, a spicy Indian pastry.

Nutritional Value

Spearmint contains significant amounts of antioxidant vitamins such as A, beta-carotene, C, and B6, folates, riboflavin, and thiamin. It also contains vital minerals such as iron, potassium, calcium, manganese, and magnesium.

Healing Properties

Throughout history, traditional physicians have used spearmint to treat fatigue, stress, stomach and digestive ailments, respiratory problems, skin irritations, and rashes. It has been applied directly to the skin for arthritis, muscle or nerve pain, and skin conditions, and directly inside the mouth to treat swelling of the gums or tongue.

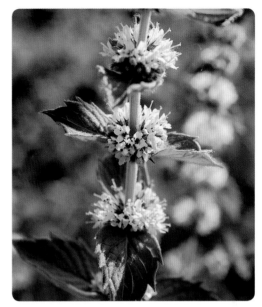

Spearmint's small pinkish or lilac flowers grow in whorls or rings on spikes in the axils of the plant's upper leaves. Butterflies and bees cannot resist the nectar of these blooms.

The plant's chemical components include alpha-pinene, beta-pinene, carvone, cineole, linalool, limonene, myrcene, and caryophyllene, which all help to ease stress and fatigue. Studies have shown that spearmint's essential oils display antifungal properties, and according to the *Journal of Chemistry,* spearmint extract has "good total phenolic and flavonoid contents" and also exhibited "excellent antioxidant activity." The journal *Phytotherapy Research* reports that spearmint tea has been used to treat embarrassing hirsutism in women—its suppressing properties are thought to reduce the blood's levels of free testosterone. Spearmint can help regulate blood sugar in diabetes patients.

History and Lore

» The mint julep (at right) is a cocktail made by muddling bourbon with spearmint. It is the official drink of the Kentucky Derby horse race.
» The mojito, a popular Cuban drink, has recently been discovered by the cocktail set. It is made with white rum, lime juice, sugar cane juice, sparking water, and spearmint.
» Sweet tea, an iced tea flavored with spearmint, is a summer tradition in the American South.

Spearmint

77

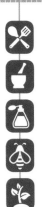

Summer Savory

Satureja hortensis

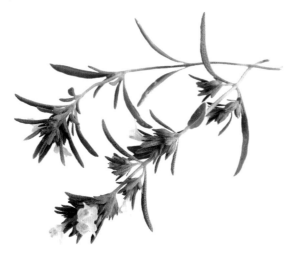

Not surprisingly, given its common name, summer savory makes a delicious addition to most recipes for savory dishes, such as meat, fish, or poultry entrees, sausages, soups, stews, chowders, and marinades. Medieval cooks even added the herb to sweet cakes and pies for a dash of peppery tang. Well before that, ancient Egyptians enjoyed the herb added to their food, while their healers used powdered versions of it as a love potion and as a medicine to relieve sore throats and intestinal disorders.

A member of the Lamiaceae (the mint or deadnettle family), summer savory is a native of southeastern Europe. It now grows almost anywhere there is sun and good soil, including planters on big-city apartment terraces.

Summer savory thrives outdoors in an herb garden, but it also grows well indoors in containers.

DID YOU KNOW?

Summer savory is a versatile plant, with culinary, decorative, aromatic, and medicinal properties. Fresh or dried leaves flavor foods, while the dried plants are used to scent potpourris.

The plant matures to approximately 18 inches tall and features many branches with soft, narrow, dark green leaves of about a half inch in length. The small pale pink or lavender flowers blossom in July, and then give way to dark brown or black, nut-shaped seeds.

Culinary Uses

Summer savory is used in a number of European and American dishes. In the Maritimes provinces of Canada, it is used to make cretonade, a thick dressing that is served with poultry. With its distinct peppery taste, its flavor has been compared to a more delicate version of marjoram or thyme. In addition to its compatibility with meat, fish, poultry, and eggs, summer savory goes well with most vegetables, especially beans, and enlivens egg dishes. In France, it is often used as an ingredient in fines herbes, herbes de Provence, and bouquet garni.

The plants dry easily: harvest just before blooming, tie the stems together, and hang the bundle in an open space for several days. Then, strip the leaves from the stems, and crush to the desired consistency. Freeze fresh summer savory in small, clean bunches inside freezer bags.

Vegetable Booster

Summer savory makes an ideal garden companion for a number of other plants. It encourages the growth of onions and garlic, and it can protect most varieties of beans from the ravages of the Mexican bean beetle *(Epilachna varivestis),* shown below, a species of voracious lady beetle that feeds on the leaves and can destroy the plants. ■

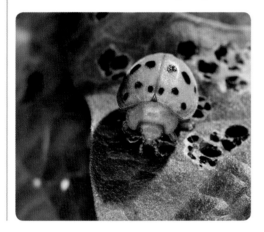

Nutritional Value

The leaves of this herb are extremely high in dietary fiber, and rich in vitamins A, C, the B-complex group, and pyroxidine. They are also an excellent source of the minerals potassium, iron, calcium, magnesium, manganese, zinc, and selenium.

Many people who are watching their sodium intake have found that this herb makes a satisfying salt substitute.

Speedy Summer Savory Sauces

To raise the taste quotient of your grilled chicken or fish, create a topping from snipped chives, lemon juice, mayonnaise, and freshly chopped summer savory. Coat one side of the meat with the sauce, grill, and then repeat on the other side.

To make a rich sauce for grilled portobello mushrooms, chop a cup of summer savory and a cup of flat-leaf parsley, and then sauté lightly in butter with a crushed clove of garlic until caramelized. Add a dash of lemon juice, reheat, and then pour over mushrooms. This sauce can also be used to top oily fish. ■

Healing Properties

The ancients used summer savory to ease a number of ailments, including stomach problems and joint pain. Nicholas Culpeper, the illustrious 17th-century apothecary, considered it to be a virtual cure-all, recommending that it always be kept on hand.

Modern medical research has revealed that the leaves and shoots of summer savory contain high levels of valuable antioxidant chemical compounds. The plant's numerous essential volatile-oil phenolics include thymol, with its antiseptic and anti-fungal properties, and carvacrol, which inhibits the growth of bacteria such as *E. coli* and *Bacilus cereus.*

History and Lore

» Summer savory was believed to be an aphrodisiac by early cultures.
» During the Middle Ages, some healers thought the herb was a cure for deafness.
» A wild cousin, *Satureja douglasii,* or yerba buena, is used by the indigenous Americans of California and Alaska as an herbal tea.

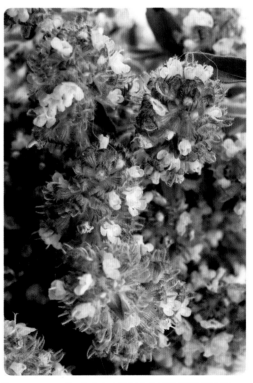

Summer savory is a fast-growing plant, with tiny white or pink flowers appearing in late summer to early fall.

Tarragon

Artemisia dracunculus

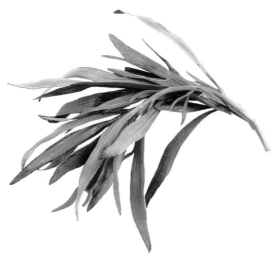

Many continental cooks consider this aromatic, woody-stemmed perennial the most illustrious of all the *Artemisias*, the one they favor for preparing béarnaise sauce, tartar sauce, and hollandaise sauce, among other classic recipes. Often called French tarragon, the plant thrives in most soil conditions providing there is sun. It grows to two or three feet in height, and produces bladelike, undivided leaves and small flowers—yellow with some black—that form round heads. Its bright green leaves differ from the other *Artemisias*, which have gray-green leaves.

The plant's specific name comes from the French word *esdragon,* after the Latin

DID YOU KNOW?

Tarragon has long been prized for its aromatic leaves, which are used both fresh and dried. A mainstay of French cuisine, it one of the herbs used in the classic fines herbes blend.

dracunculus, meaning "little dragon," possibly because it was once believed to cure the bite of poisonous serpents—as well as of mad dogs. Others believe the dragon reference was to the plant's serpentine root system.

Tarragon is a relatively "new" herb: it has only been cultivated for about six hundred years. It originated in Central Asia and was likely brought to Europe by the invading Mongols in the 13th century. Some medieval writings mention it as a pharmaceutical herb.

Culinary Uses

The peppery and slightly anise-tasting French tarragon, with its citrus-woodsy undertones, can be found in most kitchens. The Russian version (*A. dracunculoides*), which originated in Siberia, also has its advocates. It has rougher leaves and is less tart than its cousin.

French tarragon, one of the notable fines herbes of France, lends its distinctive flavor to poultry, veal, seafood, vegetables, egg dishes, salads, sauces, marinades, and rubs. It is delicious sprinkled over cheese and fresh fruit. It is also used in the pickling process and for making relishes and mustards.

Tarragon easily imparts its distinct scent and flavor to liquids, and, these days, it is increasingly popular in drinks. For a refreshing summer smoothie or sorbet, just blend lemon, water, ice, and tarragon until smooth.

Nutritional Value

This healthful herb contains high levels of vitamins A, C, B6, niacin, riboflavin, and folate. It also provides calcium, iron, copper, phosphorus, potassium, magnesium, and manganese, and is low in cholesterol and sodium.

Healing Properties

In the past, healers from many cultures employed tarragon as a cure for hiccups, worms, indigestion, rheumatism, loss of appetite, irregular menses, and water retention.

Modern researchers have discovered that this versatile plant is a powerful antioxidant with antibacterial, antifungal, anti-inflammatory, antiviral, and antiseptic qualities. Among other things, tarragon acts as a "free radical scavenger," helping the body to eliminate those harmful by-products of metabolism. It contains high levels of eugenol, also found in clove oil, a natural anesthetic that specifically relieves toothache pain. It can also be used to stimulate appetite in people who are eating poorly due to illness or old age.

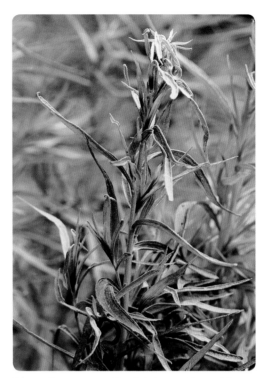

Tarragon leaves are smooth and dark green. Chopped fine, they will add an anise-like kick to savory dishes. You can also harvest the leaves in late summer to dry for winter use.

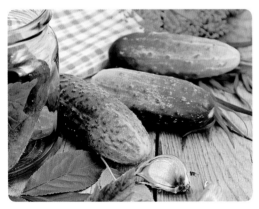

Along with garlic, pepper, bay leaves and dill, tarragon is often used in cucumber pickling spice mixtures.

History and Lore

» Medieval Catholics believed that placing tarragon in their shoes before embarking on a walking pilgrimage gave them strength.
» Seventeenth-century diarist and gardener John Evelyn said of tarragon: "'Tis highly cordial and friend to the head, heart, and liver."
» Tarragon is a member of the Composite family, closed related to wormwood. Its volatile essential oil is chemically identical to anise.

A Versatile Vinegar

Fresh tarragon loses its flavor very quickly, so the taste is best preserved in vinegar. Tarragon vinegar makes a tangy, useful addition to the kitchen condiment shelf: it can be mixed into vinaigrette, used in its own right, or included in other recipes (French chefs often mix it with mustard). Tarragon vinegar also makes a welcome gift for the home cook, especially if presented in a pretty bottle. To prepare your own, gather, wash, and dry three sprigs of fresh tarragon. Place in a jar or bottle. Heat 16 fluid ounces of white vinegar, being sure not to bring it to a boil. Add to vinegar bottle, and close tightly. Place the bottle on a windowsill and let sit for about three weeks. Store in the refrigerator or other a cool place. Use the vinegar within one year. ∎

Tarragon

81

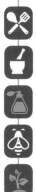

Tea

Camellia sinensis

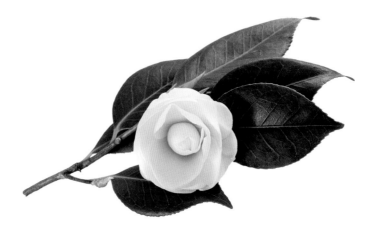

T ea, with its astringent, slightly bitter flavor, was first used as a medicinal drink. The tea plant originated in China; the Chinese, in turn, introduced it to Portuguese traders in the 16th century. It gained popularity in England during the following century, and by the Victorian era, afternoon tea was a social fixture.

Camellia sinensis is the source of all true teas. Most black tea comes from India (Darjeeling, Assam), Sri Lanka (Ceylon), and China (Lapsang Souchong). It is the basis of popular commercial blends like Earl Grey,

DID YOU KNOW?
A shrubby flowering plant, *Camellia sinensis* is the source of all nonherbal teas. Water is the only beverage that is consumed in greater quantities than tea.

masala chai, and English Breakfast tea. Black tea leaves are oxidized to achieve complexity. Black tea contains the most caffeine of any major tea, though only half as much as coffee. Oolong tea is partly fermented, giving it a red color and a sweet taste. Green tea is "pure" tea and is not oxidized; it contains only a quarter of the caffeine of coffee. White tea comes mainly from China and contains buds and young leaves. Its delicate flavor is best sampled without sugar or honey.

Culinary Use

Hot tea is typically taken with breakfast, during an afternoon break, or after dinner, often with dessert. Iced tea, first served in luncheonettes as an alternative to cold soda, has now become a consumer phenomenon, available in tall, pop-top cans all over the world.

To brew the perfect cup of hot tea, first warm up the pot and the cup by pouring in boiling water. The water for steeping black tea should be boiling, but it needs to be cooled slightly before pouring over green tea. The ideal measurement would be two teaspoons of tea leaves to eight fluid ounces of water. The leaves should be allowed to steep for two to seven minutes, according to taste.

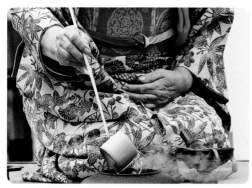

Many cultures have created intricate formalized rituals for the drinking of tea, such as the Japanese tea ceremony.

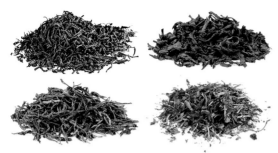

Camellia sinensis leaves are processed three different ways to produce the three major classes of tea, known as black (top left), oolong (top right), and green (bottom left). White tea (bottom right) comes from the buds and the leaves.

Tea is increasingly used for other culinary purposes, flavoring everything from meat marinades to ice creams.

Nutritional Value

Tea contains folate and is rich in manganese. It also supplies lesser amounts of magnesium, potassium, and copper.

Healing Properties

Scientific researchers have recently begun to explore the medicinal potential of tea, and already the results show that tea has a beneficial effect on the heart, the circulatory system, and the immune system.

To achieve a richer flavor, black tea leaves are fermented. This oxidation alters the tea's antioxidant polyphenols—called flavonoids—making them more complex. Flavonoids have been linked to cancer prevention, lowered cholesterol levels, and protection from heart attacks and stroke. Black tea also increases alpha brain wave activity and may lower the risk of dementia in the elderly.

The antioxidants in oolong tea can combat heart disease, and improve bone, skin, and dental health. Green tea has been linked to a lowered risk of cancer, and to weight loss and heart health. White tea contains cancer-busting antioxidant polyphenols, which also help control cholesterol, lower blood pressure, and even keep the complexion youthful by attacking the free radicals that age skin. Cold and flu sufferers appreciate its antiviral and antibacterial properties.

History and Lore

» American colonists loved their tea, but when King George III raised taxes on the brew, outraged patriots dumped an entire shipment into Boston Harbor in protest.

» Tea bags were "invented" when people received samples of loose tea in silk bags and thought they were supposed to brew the tea in them.

» In England, working-class families refer to their evening meal as "tea."

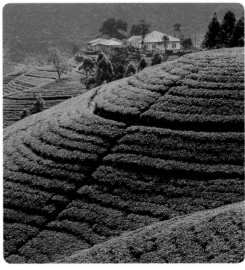

A tea plantation in Sri Lanka. Workers plant tea bushes in orderly rows so that they can harvest the tea properly. These manicured rows can stretch for miles, covering entire hillsides.

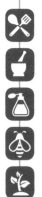

Thyme

Thymus vulgaris

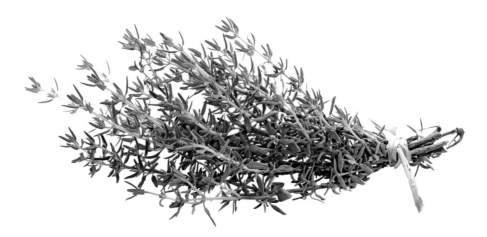

This delicate-looking plant—called English, French or common thyme—packs a powerful aromatic punch, both in the garden and on the plate.

Originally native to Asia and the Mediterranean, it was spread through Europe by the Romans, who used it to purify their chambers and to flavor cheese and liqueurs. Now found in gardens worldwide, this fragrant, woody perennial grows low and spreads, sometimes like a carpet.

The curled, elliptical leaves are small, gray-green on top, whitish below, and the purple, pink, or white flowers can be eaten when they first open. The plant is known to produce flowers that are female one day, then male the next, along with strictly female flowers. There is no scientific explanation for this, although some botanists believe the switch encourages pollinators.

The name *thyme* may have come from the Greek word *thumos* or from the Latin *fumus,* both of which mean "smoke." Both relate to the fact that thyme was often burned as a religious offering. (The Greek word *thyo* could also apply; it means "sacrifice.") There are roughly 60 species in the genus including lemon, orange, silver, creeping, caraway, wild, and woolly thyme.

Culinary Uses

Thyme is, along with parsley and bay leaf, a key component of the French bouquet garni. The herb makes an excellent accompaniment to omelets and scrambled eggs, potato dishes, tomato sauces, soups, and stocks. It works especially well in any hearty recipe made with pinto, kidney, and black beans. When poaching fish, a few springs of thyme on the fish and in the poaching liquid will blend nicely with lemon and butter.

Because of its delicate flavor, fresh or dried thyme should be added near the end of the preparation process. The herb can be purchased fresh or dried in most supermarkets all year long.

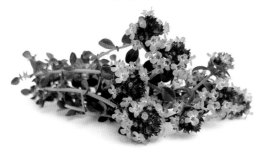

Thyme's tiny two-lipped flowers bloom in spring and summer, lighting up a kitchen garden with shades of purplish pink.

Nutritional Value

Thyme is a rich source of vitamin C, and a very good source of vitamin A. It also contains iron, manganese, copper, and dietary fiber.

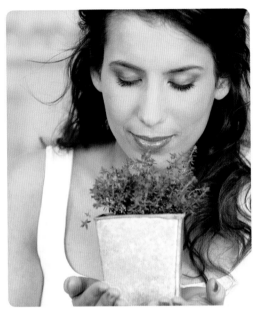

Aromatherapists use thyme essential oil, which creates a warming sensation, to treat conditions like throbbing muscles and sports injuries. Red thyme oil is currently used in perfumes and to scent soaps, cosmetics, and toothpaste.

Healing Properties

Thyme has a long history—the ancient Egyptians used the herb to embalm their pharaohs, Virgil recommended it for fatigue, and Nicholas Culpeper prescribed it to prevent nightmares. It has been associated with the treatment of respiratory ailments, such as coughing, asthma, and bronchitis, for centuries. It has been used since the 1500s as a mouthwash and topical application, as it still is today.

Modern research indicates that the herb's volatile oils, thymol, carvacolo, borneol, and geraniol, are responsible for its many beneficial qualities. Thymol (which is named for the herb), in particular, has been found to increase the percentage of healthy fats in brain, kidney, and heart membranes. The herb also contains a variety of flavonoids, establishing it as valuable antioxidant food. Its antimicrobial properties make it effective against both fungal and bacterial infections. It might also relieve the smooth muscle spasms that cause coughing.

A Cleansing Touch of Thyme

For thousands of years, herbs—along with spices—have been used to preserve foods and keep them from spoiling or becoming contaminated. Recent research published in *Food Microbiology* has shown that components of thyme or basil can not only prevent contamination, they can also actually reverse contamination in foods that have already been exposed. Researchers discovered that after lettuce was inoculated with shigella, an organism that triggers potentially harmful diarrhea, treatment with essential oil of thyme reduced the number of bacteria to a barely detectable level. With this in mind, it makes sense to include thyme and basil with the uncooked greens in your salads or to add them to your salad dressing. ■

History and Lore

» In ancient Greece, thyme was used as incense and burned in temples. It was also a symbol of courage, so the phrase "the smell of thyme" reflected honor upon a person.

» Burning thyme gets rid of insects in the house.

» In Dutch and German folklore, a bed of thyme was home to fairies, and in the Middle Ages, it was placed under the pillow as a sleep aid.

» Medieval ladies offered their chosen knight a scarf bearing an embroidered bee above a sprig of thyme.

» In Germany, thyme was named Medicinal Plant of the Year 2006.

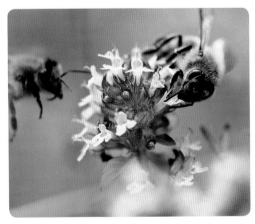

Horace wrote that the ancient Romans kept thyme exclusively for bee culture. Honeybees finds the flowers irresistible.

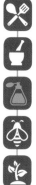

Watercress

Nasturtium officinale

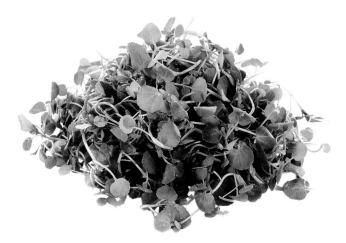

This crisp, leafy green herb with the peppery taste is a semi-aquatic plant that spreads on the banks of slow-moving streams. Watercress is part of the crucifer, or Brassicaceae family, and is a close cousin to mustard greens, arugula, and cabbage. The plant's leaves are small, scalloped, and rounded, and the tiny white flowers produce a double row of edible seeds. It is also known by the names water radish, water rocket, and hedge mustard.

Valued by ancient civilizations as both a food source and a medicinal plant, watercress has been cultivated for thousands of years in Europe and Central Asia. It might be the oldest

known green vegetable consumed by humans. It was spread to the rest of the world by European explorers, who knew that it prevented scurvy, a potentially deadly disease caused by a vitamin C deficiency. Watercress was first grown commercially in the early 19th century as its popularity increased. Currently, demand for this healthy and tasty herb inexplicably rises and falls.

Culinary Uses

Watercress can be mixed into salads, steamed or sautéed as a vegetable, or added to soups for a peppery boost. Perhaps it is most famous as an ingredient in the finger sandwiches served at a formal tea. Its seeds can be used to make a spicy mustard; they contain the same mustard oil responsible for the throaty taste of horseradish.

When shopping for watercress, look for bunches that are deep green; avoid anything that appears yellow, wilted, or slimy. To cleanse the plant, rinse it thoroughly, and then place it in a hydrogen peroxide solution (one tablespoon per quart of water) for a half hour to remove any parasites, like the larvae of the common liver fluke, or pollutants it may have picked up in the stream.

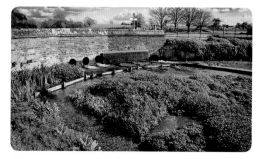

At a watercress farm, leafy beds are grown in a shallow pond. The plant's stems are hollow, which is what allows it to float.

Nutritional Value

This aquatic plant accumulates valuable minerals from the water, including potassium, phosphorus, calcium, iron, magnesium, and sodium. It also contains substantial amounts of vitamins A and C, and especially vitamin K—with 312 percent of the daily-recommended value—which protects against neuronal damage in the brain. Its B-complex vitamins, like niacin, riboflavin, and B6 boost cell metabolism, and its antioxidant flavonoids protect the body from lung and mouth cancer.

Healing Properties

As early as 400 B.C., Greek physician Hippocrates, he of the famous oath, grew watercress at his first hospital on the island of Kos. Traditional

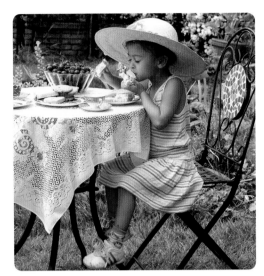

Watercress is one of the traditional fillings for the dainty sandwiches served at afternoon teatime.

healers have used the herb to relieve respiratory problems, as well as to treat baldness, constipation, parasitic worms, cancer, goiter, scurvy, and tuberculosis. It is believed to improve appetite and digestion, enhance sexual performance, kill germs, and act as a general "spring tonic." Applied directly to the skin, it is said to cure arthritis, rheumatism, eczema, scabies, and warts.

Recent medical studies suggest that the phytonutrients in the plant can help keep bones strong, fight infection, maintain healthy connective tissue, and prevent iron deficiency. A two-year research project at the University of Ulster concluded that eating watercress daily reduced the DNA damage caused by free radicals. A study at the University of Southampton focused on a compound in the herb called phenethyl isothiocyanate (PEITC), which exhibited anticancer properties, specifically for breast cancer. The researchers believe PEITC may starve tumors of blood and oxygen by triggering a "turn off" signal in the body.

History and Lore

» During the 19th century, watercress was easily found in the streams of Europe and the United States, and, because it cost nothing, it was called "poor man's bread." A bunch of leaves would be rolled into a cone and eaten for breakfast.

» Despite its genus name, watercress is not related to the popular garden plant, nasturtium.

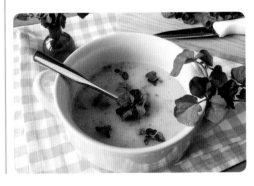

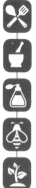

Winter Savory

Satureja montana

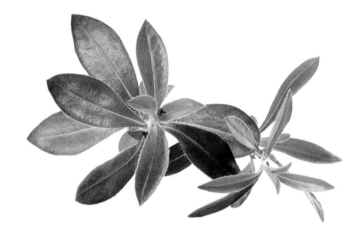

Winter savory, which is a semi-woody perennial, was originally native to the warm slopes and fields of southern Europe. After the Romans took a liking to the herb and began using it for cooking, they eventually introduced it as far north as Great Britain during their military campaigns. It has been cultivated in England since the mid-1500s, where it was popular for its peppery taste and heady aroma, and it can now be found worldwide in temperate regions.

DID YOU KNOW?

A bushy semi-evergreen perennial, winter savory is a great mixing herb, blending well with basil, oregano, and thyme.

This hardy dwarf shrub—which grows to a height of 16 inches—is woodier and bushier than its cousin summer savory and it possesses a sharper tang in recipes. Winter savory produces small, oblong, glossy green leaves and its pale purple or white flowers form terminal spikes that can bloom from late June through September. Because of its low profile, it makes a wonderful edging plant for an herb garden or perennial border.

Culinary Uses

Winter savory has been pleasing cooks in Europe and the Americas for centuries. In the 1600s, herbalist John Parkinson advised that winter savory be dried and powdered and then mixed with grated bread-crumbs, "to breade their meate, be it fish or flesh, to give it a quicker relish." Early cookbooks recommended winter savory, together with other herbs, as a dressing for trout.

Winter savory is a robust herb and works well with red meat and game. It can also stand up to beans and lentils and makes an excellent marinade or grilling rub. Yet, some cooks swear by the herb as a flavoring for more delicate chicken or turkey dishes, and it also makes a tasty addition to stuffing, bread crumbs, and bread recipes.

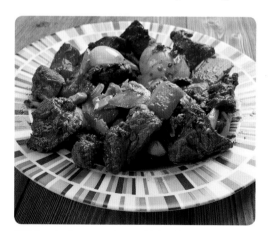

With its robust aroma and taste, this herb is best used in hearty dishes such as beef stews, duck, and venison.

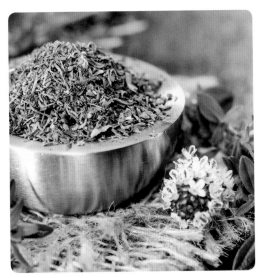

Winter savory maintains its rich, spicy scent even when the leaves are dried, making it perfect for including in spice-based potpourris and sachets.

The leaves, which are an integral part of herbes de Provence, can be used either fresh or dried. The longer fresh leaves are cooked, the less intense their flavor.

Nutritional Value

Winter savory is rich in vitamins A and C, the B-complex group, pyridoxine, niacin and thiamin, plus 100 grams of dry savory supplies more than 100 percent of the dietary fiber requirement. The same amount of the herb contains astonishing amounts of iron (474 percent of RDA, or recommended dietary allowances), calcium (210 percent), manganese (265 percent), and magnesium (94 percent), as well as zinc, potassium, and selenium.

Healing Properties

While traditional healers often employed summer savory, they used winter savory less often. Famed 17th-century English botanist Nicholas Culpepper nevertheless claimed that the herb was a good remedy for colic, and a tea made from winter savory proved effective for treating intestinal disorders including cramping, indigestion, diarrhea, nausea, and gas. It was also thought to relieve coughs and sore throats, reduce sex drive, and act as a tonic.

Current research shows that the herb's leaves contain various beneficial essential oils, such as carvacrol and thymol, which have antifungal and antibacterial properties. And the tea, which is a powerful antiseptic, actually does relieve digestive problems and sore throats. The tea can also improve the functioning of the liver and kidneys. Both the shoots and leaves contain antioxidant compounds, which can prevent certain diseases and promote general well-being.

History and Lore

» The Roman god Mercury claimed dominion over winter savory.

» In German, the word for savory is *Bohnenkraut,* meaning "bean-herb," because the Germans use it to flavor bean dishes.

» American colonists brought savory from England and valued it as a digestive aid.

» Rubbing a sprig of winter savory on a bee sting can ease the pain.

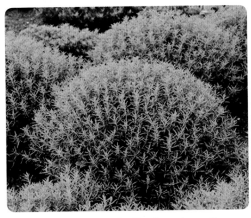

Mounds of winter savory make attractive and aromatic additions to an herb garden. In Shakespeare's day, winter savory was prized for its appealing smell. In fact, it was considered one of the most fragrant herbs and was often planted near beehives to lend its flavor to honey.

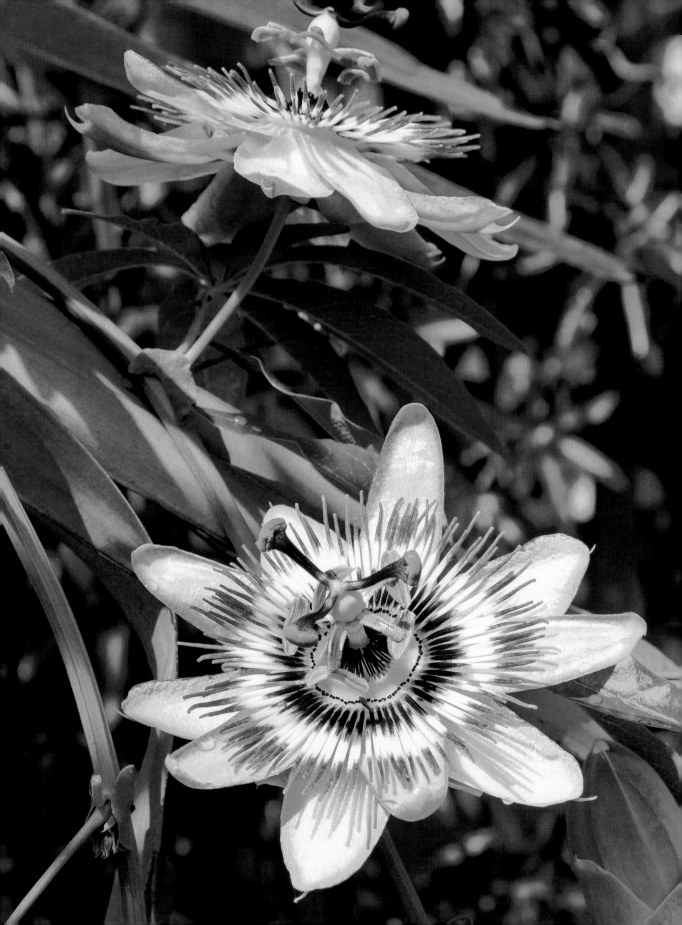

CHAPTER TWO

MEDICINAL HERBS

Opposite: **Passionflower**

Nature's Pharmacy

HARNESSING THE HEALING POWER OF HERBS

It is likely that one of the first things early man figured out was that if he ate something that made him feel unwell, early woman could find something growing somewhere that would make him feel better. (It would not be surprising to discover that humans learned this behavior from observing animals: dogs and cats, especially, eat grass or weeds to ease gastric distress.) And such may have been the inauspicious beginning of herbal medicine.

Still, it took humankind thousands of years to develop an understanding of plants and herbs and to learn which ones were beneficial as healing agents and which ones to avoid. The study of natural medicine was practiced by many cultures, beginning at the dawn of civilization. One of the earliest books on the subject, cataloging hundreds of medicinal plants and their uses, was the Indian *Rig Veda,* which dates back to a period from 4500 to 1600 B.C.

SIGNS IN NATURE

Superstition, and the notion that the natural world revolved around humans, did sometimes lead to a wrong turn. From the days of ancient Greece and Rome until the end of the 17th century there existed a curious belief, called the "doctrine of signatures," that proclaimed that an herb's appearance—its resemblance to a body part, animal, or other object—revealed its

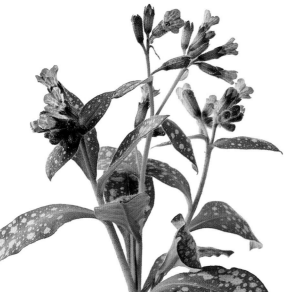

Pulminaria officinalis, or lungwort, is so named because it was once believed to cure lung ailments.

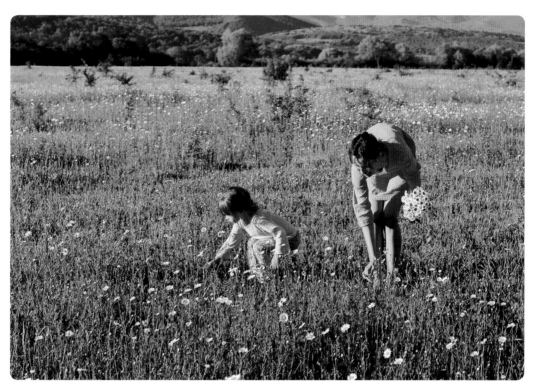

Nature provides many healing herbs, such as German chamomile, that you can grow in your garden or collect in the wild.

medicinal value. In other words, tarragon, with its serpentine roots, was thought to cure snakebite, and the spotted oval leaves of the lungwort plant were thought to resemble diseased lungs, and so were used to treat pulmonary infections. Botanist William Coles explained it simply—God wished us to see what each plant was useful for by offering us a sign or "signature."

> "All that mankind needs for good health and healing is provided by God in nature . . . the challenge of science is to find it."
>
> —*Paracelsus*

HERBS TODAY

In modern times, many manufactured medicines are distillations, variations, combinations, or reproductions of substances found in nature, and so it is never a good idea to dismiss an herbal remedy without some scientific investigation. The broad claims made by certain traveling healers for their various herbal concoctions and plant potions were sometimes exaggerated, but a surprising number of herbs have more than lived up to their early reputations as agents for easing pain and treating disease. Today's "flavor of the month" herb among traditional healers and practitioners could easily become tomorrow's cure for cancer.

Alfalfa

Medicago sativa

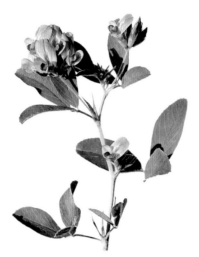

Used as fodder for livestock since the time of the early Persians, alfalfa has also been employed as a healing herb for 1,500 years or more. Although the name *alfalfa,* which comes from the Arabic *al-fac-facah,* or "father of all foods," is widely used, the plant is called lucerne in the United Kingdom, New Zealand, and South Africa. It is a member of the pea family Fabaceae, a legume that returns nitrogen to the soil.

The plant was originally native to the Mediterranean and Middle East, but it can now be found in most temperate parts of Europe and the Americas. When in bloom, alfalfa bears a distinct resemblance to clover, with its clusters of delicate purple flowers. It is a perennial with a lifespan of 5 to 8 years, although some specimens have lived 20 years or more. Once it is

---

DID YOU KNOW?

Grown throughout the world for its use as livestock forage, alfalfa also has other important medicinal and culinary uses.

---

established, the plant forms a tough crown with many shoot buds that enables it to regrow after repeated harvesting. Its roots can grow 20 or 30 feet into the ground, allowing the plant to draw many nutrients from the soil. It is most often cut as hay, used as silage (fermented fodder for cud-chewing ruminants), or for grazing. It not only has a high yield per acre, it also has the highest feed value of any of the common hay crops.

Healing Properties

This is a plant with an ancient pedigree—remains of alfalfa leaves have been found in Persian ruins dating back to 4000 B.C., and it is mentioned in Turkish writings from 1300 B.C. Chinese apothecaries used the plant to stimulate the appetite and relieve ulcers, while Ayurvedic healers in India use it as a diuretic and to treat arthritis. American colonists employed it to treat scurvy, urinary and menstrual problems, and arthritis. Native Americans made a thickening paste from the seeds and used them as a nutritional additive. In 19th-century America, traveling healers incorporated alfalfa into their spring tonics.

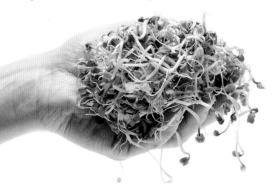

Alfalfa sprouts make a healthy addition to a sandwich.

MEDICINAL HERBS

Traditional healers find it useful for treating morning sickness, nausea, kidney problems, and urinary discomfort. It can cleanse the liver and bowel, help reduce bad cholesterol, and support healthy circulation and the immune system. As a poultice, it eases the pain and itch of insect bites. With all these benefits, it's not surprising that alfalfa is often mixed with other botanicals.

Nutritionally, the leaves are a good source of vitamins and minerals, including the full spectrum of the B vitamins, A, C, D, E, and K, as well as iron, niacin, biotin, folic acid, calcium, magnesium, phosphorus, and potassium. Alfalfa also supplies chlorophyll and beta-carotene, plus high levels of protein and amino acids compared to other greens.

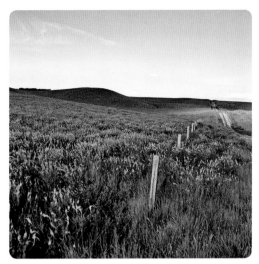

A crop of alfalfa growing in Saskatchewan, Canada. Alfalfa is an autotoxic plant, meaning new seeds have difficulty taking root in an existing field. Most farmers rotate alfalfa fields with other grass and grain crops like wheat or corn.

History and Lore

» Other names for the plant include *erba medica,* lucerne grass, purple medic, buffalo grass, and Chilean clover.
» A home remedy for thick, healthy hair recommends mixing the juice of alfalfa along with lettuce and carrot juice and consuming it on a daily basis.

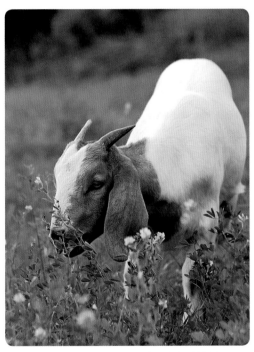

A Boer goat grazes in a field of alfalfa. This healthful legume is often used as a forage food for goats, sheep, and cattle.

Culinary Uses

During the advent of New Age thinking in the 1980s, alfalfa sprouts became available in health food stores and quickly caught on as a crisp, zesty source of nutrition in salads or sandwiches. They can now be purchased in most supermarkets or sprouted at home from a kit. The mild-flavored leaves can be taken straight from the field for use in salads, soups, casseroles, and stews.

CURIOSITIES

Head-Bumping Bees

Alfalfa has become a "special needs" plant when it comes to pollination. Nature has shaped its flowers in a way that causes bees to hit their heads on the pollen-carrying keel when they enter the flower, forcing pollen to shower down on them. The trouble is that western honeybees, the pollinators most commonly used, don't appreciate repeatedly getting their heads bumped, and many have learned to retrieve nectar from the side of the flower, which means they never gather any pollen. So now, whenever fields of alfalfa need pollinating, beekeepers use young bees that have not yet learned the aversion technique of feeding from the side. Recently, the alfalfa leaf-cutter bee has also been recruited for this task. They do not form colonies or make honey, but they are very efficient pollinators—and don't seem to mind a bump on the head. ■

Aloe

Aloe vera

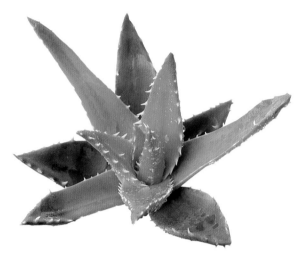

loe, or aloe vera, is a succulent plant native to Africa, Madagascar, and Jordan. Lauded by the ancient Egyptians, Greeks, and Romans for its healing powers, aloe is also mentioned in Indian and Chinese writings. Perhaps the earliest record of aloe is on a Sumerian tablet dating back four thousand years. A popular houseplant and garden ornamental today, aloe is known for the clear, jelly-like substance produced in the leaf, which is used to ease the pain of burns. Aloe also produces a form of yellow latex in the cells just below the skin.

The green or gray-green plants, which average two to three feet in height, have no stem or a very short stem, and serrated, fleshy, lance-shaped leaves. The showy orange or pink flower resembles a firecracker and grows on a tall stalk, or scape. Aloe flourishes in dry climates, and, although it looks like some type of cactus, it was once classified as a lily. It has lately been reassigned to the tropical Xanthorrhoeaceae family.

DID YOU KNOW?
Found only in cultivation, *Aloe vera* has long been appreciated as both an ornamental and as a source of the healing gel obtained from the plant's leaves.

Aloe manages to stay plump and juicy when other plants dry out and die by closing its pores to prevent moisture loss.

Healing Properties

There are more than 400 species of aloe, but *A. vera* (often called *A. barbadensis*) is the one known as the "burn plant" or the "miracle plant." Although there are countless aloe-based products for treating burns, many people still prefer to apply the gel fresh from the plant.

The aloe leaf contains four layers: The rind is the outer layer; the sap is a bitter fluid that helps protect the aloe from animals; the mucilage gel is the part of the leaf that is used to make aloe vera gel; aloe vera is the inner gel, which contains eight essential amino acids that our bodies cannot manufacture. Healers from many cultures have used aloe for treating asthma, constipation, ulcers,

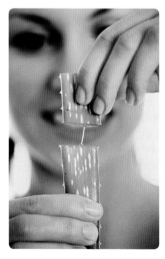

Aloe gel is the clear, jelly-like substance found in the inner part of the aloe plant leaf. This gel can be used straight from a leaf to soothe and heal irritated skin.

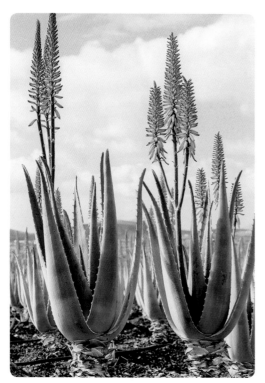
An aloe field in the Canary Islands

Aloe and Agribusiness

Aloe is nothing if not adaptable, and it can be found in many warmer regions of the world. The Canary Islands produces a particularly high-grade aloe. In the United States, it is farmed commercially for its gel extract, which is used in hundreds of products, from sunscreens and moisturizers to cosmetics and alternative medicines. In 1912, Colonel H. W. Johnston established the first aloe vera farm in the country, in Florida. Today, aloe is grown in the Rio Grande Valley of Texas, in California and Florida, and in specially built greenhouses in Oklahoma. ■

Culinary Uses

Both the leaves and seeds of the aloe plant can be eaten, but aloe alone has a bitter flavor. It is typically combined with other foods or fruit juice to make it more palatable. In Japan, it appears in a commercial brand of yogurt, while beverages that include aloe vera are sold around the world. In the Tamil Nadu state of India, aloe is used an ingredient in curry.

History and Lore

» Egyptian queens used aloe as part of their daily beauty routine. It is possible that after aloe is absorbed, it stimulates fibroblast cells and causes them to regenerate faster.
» Ancient Egyptian stone carvings of aloe refer to it as the "plant of immortality."
» Legend claims that Alexander the Great conquered Socotra, an island in the Indian Ocean, to secure the aloe growing there to treat the wounds of his soldiers.

diabetes, headaches, arthritis, and coughs. Even now, in the Philippines, the juice is blended with milk and used to treat kidney infections.

Contemporary researchers report conflicting results on the medical usefulness of aloe. Natural Medicines Comprehensive Database, which rates effectiveness based on scientific evidence, found that aloe did reduce the size of first- or second-degree burns. They also found it "possibly effective" for treating constipation, cold sores, itchy mouth rashes, and psoriasis. There is some indication that a dose of aloe and honey three times a day helped lung cancer patients on chemotherapy to heal completely or partially, or take better control of the disease, compared to those on chemotherapy alone.

Aloe has not proven effective for treating HIV, skin damage caused by cancer radiation treatments, or sunburn. On the other hand, in a clinical trial by the Royal London Hospital and the John Radcliffe Hospital in Oxford, when 44 patients suffering from ulcerative colitis were treated with aloe vera, there was improvement in 38 percent of patients as opposed to 8 percent in the placebo group.

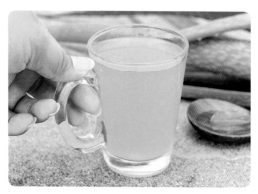
Aloe juice can be a healthy beverage, but be sure that you buy aloe vera that is made for internal consumption.

Aloe

97

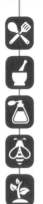

Angelica

Angelica archangelica, A. sinensis

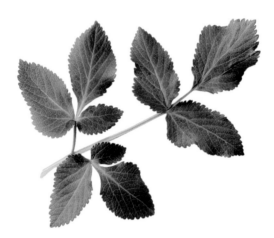

This graceful, biennial member of the umbellifer family is an herb of great antiquity and one of the most treasured tools of the healer's art. Although angelica is believed to have originated in arid Syria, it can now be found growing wild in many temperate to subarctic regions, even as far north as Iceland and Lapland.

The plant presents an impressive profile in garden or field, with the stout, hollow stalks reaching five feet in length, the leaf stems reaching three feet including footstalks, the leaves themselves a profusion of serrated green spearheads. The tiny yellowish flowers, which blossom in July, form large, nodding umbels.

DID YOU KNOW?

Cultivated for the edible stems and roots that are used in cooking, as well as used medicinally, angelica gives off a pleasant fragrance that also makes it useful in aromatherapy.

It is commonly called garden angelica, wild celery, and Norwegian angelica. One possible explanation for the plant's name is that, according to legend, an angel appeared to a monk in a dream and proclaimed that the herb could cure the plague. Another possibility is that the plant flowers around May 8, the holy day of St. Michael the Archangel. Such was angelica's purported power that it could stand against evil spells, enchantments, and witchcraft. It eventually came to be known as the "root of the Holy Ghost."

Healing Properties

Of the roughly 60 species of angelicas, *Angelica archangelica* was the one most relied on by healers in England and on the Continent for centuries. In 1629, English botanist John Parkinson elevated angelica above all other herbs in his book *Paradisi in sole paradisus terrestris,* and it remains a staple of the modern herbal healer. Chinese apothecaries employed many species of angelica—Chinese angelica (*A. sinensis*), called dong quai or female ginseng—as treatment for female disorders and fertility problems.

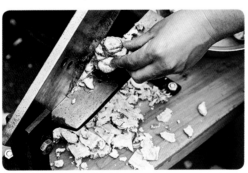

The root of *A. sinensis,* called dong quai, being sliced in a Chinese herb market. There are about 60 species of angelica.

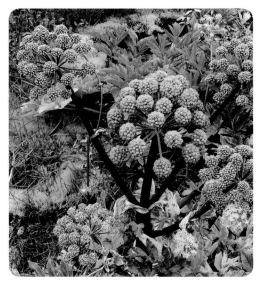

A. archangelica produces puffy pinwheels of yellow-green flowers, which attract honeybees that feed on its on pollen and nectar. It is a biennial plant and during its first year grows only leaves, which are composed of numerous small finely toothed leaflets, divided into groups (see opposite page).

The essential oil of *A. archangelica* is sometimes used as a digestive, expectorant, diuretic, stimulant, and carminative. European healers have long used it to treat colds, indigestion, and coughs and bronchial ailments, as well as to calm the nerves and stimulate the appetite.

Modern medical research has found that angelica contains carotene, used by the liver to produce vitamin A; valeric acid, which has a calming effect on the nerves; and plant steroids, which are key to the processes of the immune system. The herb also contains pectin, an enzyme essential for proper food digestion, and about 5 percent copper salts.

Culinary Uses

Although it is not thought of as a culinary herb, angelica has a pleasant taste. The stems can be candied and used to decorate cakes, while the dried root is used to flavor bread and the seeds to flavor pastry. Angelica is also used commercially as a flavoring agent in honey, alcohol—possibly part of the secret recipes for Benedictine and Chartreuse—and other beverages.

Aromatic Qualities

Unlike other umbellifers, such as fennel, anise, or chervil, angelica gives off a pervasive, peppery-sweet aroma, one that has been compared by early writers to the scent of musk or juniper. Even the plant's rhizomous roots are aromatic. In the practice of aromatherapy, angelica is used to treat psoriasis, skin irritations, indigestion, rheumatism and gout, bronchitis, colds, and stress. The herb is used to scent lotions and soaps, and its essential oil is especially prized by the perfume industry for creating exotic, oriental-inspired scents.

History and Lore

» During the 14th century, Norwegians traded angelica with much of the known world.
» In America, the herb was used by the Iroquois and other tribes in ceremonial medicine.
» In Spain and France, candied angelica stalks are considered a delicacy.

CULTURAL CONNECTIONS

Sustaining the Sámi

For the Sámi, the indigenous people of northern Scandinavia, angelica was long both a source of food and a medication. They dried the root in the fall and ate it as a vegetable during the long winter months. In a largely meat-based culture—the Sámi were (and many still are) skilled reindeer herders—this therapeutic plant was helpful in aiding digestion and curing any stomach-related problems. The root also contains a number of vital nutrients: vitamin B12 and trace minerals such as thiamin, magnesium, iron, riboflavin, and potassium. ■

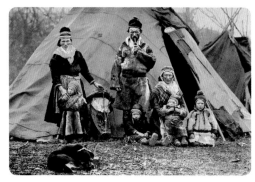

A Sámi family in Norway, circa 1900. As well as using *Angelica archangelica* as a food source, the Sámi also fashion the fadno, a reed pipe instrument, from the plant's stems.

Angelica

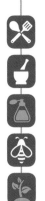

Annatto

Bixa orellana

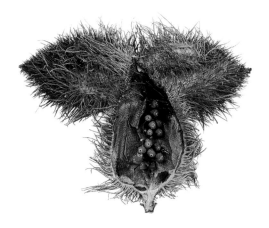

Annatto, also called roucou or achiote, is best known as a commercial dye, a healing agent, and both a colorant and a flavoring for food. Annatto comes from the seed pulp of the achiote tree, an evergreen shrub indigenous to the tropic and subtropic zones of the Americas. The tree is cultivated commercially for the valuable annatto pigment in Bolivia, Brazil, Colombia, Ecuador, India, Jamaica, Kenya, Peru, Mexico, Puerto Rico, the Dominican Republic, and Southeast Asia, where the Spanish introduced it in the 17th century.

The plant's specific name comes from Spanish conquistador Francisco de Orellana, who explored the Amazon region. The tree reaches a height of eight to ten feet and produces exquisite pink, five-lobed flowers that mature into brick red hairy fruit. The fruit is inedible, but the reddish pericarps that surround the seeds contain the annatto, also

> **DID YOU KNOW?**
> Long valued for the yellow-to-red dye produced from its seeds, antioxidant-rich annatto is increasingly harvested for its medicinal properties.

called bixen, which can be extracted by grinding the seeds or stirring them in water. The resulting dye, orange to deep red, is used to color cheese, fish, chorizo sausage, popcorn, salad oil, margarine and butter, rice, snack foods, custard powder, and breakfast cereals. As a natural substitute for synthetic dyes, annatto's popularity keeps increasing.

Healing Properties

In Brazil, where the tree may have originated, herbalists recommend annatto to ease heartburn and stomach distress, prevent sunburn, repel insects . . . and possibly ward off evil. In Colombia, folk healers have traditionally prescribed annatto to treat microbial infections. Research shows that extracts of the leaf do, indeed, possess antimicrobial activity against Gram-positive microorganisms. The leaves have also been used to treat malaria and Leishmaniasis, an ulcerative disease caused by protozoan parasites.

Annatto is nutrient rich, containing amino acids, vitamins B2 and B3, calcium, iron, and phosphorus, as well as the powerful antioxidants beta-carotene and vitamin C. It also supplies phytochemicals, compounds found in plants that help to prevent and treat disease.

Most often commercially grown, achiote, the tree that yields annatto, can also be used as a garden tree that flourishes in containers, showing off its delicate pink and white flowers in summer.

The Lipstick Tree

Rainforest tribes and Caribbean natives found many uses for annatto—as a food source, a medicine, a sunscreen, and an insect repellent. They also applied the dye as body paint, especially on their lips, which led to the achiote being called the lipstick tree. Some historians believe this practice of painting the body with ruddy dyes might be the origin of the word "red-skins," a derogatory term some Europeans and colonials used for indigenous tribes. ■

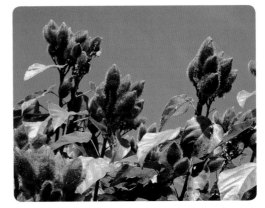

After the flowers fade, annatto puts on a show with its bright red spiny fruits, which contain red seeds. Annatto seeds are often described as resembling "little puppy teeth."

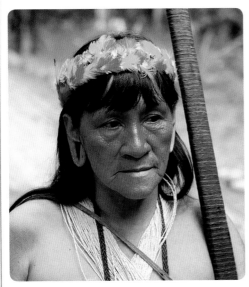

An Amazon indian woman dons annatto face paint.

Culinary Uses

Annatto's taste has been described as musky, earthy, peppery, and slightly sweet. Many believe that the taste recalls primitive foods, harking back to pre-Columbian eras. The ground seeds, which give off a faint floral or peppermint scent, are used to add color and subtle flavor to the cuisine of Latin America, Jamaica, Cameroon, and the Philippines. Annatto is also added to *tascalate*, the pine nut and chocolate drink served in Chiapas, Mexico. Achiote paste, made from red annatto seeds ground with other spices, is popular in the Yucatan, Oaxaca, and Belize. When dissolved in oil or vinegar, it makes a tangy meat marinade or grilling rub. Puerto Rican cooks make *sazon*, a special seasoning, by crushing annatto, cumin, and coriander seeds, adding garlic powder and dried cilantro, and then spread the mixture over fish or meat. Annatto is even sometimes used in place of precious saffron.

Annatto might be a little exotic for your local grocery; it is best located online or at ethnic markets that specialize in Latin, Mexican, or Caribbean herbs and spices. You can usually choose from whole seeds, powder, or flavored oil. Sazon is often available in the Latin foods aisle.

History and Lore

» In India, annatto is known as *sindoor*. It is considered auspicious for married women, and many apply it to their foreheads next to the hairline to indicate their marital status.

» In the Philippines, it is called *atsuete*, and it is used as food coloring in traditional dishes.

» The Aztecs added annatto to their chocolate drinks to deepen the hue.

» In 16th-century Mexico, the intense pigment was used for manuscript painting.

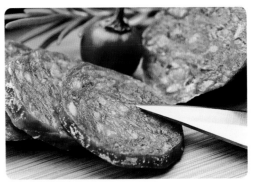

Annatto gives Spanish chorizo sausage its rich red color.

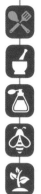

Arnica

Arnica montana

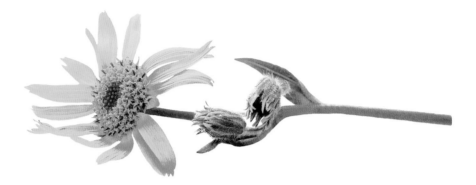

Arnica has been an important topical healing herb since the 15th century. It is a member of the large and varied Asteraceae, or Composite family, along with sunflowers, daisies, lettuce, and chicory. This perennial herb originated in the mountains of Europe and Siberia, and is now widely cultivated in North America.

The plant's genus name derives from *arna,* Greek for "lamb," because of the soft, fleecy hair on its green leaves. It reaches an average height of one to two feet and produces daisy-like yellow-orange flowers that begin to bloom in May.

Healing Properties

Arnica's flower heads, either fresh or dried, are the base of creams, salves, ointments, liniments, or tinctures that are applied to the skin to treat muscle aches, sprains, strains, and bruises. Arnica can also be useful in treating superficial phlebitis, inflamed insect bites, and swelling from broken bones. There are studies that suggest it might be useful in treating burns. It is not recommended for use on any open wounds.

In a high-profile testimonial on the herb's effectiveness, Memorial Sloan-Kettering Cancer

> **DID YOU KNOW?**
> For centuries, arnica has been a mainstay of the traditional healer's supply of remedies, used to make liniments and ointments to soothe strains, sprains, and bruises.

Center states: "A few clinical trials suggest benefits of topical arnica for osteoarthritis and for affecting significant reduction of bruising compared to placebo or low-concentration vitamin K ointments." On the other hand, a small study reported that topical arnica increased pain in subjects 24 hours after calf exercises.

Several species of arnica, including *A. Montana,* contain two sesquiterpene lactones: helenalin and dihydrohelananin, which help reduce inflammations and ease pain. Arnica also contains inulin, a compound somewhere between sugar and starch, that plants store underground as a source of energy and that diabetics can use as a natural sweetener.

Arnica has several uses outside the realm of sprains and bruises. Swiss mountain guides chewed the herb to avoid fatigue while climbing. The dried leaves can be used like tobacco—the herb is even sometimes referred to as mountain tobacco—while the dried flowers mimic snuff and produce sneezing.

Minerals found in arnica include selenium and manganese, both powerful antioxidants. Manganese is important for maintaining healthy bones, healing wounds, and metabolizing proteins, carbohydrates, and cholesterol.

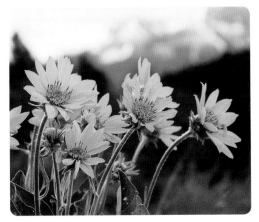

The plant's species name, *montana,* is Latin for "from the mountain." Arnica can flourish in poor mountainous soil.

Arnica is a favorite medication of homeopathic practitioners, and it is widely marketed and praised for its healing powers. Yet, clinical trials indicate that when heavily diluted homeopathic arnica—typically at a strength of one part per million—is prescribed, it is no more effective than a placebo. (Arnica can be toxic in high doses, and undiluted extracts should never be taken by mouth.)

Aromatic Qualities

Arnica is not a heavily scented herb, and most arnica products are very lightly fraganced or fairly scent neutral. Arnica is a sub-alpine plant; it is used to growing in nutrient-poor soil and thrives in sunlit mountain meadows ten thousand feet up or higher. Although the flowers normally do have a light grassy or dusty scent, the higher the altitude the plants reach, the more intense their aroma becomes.

History and Lore

» With popularity comes problems. Over-harvesting has depleted wild arnica populations in many areas. The World Wildlife Fund (WWF) and other conservation groups publicized this issue, resulting in protective legislation in most of Europe.

» *Arnica montana* is sometimes called leopard's bane or wolfsbane, although the latter name is more often applied to aconite, a European flowering herb with a poisonous root.

» Arnica flowers mixed with safflower oil makes an anti-inflammatory massage oil that may ease the pain of sports injuries.

FOR YOUR HEALTH

The Memory of Water: Homeopathic Medicine

Unlike traditional healers, who use time-tested natural cures, there is a separate school of thought, called homeopathic medicine, that believes if a substance causes a symptom in a healthy person, it will cure that symptom in an ailing person. The word derives from the Greek *homolos,* or "like," and *pathos,* "suffering." In 1796, German physician Samuel Hahnemann founded the movement on the premise that "like cures like." This belief supposedly began with Hippocrates, who prescribed a small amount of mandrake root to treat mania, when large amounts were known to *cause* mania. The ingredients in homeopathic remedies are diluted to such an extent, however, that often no molecules of the original medication remain. Yet, followers insist on the "memory of water"—that water can recall and then transmit the medicines that were mixed with it.

Homeopathy is considered a pseudoscience, and studies confirm most medications have no more effect than a placebo. Still, the concept was very popular in the 19th century, and its possibilities were even investigated in the 20th century by Nazi scientists. In the 1970s, America saw a resurgence of homeopathic medicine, perhaps linked to the emerging New Age movement. ■

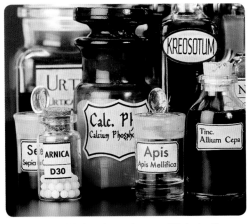

Arnica is one of the best-known homeopathic herbs. The whole plant is used to make the homeopathic remedy.

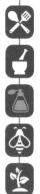

Burdock

Arctium lappa, A. minus, A. tomentosum

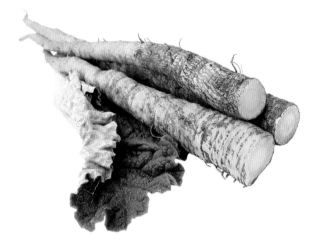

If you have ever come home from a tramp in the woods to find cockleburs clinging to your coat or jeans, chances are you have picked up burdock seeds. Burdock is not only adept at spreading its seeds, it is also a traditional treatment for skin diseases and other ailments. Originating in Europe, burdock was carried—possibly literally—to the New World by French and English settlers.

A tall, dense, pale green plant, burdock grows to about four feet in height and produces large wavy leaves and purple flowers that form round, thistle-like heads. The root are roughly an inch wide and are typically a foot long, though some can grew to three or four times that length.

DID YOU KNOW?

The inspiration for hook-and-loop fasteners, burdock also has a long history as a medicinal herb.

The genus name, *Arctium*, comes from the Greek *arktos*, meaning "bear" and referring to the roughness of the burrs, while the specific name, *lappa*, is derived from a word meaning "to seize." In the common name, "bur" is from the French *bourre* by way of the Latin *burra*, a clump of wool caught on a plant, and "dock" from its large leaves. Typically, only donkeys will graze on the prickly plants, though they also attract honeybees.

Healing Properties

European, Far Eastern, and Indian herbalists have relied on this plant for centuries and most often employ the dried roots, which are dug up after a year's growth. Burdock is believed to be effective as a blood purifier, a diuretic, and a treatment for psoriasis. It is also an antiscorbutic that can treat scurvy, boils, and rheumatism. In Japan, burdock is used to cleanse the body of toxins and improve liver function, and in China and India, is it used to treat colds and flu.

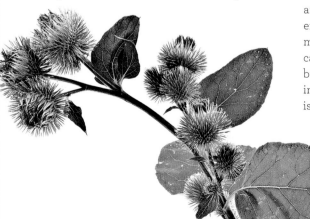

Greater burdock *(Arctium lappa)*. Dried burdock burrs easily catch on to animal fur, providing the plant with an excellent mechanism for dispersing its seeds.

Velcro: Sticking to It

One day after taking his dog for a walk, Swiss inventor George de Mestral noticed the barbed burdock burrs stuck in his pet's fur. Curious about how they clung, he studied them under the microscope and saw the hook-and-loop system that they used to grab on to passing animals. After replicating this "seizing" effect in synthetic materials, he introduced Velcro to the world in the early 1940s. It was an immediate hit. ■

The leaves can be prepared as an infusion to soothe the stomach and formed into a poultice to relieve gout, bruises, swelling, inflammation, or heat. A tincture made from the fruit (often referred to as seeds) makes an effective treatment for chronic skin diseases. Nicholas Culpeper wrote: "The seed is much commended to break the stone," referring to gallstones and kidney stones. Those who subscribed to the doctrine of signatures believed the stone of a plant—its seed—could be used to break up the calcified stones inside a human body.

The plant's components include significant inulin, with its proven anti-inflammatory properties, as well as mucilage; sugar; a bitter, crystalline glucoside; flavonoids; resin; fixed and volatile oils; vitamins A and B12; and tannic acid. The phytosterols in the plant are believed to stimulate natural hair growth.

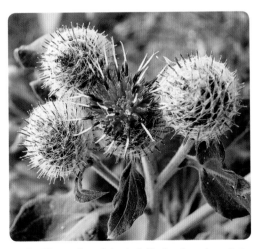

The floral bracts of woolly burdock *(Arctium tomentosum)* are covered in cobweb-like hairs below their hooked tips. Also known as downy burdock, this species is also used medicinally.

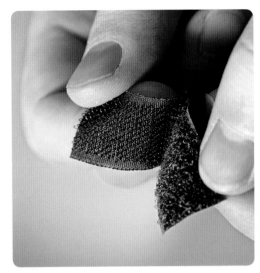

Burdock inspired Velcro, with hooks and loops that seize together to form a strong and stable closure or joining.

Culinary Uses

The root has the firm texture of any root vegetables and a sweet, somewhat mucilaginous flavor similar to artichoke hearts. In Japan, it is called *gobo*. Roots can be found in many Asian groceries, and while some farmers only harvest burdock in the spring or fall, the Japanese export the root all year long. Scrub each root lightly (the light brown color is natural, not dirt) and do not peel, because that is the plant's source of nutrition.

If the stalks are cut before the flower is open and stripped of their rind, they can be served as a delicate vegetable.

History and Lore

» Burdock is known by a host of other names, some of which date from the Middle Ages or earlier: lappa, fox's clote, bardona, thorny burr, beggar's buttons, cockle buttons, love leaves, philanthropium, personata, happy major, clotbur, and *niu bang zi* in China.

» As a nitrogen fixer, burdock is a great plant to leave on depleted soil. Cover plants with cardboard or hay to smother them, and they will die back, leaving viable nutrients in the earth.

» Leo Tolstoy noted of the herb: "It asserts life to the end, and alone in the midst of the whole field, somehow or other had asserted it."

» Native Americans used burdock medicinally and boiled the stems of the plant in maple syrup to make a tasty candy.

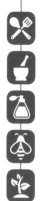

Calendula

Calendula officinalis

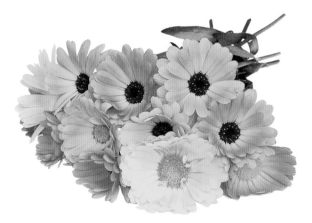

Also called pot marigold, calendula is a plant of many facets, thriving and continuously blooming in the garden, and useful in herbal medicine and in the production of dyes and cosmetics. A member of the daisy or Composite family, Asteraceae, calendula is probably native to southern Europe—although its precise origins are uncertain—and it has naturalized in other parts of Europe and in many warm, temperate regions of the world.

The mature plant reaches 30 inches in height and produces oblong, hairy leaves, either wavy or toothed, of 2 to 7 inches in length. The clustered golden yellow flowers, or inflorescences, form a lush head surrounded by double rows of hairy bracts. This perennial is typically treated like an annual in cooler zones.

The Latin name derives from when the plant was once thought to bloom: the "calends," or first days, of each month. The common name pot marigold derives from the Anglo Saxon *merso-meargealla*, which was the term for marsh marigolds.

Healing Properties

The ancient Greek, Roman, Middle Eastern, and Indian cultures all utilized calendula flowers for medicinal purposes, as well as for dyes

DID YOU KNOW?
Since ancient times, calendula flower petals have been used for medicinal purposes.

used on fabrics and in foods, and cosmetics. Calendula remained popular with healers throughout the Middle Ages, when the petals were applied to cuts and wounds to stop bleeding, prevent infection, and speed healing. The flowers were also used to treat skin conditions, boils, ulcers, colitis, fevers, vomiting, and female reproductive ailments. During the mid-20th century, the Russians believed that the plant could cure smallpox and measles, and, as a result, so much was grown there that pot marigolds became known as Russian penicillin. The Shakers, an American religious sect, once believed that calendula could cure gangrene.

The flower's components include flavonol glycosides, saponins, a sesquiterpene glucoside, triterpenoid esters, and the carotenoids flavoxanthin and auroanthin (antioxidants and the source of the gold-yellow coloration). The leaves and stems contain additional carotenoids, mainly lutein, zeaxanthin, and beta-carotene. The plant's saponins, resins, and essential oils make it valuable in the manufacture of cosmetics.

Contemporary pharmacological studies suggest that calendula extracts have antiviral, antigenotoxic (countering the effects of genotoxins on DNA), and anti-inflammatory properties in vitro.

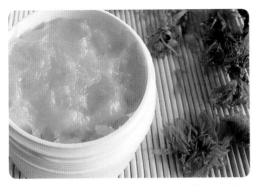

Calendula's blossoms are common ingredients of homemade cosmetics. Mildly antiseptic and anti-inflammatory, the plant's extracts are also used to make an alternative to peppermint-flavored toothpaste that cleans and soothes the gums.

Culinary Uses

For centuries, cooks have put calendula to good use in their kitchens. The petals, with their aromatic bitterness, have been added to fish and meat soups and rice dishes, dried to use in broths, mixed into salads, and added to dishes simply for color. They have even been used in place of saffron. The flowers are found in German soups and stews (where the term "pot" marigold came from), they once added color to butter and cheese, and they are still used in a number of traditional Mediterranean and Middle Eastern dishes.

The flowers can be chopped up and placed in custards or baked puddings. A tea made from calendula is both healthful and tasty.

Aromatic Qualities

Every part of the plant is highly scented, making calendula attractive to bees. Hover flies that are drawn to the plant by its aroma eat the aphids that may infest it.

History and Lore

» The golden flowers were once used to make fabric dyes. A whole range of yellows, oranges, and browns could be obtained by using different mordants, or setting agents.

» In the Middle Ages, calendula symbolized jealousy. The whole flower was often used as a decorative garnish.

» The flowers typically open from nine in the morning until the sun goes down.

» The larvae of many Lepidoptera used calendula as food plants, including the cabbage moth, the Gothic moth, the large yellow underwing, and the setaceous Hebrew character.

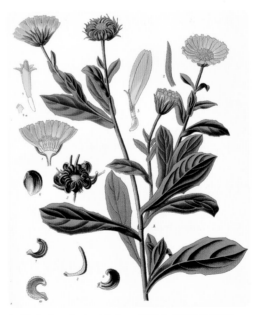

An illustration of calendula from *Köhler's Medicinal Plants*, published by Franz Eugen Köhler in 1887. Calendula is often called pot marigold, although it is not in the same genus as the common marigold, *Tagetes*. Both are in the aster family.

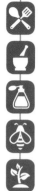

Catnip
Nepeta cataria

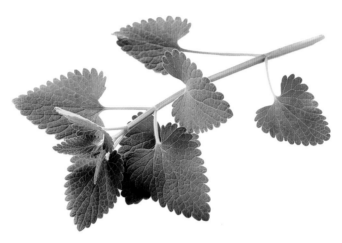

T his familiar plant offers endlessly intoxicating amusement to our pet cats, but it also has a host of other uses. The early Romans used catnip for both culinary and medicinal purposes, and, during the Middle Ages, steeped catnip was a popular hot drink before black tea became available.

A member of the widespread mint family, Lamiaceae, catnip was native to Europe and Asia and was brought to North America by early settlers, who introduced the herb to Native American tribes. The Latin name possibly comes from the ancient Etruscan town of Nepete or Nepta, combined with the Latin word for "cat."

The root of this perennial plant sends up erect branch stems that reach two to three feet in height; the downy, toothed, heart-shaped leaves have white undersides, giving the whole plant a slightly dusty look. The white or pale purple

DID YOU KNOW?
The true catnip loved by house cats, *Nepeta cataria,* known as catnip, catswort, or catmint, has a history of medicinal use by humans, too.

flowers grow in dense whorls that form a spike and bloom from July to September. In the garden, catnip makes an attractive border plant.

In manufacturing, *Nepeta cataria* is used as a pesticide and insecticide. Research indicates that nepetalactone, the substance that causes the feline high, is about ten times more effective at repelling mosquitoes than DEET, the active ingredient in most insect repellents. The herb reportedly also repels cockroaches, rats, and mice.

Healing Properties

Healers use the flowering tops of catnip, which are harvested in August, when the plant is in full bloom. Catnip should always be infused as a remedy, never boiled. It has been used to treat insomnia, anxiety, migraine, colds, coughs, and respiratory infections, hives, worms, bruises, colic, cramping, and gas. It was made into an ointment to ease boils, scabs, scurf, and other skin problems. Applied directly to the skin, catnip has reportedly relieved arthritis pain, hemorrhoids, and swelling. Catnip can also be smoked medicinally for respiratory conditions.

Catnip leaves contain vitamins C and E, which are both powerful antioxidants.

Its fragrant pale violet flowers growing in whorls on a tall, square stem attest to catnip's mint family lineage.

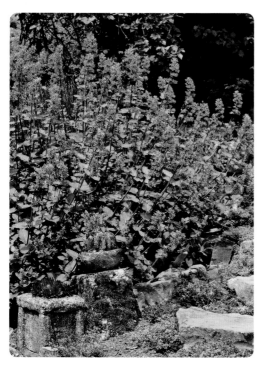

When planted in a backyard garden, catnip makes a tall and striking display. Be sure to keep an eye on the plant, though, because it spreads easily and can eventually choke out other less hardy plants.

CURIOSITIES

The Feline Allure of Catnip

Most cats completely lose their dignity when exposed to catnip, quickly becoming pixilated by the herb. The component responsible for this mostly mellow high is called nepetalactone, an essential oil found in the leaves and stems. This oil causes a hallucinogenic reaction in cats, possibly similar to that of LSD. The effects are mediated through the olfactory system, and when cats inhale the herb the results can include sniffing, chewing, licking, head shaking, chin, cheek, and body rubbing, rolling on the ground, stretching, drooling, and hyperactivity or aggression. The high typically lasts five or ten minutes, followed by an hour refractory period.

While 50 to 60 percent of adult cats respond to catnip—the trait has to be passed by at least one parent—young kittens are not affected by it. Big cats such as lions and jaguars are not immune to the lure, however, and can smell one part per billion of the "nip in the air." ■

Culinary Uses

Although it is not as popular in the kitchen as some other members of the mint family, this aromatic herb is sometimes added to soup recipes and salads. In France, the young leaves and shoots are gathered for use as a seasoning.

Catnip makes a soothing tea that can calm your stomach or help you to sleep. It is also believed to bring down a fever. To prepare catnip tea, place one or two teaspoons of the dried herb in a cup of hot water, steep for ten minutes, strain, and drink with honey or lemon.

Aromatic Qualities

Some herbalists say this plant's distinctive aroma is reminiscent of both mint and pennyroyal, while other compare it to citronella with light minty undertones. The essential oil of catnip is extracted by steam distillation.

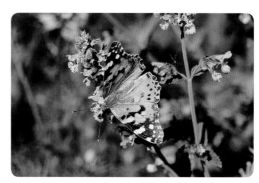

A painted lady butterfly (Vanessa cardui) alights on a catnip blossom. For anyone wanting a butterfly garden, catnip is a perfect choice, especially if it is planted in a container.

History and Lore

» Legend tells of a conscience-stricken hangman who could not carry out his duties until he ingested catnip—which lowered his anxiety so he could complete his gruesome task.

» Catnip gets a mention in literary works by Washington Irving, Harriet Beecher Stowe, and Nathaniel Hawthorne.

» In the practice of Wicca, the herb is associated with the female deities Bast, Sekhmet, and Venus.

APOTHECARY TOOLKIT

Create your own healing remedies at home.

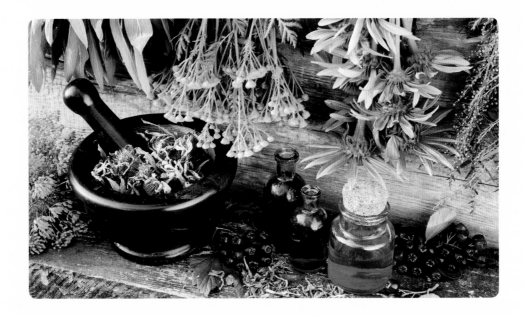

Imagine preparing your own herbal medicines and having them at hand whenever you require a tonic, treatment, or cure. Your workshop can be as basic or complex as you choose, but start with a simple setup and then expand from there.

Initially, you will need a selection of medicinal herbs, some essential oils, and various carriers (usually oils, but also anything that holds an herbal preparation), and, before long, you will be creating your own customized teas, salves, tinctures, syrups, pillows, sachets, and infused oils. Experiment with various herbs, mixing them to blend their respective healing properties or to achieve stimulating or soothing scents.

Create an area dedicated to your herbal workshop. Hang a wooden shelf above your prep area so that your ingredients are within easy reach, and use large tins or wooden boxes to store your fabric, strainer, measuring tools, and spare carriers.

Herbs to Have at Hand

You can use fresh or dried plants. Sage, lavender, rosemary, thyme, marjoram, chamomile, ginger, calendula, peppermint, spearmint, fennel, elderflowers and berries, and milk thistle are all great herbs to have on hand.

Essential Oils Are Essential

These are not cheap, but only small amounts are required, and most can be purchased at health food stores. Look for lemon, orange, grapefruit, clary sage, rosemary, lavender, peppermint, spearmint, eucalyptus, and tea tree oils.

Carriers and Storage

Most carriers are reasonably priced and easy to find: olive oil, jojoba, sweet almond oil, or other vegetable oils are traditional. You can also use vodka, unscented castile soap, or absorbent foods like rice or beans (for eye or muscle pillows). Your carriers will also include storage devices such tea balls, cotton fabric (for sachets), lidded jars, tubes, and glass bottles.

Other Things You'll Need

Keep on hand an eye dropper, measuring cups and spoons, strainers and cheesecloth, mixing bowls, and a mortar and pestle. Naturally, you will also need a collection of guidebooks on how to prepare herbal remedies and how to safely store them. Your local health food store should be able to steer you toward some tested options.

Quick and Easy Herbal Remedies

Stomach-Easing Syrup: A teaspoonful of this syrup will soothe digestive upsets. Combine one teaspoon each of sage, marjoram, rosemary, and thyme in a tea ball and immerse for five minutes in a cup of boiling water. Add one teaspoon honey, and stir. Cool, and store it in airtight container.

   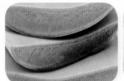

SAGE   MARJORAM   ROSEMARY   THYME

Relaxation Eye Pillow: Create a fabric pouch roughly the size of an eyeglass holder, stitch up three sides and fill with dried beans. Add a tablespoon of lavender flowers and 20 drops each of lavender oil and spearmint oil, and stitch closed. Warm in microwave or freeze. Lie back, place over eyes, inhale, and relax.

LAVENDER FLOWERS   LAVENDER OIL   SPEARMINT OIL

Cooling Massage Gel: Treat yourself to a neck or shoulder massage after exercising or to ease the fever and aches of a cold. Add two or three ounces of aloe vera gel to 15 drops of any essential oil, and mix together in a jar until the gel turns cloudy. Mint oil works well and has an invigorating scent.

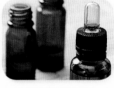

ALOE VERA GEL   ANY ESSENTIAL OIL

Restorative Tea: This tea is especially welcome after a stressful workday or a weekend of over-indulgence. Mix a quarter cup each of dried milk thistle (promotes liver function), fennel (eases the stomach), and peppermint (soothes headaches) in a bowl, and transfer to disposable tea bags or a lidded jar. Steep for about five minutes. ■

MILK THISTLE   FENNEL   PEPPERMINT

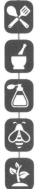

Chamomile

Matricaria chamomilla, Chamaemelum nobile

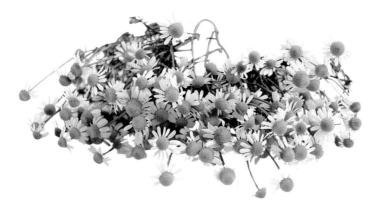

P erhaps best known as the source of a soothing tea, the herb called chamomile is actually two different herbaceous plants: German chamomile (*Matricaria recutita*) and Roman chamomile (*Chamaemelum nobile*). From the days of ancient Egypt, Greece, and Rome to the Middle Ages, both chamomile species have been employed by healers, for their anti-inflammatory properties, as well as their own additional benefits.

A member of the daisy or Composite family, Asteraceae, these herbs were originally native to many European countries, and are now cultivated in Germany, Egypt, France, Spain, Italy, Morocco, and Eastern Europe. Although both are daisy-like, the two plants

differ in appearance and require different growing conditions. Roman chamomile is a perennial that hugs the ground and produces small white or yellow flowers. It tastes bitter when used in teas. German chamomile, an annual that is also called scented maywood, has a sweeter taste and features fernlike foliage and white flowers that resemble daisies on leggy, drooping stalks.

The common name of both species comes from the Greek *chamos*, "ground," and *melos,* "apple"—probably in reference to the plants' apple-like scent.

Healing Properties

Often described today as the European version of Chinese ginseng, chamomile was once used to treat asthma, colic, fevers, inflammations, nausea, nervous complaints, children's ailments, skin diseases, and cancer.

The plant's healthful components are found in its flowers and include volatile oils (including bisabolol, bisabolol oxides A and B, and matricin) as well as flavonoids (especially a compound called apinegin) and other beneficial substances. Over the past 20 years, extensive research has confirmed the herb's legitimate usefulness in treating

German chamomile. Keep regularly harvesting these daisy-like yellow-and-white flowers as they blossom, otherwise the plants stop producing new buds.

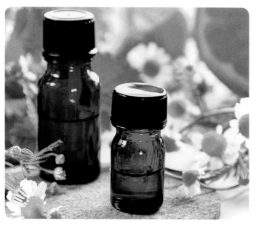

The compound azulene gives German chamomile oil its characteristic blue color. Both varieties of chamomile oil are said to have very good antiseptic and antibiotic properties.

Culinary Uses

While not a culinary herb, per se, chamomile has challenged home cooks to come up with creative ways to use the plant in the kitchen. Some cooks add the dried flowers to oatmeal, lemonade, or fruit-crisp toppings, or infuse them in jam. There are even recipes for a honey-chamomile soda.

Aromatic Qualities

The sweet, crushed-apple scent of chamomile's essential oil can be inhaled as a form of aromatherapy to relieve depression, soothe agitated nerves, and ease headaches. In earlier times chamomile was a "strewing herb," meaning it was scattered on bare floors so that people would tread on it and release its pleasing odor.

a wide spectrum of problems and validated its anti-inflammatory, antibacterial, antispasmodic, muscle-relaxant, antiallergenic, and sedative properties. Chamomile can be used as a tea for lumbago and rheumatic problems, as a salve for hemorrhoids and wounds, and as a vapor for colds or asthma. It can relieve allergies, morning sickness, menstrual cramps, gastritis and colitis, skin rashes, sunburn, eye inflammations, mouth and gum sores, as well as ease teething problems and colic in young children.

History and Lore

» In Ecuador, babies are bathed in chamomile tea made of the flowers and stems—it soothes skin irritations like prickly heat and diaper rash.
» In Beatrix Potter's classic *The Tale of Peter Rabbit*, his mother makes Peter chamomile tea and sends him to bed after he raided Mr. McGregor's garden.
» German and Roman chamomile are also called Hungarian or English chamomile, respectively.

FOR YOUR HEALTH

The Sleepy-Time Herb

Herbal teas, which contain no caffeine, became widely popular in the late 20th century after scientific research reported that the caffeine in black teas could aversely affect blood pressure, glucose metabolism, sleep centers, digestion, and fertility. Herbal teas had been a mainstay of alternative medicine for centuries, and chamomile, one of the most dependable of these, quickly caught on everywhere. This tea promotes a welcome sense of relaxation and also relieves stress, making it perfect nightcap for the driven, high-powered careerists of the late 1990s. Animal studies showed that this effect is due to the apigenin, the calmative agent in chamomile, binding to the same receptors in the brain that some anti-anxiety medications do. The herb's muscle-relaxing, mildly sedative qualities have helped many of those who suffer from insomnia to fall asleep more easily. ∎

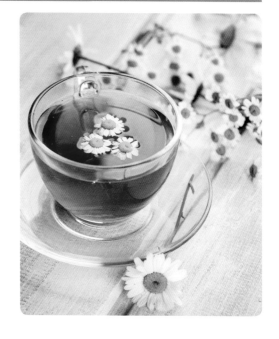

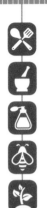

Clary Sage

Salvia sclarea

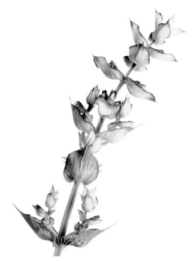

Clary sage is an ancient herb that has been used by many cultures to medicate the eyes and treat a variety of diseases. This biennial member of the mint family, Lamiaceae, is native to the northern Mediterranean, parts of North Africa, and Central Asia. It is now a commercial crop in the Mediterranean, Russia, the United States, England, Morocco, and Central Europe, cultivated primarily for its essential oils. It still grows wild in many places.

The plant begins as a rosette, and, by its second year, produces strong, hairy stems that reach an average height of three feet. The large, downy green leaves are paired and show a hint of purple. The herb produces lush spikes of lilac or blue flowers that bloom from spring to mid-summer and attract bees and other pollinators.

Healing Properties

Written records of the herb's healing powers go back to Theophrastus in the fourth century B.C., and Dioscorides and Pliny the

DID YOU KNOW?

Clary sage, prized for its many healing properties, is also used to make fragrances and fixatives in detergents, soaps, and cosmetics.

Elder in the first century A.D. By the Middle Ages, clary sage was cultivated almost exclusively for the perfume trade, but healers still relied on it for treating digestive issues and renal complaints. In modern times, it has begun to regain some of its medicinal popularity.

The herb is notable for one specific medical attribute—a seed placed in an irritated eye will soon turn to mucilage and carry out any irritants. This practice of clearing the eye gave rise to the herb's name—from the Latin *clarus,* for "clear." Clary sage is still used today to brighten the eyes, improve vision, and slow down the ocular aging process.

In Asian medicine, clary sage oil is thought to circulate and strengthen *qi* energy that has become "stuck." *Qi* is considered the life force that flows through our bodies and sustains our physical being. In Jamaica, the herb was once used to soothe ulcers, while a decoction of the leaves boiled in coconut oil was thought to cure scorpion stings.

Traditional healers also use it to treat bronchitis, high cholesterol, high blood pressure, hemorrhoids, circulatory problems, digestive distress, muscle aches, kidney disorders, and hair loss, and as an aphrodisiac. By acting on the

Clary's large, aromatic leaves can be used like common sage to season food or to make sachets and potpourri.

The Woman's Helper

Clary sage is called the "woman's helper" because of a long history treating female reproductive complaints, from the onset of menstruation—cramps and PMS—through to menopause—night sweats, hot flashes, and mood swings. The herb contains sclareol, a compound with a chemical structure similar to estrogen; this allows clary sage to mimic the effects of estrogen if there is a deficiency and to help restore hormonal balance. The herb should be avoided during the first trimester of pregnancy. ∎

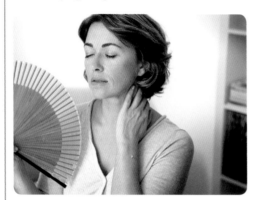

Clary sage can help alleviate hot flashes, night sweats, and mood changes, along with other effects of menopause.

"primitive" hypothalamus in the brain, clary sage produces a euphoric effect when used for anxiety or depression. It can heighten the effects of alcohol, so should not be combined with drinking.

It is one of only a few herbs with a high proportion of esters—gentle chemical compounds with anti-inflammatory properties. The other two are lavender and petitgrain, or bitter orange.

Culinary Uses

If harvested early, the leaves can be eaten raw or added to most recipes that call for sage. The older leaves turn bitter, so use only tender, young leaves. The flowers can also be eaten and make a tasty addition to salads or, dried, can be steeped in a tea.

Aromatic Qualities

The scent of clary sage has been described as sweet-spicy, floral, grassy, tea-like, somewhat nutty, and similar to ambergris. The essential oil is extracted from the buds and leaves by steam distillation and is used as a perfume fixer, in cosmetics, and as a flavoring—mimicking the taste of muscatel wine—in vermouths, wines, and liqueurs. In aromatherapy it is used to relax the mind, aid sleep, and to relieve PMS and cramps. The essential oil can be applied topically, used as a compress, massaged into the skin, placed in a warm bath, or directly inhaled or diffused. It is not ingested.

History and Lore

» In the Middle Ages, clary sage was called *Oculus Christi* or Christ's Eye.
» In 16th-century England, the herb was sometimes substituted for hops as a flavoring in the production of beer.
» Clary sage is said to enhance the ability to dream and to recall the dreams accurately.

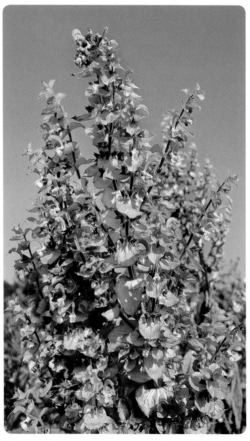

Clary sage flowers change color, depending on the lighting conditions, from white through cream, ivory, pink and purple. The flowering stems yield an essential oil that blends particularly well with sandalwood, juniper, lavender, pine, geranium, jasmine, frankincense, and many citrus oils.

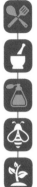

Comfrey

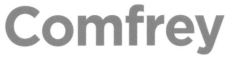

Symphytum x *uplandicum, S. officinale*

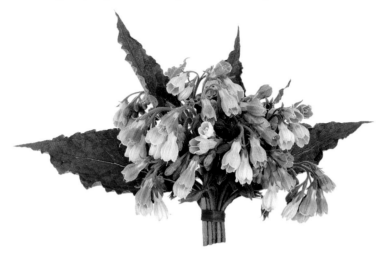

Comfrey is a versatile herb that offers both healing benefits to humans and regeneration to the garden. True, or common, comfrey is native to Europe and Asia, and can be found growing in damp, grassy areas—especially riverbanks, ditches—and even waste spaces. More widely cultivated is a hybrid between *Symphytum officinale* and *S. asperum* called Russian comfrey, *Symphytum* x *uplandicum*. The most popular cultivar is called 'Bocking 14', which was developed in the 1950s after trials in the town of Bocking, in Essex, England. 'Bocking 14' is sterile and must be propagated through root cuttings.

Comfrey is a perennial, part of the family Boraginaceae, and features deep, black, turnip-shaped roots; broad, rough-textured green leaves; and small bell-like flowers of purple, blue, or cream on coiling racemes.

DID YOU KNOW?

Renowned as an essential first aid plant, comfrey also produces beautiful bell-like flowers that are much loved by bees.

Healing Properties

Herbalists have prescribed comfrey for centuries, both internally and topically, to treat coughs and asthma, to soothe irritated throats, to ease ulcers, relieve digestive problems, and to treat cuts, burns, shingles, boils, and other skin ailments. It was also believed to have the ability to mesh broken bones. Not surprisingly, its folk names were boneset and knitbone, and its genus was named *Symphytum,* from the Greek *symphia,* "bones growing together," and *phytum,* "plant." Even the name *comfrey* derives from the Latin *confera,* or "knitting together." Dioscorides, the respected author of one of the oldest herbal texts, *De Materia Medica,* written between A.D. 50 and 70, himself recommended the herb for healing broken bones. It's clear that comfrey was thought to have extraordinary powers.

Recently, however, a controversy has arisen over the oral use of this herb, and after some study, the federal Food and Drug Administration has banned any internal use of comfrey, claiming it contains dangerous amounts of hepatoxic pyrrolizidine alkaloids, or PAs, which can affect

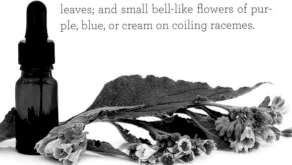

Essential oils are made from a blend of both the dried leaves and dried roots or either the leaves or roots of comfrey alone.

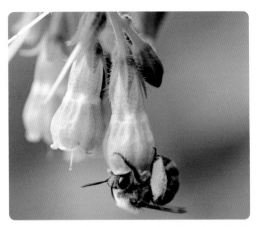

The flowers of comfrey range in color from the palest pinks to intense cobalt blues. All of them make great forage for bees.

the liver. Many herbalists question this ruling, pointing out that the tests did not take all dietary, physiological, and pharmacodynamic factors into consideration. There is some evidence that drying the leaves removes most, if not all, traces of the harmful alkaloids.

Even used topically, the herb has many health benefits. Allantoin, a chemical compound found in the plant, is believed to help replace and repair cells in the body. The mucilage it produces will soothe and coat irritated tissues. Used for skin wounds or infections, comfrey can reduce inflammation and lessen scarring. As for the knitbone claims? Medical science confirms that comfrey in an ointment or poultice can relieve joint, muscle, or back pain—even if it cannot quite mend broken bones.

Nutritionally, the plant's deep-diving roots pay off in spades. Comfrey contains vitamin A (28,000 IU per 100g), a wide spectrum of the B vitamins, and vitamins C and E, plus the essential minerals calcium, phosphorus, potassium, chromium, cobalt, copper, magnesium, iron, manganese, sodium, boron, lead, sulfur, molybdenum, and zinc.

History and Lore

» An old folkloric belief that carrying comfrey protects travelers still persists today—you can buy comfrey dried just for that purpose online.

» Folk wisdom maintains that with comfrey "a leaf a day keeps illness away."

» Farmers have been using comfrey as livestock fodder for centuries.

Getting Down and Dirty

Comfrey has a host of uses in the garden, especially when it comes to restoring soil. It is rich in nitrogen and potash, two things most gardens crave, and the leaves are virtually fiber-free, which makes them break down quickly.

• Comfrey becomes a powerful fertilizer if allowed to rot and liquefy in rainwater for five weeks. Add this "comfrey compost tea" to tomatoes to raise the acid levels in the soil and make them thrive.

• As a mulch, the leaves can be laid inches thick at the base of plants; they will add potassium to the soil as they break down.

• As a compost activator, comfrey clippings add nitrogen to the compost pile and help to heat it.

• This herb is a dynamic accumulator, which means that its deep root system gathers nutrients and minerals from the soil and transfers them to the leaves.

• Comfrey makes a good companion planting for many trees and other perennials.

• Create a rich potting mixture suitable for general use by layering well-decayed leaf mold with chopped comfrey leaves in a black garbage bag. Add a bit of dolomite limestone and store the mixture for two to five months until the comfrey has completely broken down. ■

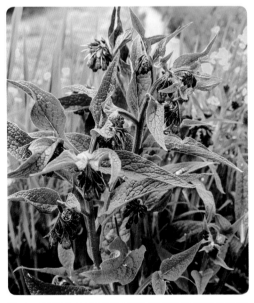

Place comfrey in a sunny spot with rich soil. It can be planted spring, summer, or fall—any time the soil can be worked.

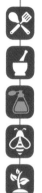

Echinacea

Echinacea purpurea, E. angustifolia, E. pallida

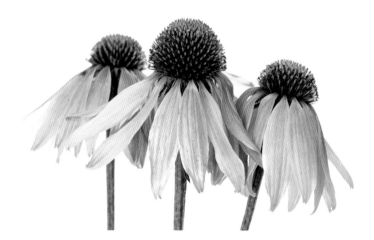

Echinacea zoomed up the herbal remedies "must have" list several decades ago and has not given up its favored spot since then. The genus *Echinacea* belongs to the daisy family, Asteraceae, and has nine species, with the most popular probably being purple coneflower, *E. purpurea*. Unlike many other herbs that are transplants from Europe or Asia, this genus is native to eastern and central North America only. These hardy, drought-resistant perennials can be found in moist, open woodlands and sunny meadows, as well as arid prairies. The plant was acclimated in Europe starting in the 16th century, where it eventually became a cornerstone of their herbal pharmacopoeia.

Mature echinaceas can reach as high as four feet, making them back border plants. The stems and leaves are usually covered with small hairs, and the flower heads consist of a single or double row of petals and raised, prickly spines on a conical seed head. Colors range from pink, purple, red, and burgundy, to white, yellow, orange, salmon, and gold. The name comes from the resemblance of the spiny cone to a sea urchin, *echino* in Greek. Echinacea offers an extended

DID YOU KNOW?
Endemic to eastern and central North America, *Echinacea* is a genus of herbaceous flowering plants commonly called coneflowers.

bloom time—flowering from early to late summer—when it regularly lures bees; in fall, the seeds attract finches.

Healing Properties

Native Americans were using the echinacea plant as a healing and analgesic herb since before Europeans settled the New World. Colonists used it as a remedy for scarlet fever, malaria, blood poisoning, diphtheria, and syphilis. More recently, it has been used to ease the effects of the common cold and flu, to soothe sore throats, and to reduce fevers, even to treat depression. Both the root and the upper plant are used in herbal preparations.

Echinacea has long been heralded for its ability to strengthen the immune system, especially during a head cold or flu. Recent research studies have concluded that purple coneflower, *E. purpurea*, actually does possesses chemical compounds that help boost the activity of the immune system, as well as alleviate pain and reduce inflammation. These compounds can also activate positive hormonal, antiviral, and antioxidant changes.

Echinacea is always more effective if taken at the early signs of illness. Take it as a tea or tincture to boost immune-system function.

Native American Natural Healing

Several Plains Indian tribes used echinacea as a cure for snakebites, insect bites, and anthrax. The Indians also discovered that it eased pain by observing elk—whenever the animals sustained a wound or were ill, they would seek out coneflowers and consume them. The Lakota Sioux called the herb *Ichahpe hu,* and they used the root to poultice wounds and chewed the roots and seeds to ease toothaches and sore throats. The Kiowa and Cheyenne used the flower for coughs and sore throats, while the Pawnee found it effective for headaches. ■

There are other studies, however, that were unable to substantiate echinacea's claims. One reason some studies remain inconclusive might be that botanicals derived from echinacea can come from different species—which have different medicinal properties, or the supplements might use different parts of the plant, such as the roots or flowers, or be made up as different preparations, extracts, or juices, for instance. Until there are standardized, well-controlled trials, it remains to be seen if echinacea is an immune-boosting miracle herb. Still, plenty of herbalists, especially those in Europe, stand by its reputed powers.

Echinacea can be purchased commercially in pill form, standardized extracts, tinctures, and teas. Pills often contain the most reliable dosage of the product.

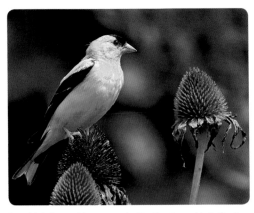

Songbirds love echinacea seeds. To attract songbirds like the American goldfinch *(Spinus tristis)* to your garden during the summer and fall, leave coneflower seed heads on the stalks.

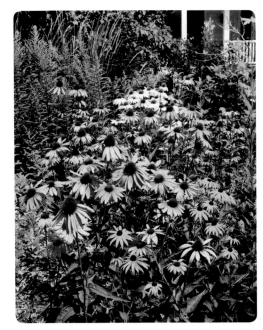

Echinacea comes in an wide array of colors, including pinkish purple and paper white. For a striking summer display in a garden border, mix various colors of echinacea with golden yellow black-eyed Susans *(Rudbeckia hirta)*.

Culinary Uses

Echinacea leaves can easily be made into a beneficial tea. Use two teaspoons if the leaves are dried, a quarter cup if they are fresh. Place leaves in a small, cheesecloth-lined sieve, then place the sieve in a mug and pour boiling water over the leaves. For best results, allow them to steep for five minutes. Drink tea with lemon or honey. Two teaspoons of seeds can also be added to the mix.

Aromatic Qualities

Although coneflowers in the wild are not notable for their aroma, several new cultivars feature attractive fragrances, among them: 'Fragrant Angel', a white, scented echinacea; 'Orange Meadowbrite', the first truly orange-colored echinacea, with a sweet, orange tea fragrance; and 'Twilight', cherry red with an intoxicating scent.

History and Lore

» An echinacea tincture, made by crushing the flowers and mixing them with alcohol, can be used as part of a homeopathic therapy called the "Bach Flower Remedies."

» Stately echinacea is sometimes called the Queen of the Daisies.

Echinacea

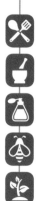

Elder

Sambucus nigra

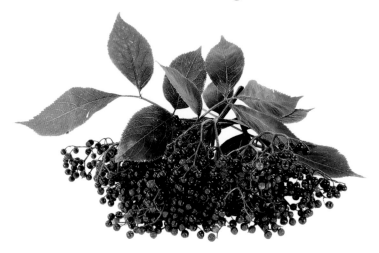

This perennial shrub, *Sambucus nigra*, produces tasty black berries each fall, but it has also been used by healers throughout Europe, North Africa, Asia, and North America for millennia. Archaeologists found elder seeds in a Neolithic dwelling in Switzerland, Greek physician Hippocrates wrote of the elderberry in the fifth century B.C., and during the Middle Ages it was prescribed as a longevity tonic. In America, Native Americans used another species, the American elder (*S. canadensis*), to treat rheumatism and fever.

A member of the Adoxaceae family, the elder grows in urban landscapes as well as in country meadows. The plant, which can reach six to ten feet, produces pinnate, serrated leaves and saucer-sized clusters of lacy, five-petaled white flowers that mature into black or blue-black drupes, which are fleshy fruit with a

Elderflower. After flowering, an elder produces drooping clusters of tiny green berries that ripen to a glossy dark purple to black in late autumn (shown above).

DID YOU KNOW?

The ancient elder is a versatile plant that yields flowers and berries with a multitude of both medicinal and culinary uses.

---

single seed. The name *elder* comes from the Anglo-Saxon word *aeld*, or "fire," possibly because the twigs were used as kindling.

Healing Properties

The black elder of Europe was called the "medicine chest of the country people," used for centuries to combat colds and the flu. Studies have tried to pinpoint why the plant is so effective against the latter, potentially deadly, disease, which in 1918 wiped out 25 million people worldwide. According to a study by the American Botanical Council, 90 percent of flu patients taking elderberry eliminated their symptoms in three days, versus six days for the placebo group. Possibly one of elderberry's constituents, free radical scavengers called anthocyanins, are able to inhibit the production of hemagglutinin, the tiny protein spikes that the flu virus uses to attach itself to—and invade—healthy cells. Elderberry then promotes production of lymphocytes, which defend the immune system from attack.

Herbalists have also used elderberry to lower cholesterol levels, improve heart health and vision, and to boost the immune system. Elderberry has no side affects and no drug

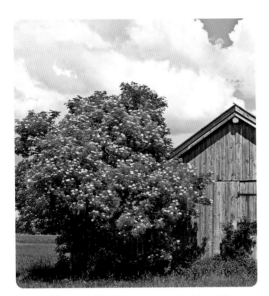

Masses of fragrant white blossoms cover an elder in bloom. The flowers of this woody shrub or small tree can be made into a tasty wine. The close-grained wood of older trees is often used to make various turned articles, such as tops for angling rods and musical instruments like flutes.

interactions, and, as a natural food source, it is safe to ingest, as long as the berries are fully ripe.

Other beneficial components of elderberry include organic pigments, tannins, amino acids, carotenoids, and substantial amounts of vitamins A, B, and C, calcium, and phosphorus. Elderberry stimulates the kidneys, lungs, colon, and skin to encourage the body to release toxins.

Culinary Uses

Americans have used elderberries to make jellies, jams, pies, tarts, and syrups since the time of the pioneers. Sometimes called the "Englishman's grape," the elderberry has also been used for centuries in Europe to make wine. Elderberries age well in oak and if the proportions are correct—if neither too few berries were used nor too much tannin was produced—the wines they make can be exceptional, either alone or added to grape wines. The blossoms can also be used to make elderflower wine.

Aromatic Qualities

Elderberries lend their sweet scent to artisan beers and ales, and herbal teas. As most gardeners who grow this plant could attest, elderflowers can seduce the unwary with their delicious mixture of lemon, anise, and lilac aromas.

History and Lore

» Legends claim that Judas Iscariot hung himself on an elder tree and that the cross of Calvary was made of elder. These tales led elder to become a symbol of sorrow and death.

» European folklore insisted it was bad luck to cut down an elder tree or remove the branches, because this would displease the spirit of the tree.

» In the Harry Potter series, the Elder Wand was one of the Deathly Hallows—along with the Cloak of Invisibility and the Resurrection Stone—three magical artifacts that would make their owner invincible.

» Native Americans made baskets from elder twigs and arrows from the branches.

IN THE KITCHEN

Traditional Elderberry Jelly

This time-tested recipe produces a clear, ruby-hued jelly that is wonderful on croissants, scones, muffins, crepes, or pancakes.

Ingredients
- 3 pounds of elderberries
- juice of 1 lemon
- 1 box fruit pectin
- 4½ cups sugar

Directions
Heat the berries over a low flame until they begin to break down, then simmer for 15 minutes. Strain through a double sheet of cheesecloth into a large bowl. Add lemon, and then enough water to make three cups of fluid. Add the box of pectin and bring to a boil before stirring in the sugar. Return to the boil for a minute. Pour into prepared jars and seal with paraffin. ■

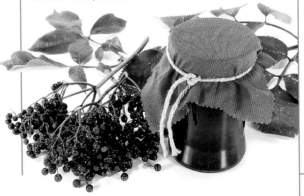

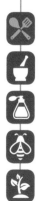

Evening Primrose

Oenothera biennis

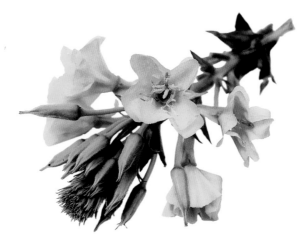

Evening primrose is an attractive wildflower that possibly originated in Mexico and Central America and eventually spread to North and South America. Today, this member of the Onagraceae family can be found naturalized all over the world. The plant is not choosy about where it spreads it seeds, and you can frequently spot these showy flowers flourishing in vacant lots, sand dunes, and on other rough ground.

Oenothera biennis is a biennial plant with an upright stem and narrow, lance-shaped leaves that grow in a tight rosette the first year, and then spiral up the stem the second year. The leaves can reach a length of more than seven inches. The plant flowers in spring, with bright yellow blossoms that open in late afternoon and die back the next day, giving it its "evening" appellation. The flowers typically

> **DID YOU KNOW?**
> With vivid yellow blossoms that last from late spring to late summer, evening primrose is an imposing wildflower with multiple health benefits.

Evening primrose seeds provide food for many bird species during the winter months.

exhibit a large X-shaped pistil, which projects noticeably beyond the stamens, and they attract active pollinators like hawkmoths and possibly hummingbirds. Subspecies occur in different regions of the country, mostly east of the Rocky Mountains.

Several Native American tribes, including the Cherokee, Iroquois, Ojibwa, and Potawatomi, used nearly the entire evening primrose plant as a source of food, eating the roots raw or boiling them as a potato-like vegetable and cooking young leaves to serve as greens. They also found a number of medicinal applications. They made poultices from the whole plant to heal bruises and decoctions of the roots to alleviate hemorrhoids. They used the leaves to treat wounds, digestive complaints, and sore throats. Yet, it was not until the 1930s that other herbal healers began to take an interest in the plant.

Healing Properties

Evening primrose oil (EPO) has been hailed by its advocates as the biggest breakthrough in natural medicine since the benefits of vitamin C were discovered. This herb contains one of the highest concentrations of the fatty acid GLA

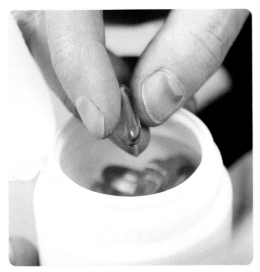

Evening primrose seed oil, high in omega-6 fatty acids, is sold as a dietary supplement. It is also added to skin preparations.

(gamma-linolenic acid), and some healers believe this gives the oil the ability to treat aging problems, rheumatism, alcoholism, acne, eczema, heart disease, hyperactivity in children, symptoms of menopause, multiple sclerosis, weight control, obesity, PMS, and schizophrenia.

According to natural healers, the GLA, linoleic acid, and other nutrients in the oil are critical for strengthening cell structure and improving skin elasticity; they help regulate hormones, which contributes to healthy breast tissue, and improve nerve function. They can even nourish the hair, scalp, and nails. Evening primrose also contains a pain-relieving compound, phenylalanine, which makes it useful for treating chronic headaches.

The Natural Medicines Comprehensive Database is less enthusiastic, however. They found EPO "possibly effective" for treating breast pain, but ineffective against PMS, ADHD, eczema, and menopausal symptoms and recommended further testing on the herb's host of other claims. Still, many individuals swear by the oil, for instance, insisting in testimonials that EPO in capsule form has an almost instant softening effect on dry skin, especially on the face.

Aromatic Qualities

The herb and its corresponding oil have a light, sweet aroma. Although it is not itself typically used in aromatherapy, EPO is a popular carrier for the other herbal essential oils that are used.

History and Lore:

» The origin of the genus name is cloudy: it could mean "donkey catcher" or "wine seeker" from the Greek, or "plant with juice that causes sleep" from the Latin.

» Other common names include fever plant, suncup, and Ozark sundrop.

» *Oenothera* is used as a food plant by the larvae of the flower moths, *Schinia felicitata,* and *S. florida,* with the former feeding exclusively on *O. deltoides.*

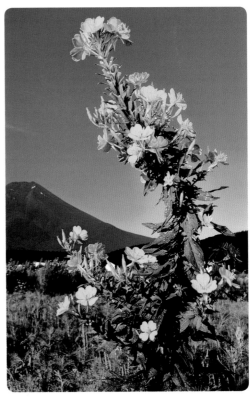

Evening primrose has a commanding presence when in full bloom, but it can be an invasive plant, taking over a garden.

FOCUS ON

SKIN-CARE SOLUTIONS

Herbal beauty aids feature an anti-aging bonus.

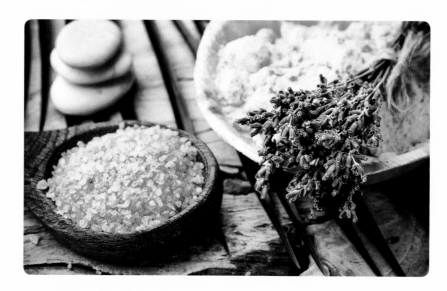

As we age, free radicals and inflammation can contribute to the loss of youthful tone in the face and skin. The good news is that many herbs contain antioxidants and other beneficial compounds that help combat these aging factors.

Women have been using herbal treatments to achieve silky skin since the time of Queen Nefertiti in ancient Egypt. Today's modern herbal skin-care products offer a variety of applications, from basic cleansing and maintenance to enhancing natural beauty to targeting specific problems. Some herbs contain protective chemicals, like tannins, that can reverse the harsh effects of sunlight, pollution, and stress, while others have moisturizing qualities.

The skin-protecting herbs include basil, ginkgo, green and black tea, rosemary, milk thistle, nettle, patchouli, and sage. Skin soothing, anti-inflammatory herbs include calendula, witch hazel, and rose, while herbs for dry or mature skin include fennel, jasmine, licorice, and rose. For oily skin, try rosemary, sage, thyme, yarrow, and lavender.

Customize Your Skin Care

While there are plenty of herbal skin-care choices in health food stores, why not try creating your own? Once you have mastered a few basic recipes, you can customize your own lotions by substituting other herbs based on their scents or beneficial qualities.

MEDICINAL HERBS

Homemade Herbal Lotions and Scrubs

These easy-to-follow recipes from herbalist Kelley Edkins are intended to produce multiple jars—perfect for giving to friends and family.

Patchouli Aphrodisiac Cream

This healing face and body cream offers the sensual essence of patchouli flowers and essential oil. Yields eight ½-ounce jars.

Ingredients
- ½ cup patchouli flowers
- ½ cup organic grape-seed oil
- ⅓ cup beeswax
- 10 teaspoons hemp seed oil
- 5 teaspoons organic raw honey
- 40 drops patchouli essential oil

Directions
Place fresh or dried patchouli flowers in an airtight jar, add grape-seed oil, seal, and let stand for at least two weeks. Strain oil into a 2-cup glass measuring cup, and place in a small saucepan of water, making sure the water will not slosh into cup. On low heat, add hemp seed oil, beeswax, and honey. Let beeswax melt slowly while mixing occasionally with a chopstick. Pour mixture into 1/2-ounce jars. Add five drops of patchouli essential oil to each jar before mixture hardens. Seal jars. and let sit for 24 hours.

Lavender-Rose Salt Scrub

Perfect for exfoliating and softening the arms and legs, especially during the drying, cold-weather months. Yields four 4-ounce jars

Ingredients
- 1 cup Himalayan pink salt
- 1 cup cheltic sea salt
- ½ cup organic grape-seed oil
- ½ cup organic coconut oil
- 10 sprigs freshly dried lavender
- 5 dried roses
- 9 teaspoons organic raw honey
- 10 drops organic water-distilled lavender essential oil

Directions
Mix salt in a large bowl. Crush lavender into a powder with a mortar and pestle. Using a fine strainer, add the lavender to the salt, and then add oils. Mixture should be moist, not oily. Add honey, and mix well with a wooden spoon. Scoop mixture into 4-ounce glass jars. Add ten drops lavender essential oil to the top; do not mix. Place rose petals and a lavender flower on top, seal jar, and let sit for 24 hours.

Honeybee Body Butter

Use on both face and body as a moisturizer and anti-inflammatory agent. Yields eight 1-ounce jars.

Ingredients
- ½ cup fresh or dried St. John's wort flowers
- 1 cup organic sunflower oil
- ½ cup dried nettle leaf and flower
- 5 teaspoons organic raw honey
- ½ cup beeswax
- 1 cup coconut oil
- 10 drops camphor essential oil
- 10 drops peppermint essential oil

Directions
Place St. John's wort flowers in a lidded jar. Pour in sunflower oil, and seal the jar. Store for six weeks or until the oil turns red. Strain into a 4-cup glass measuring cup. Powder the nettle with a mortar and pestle, and add to oil using a strainer. Submerge measuring cup in a saucepan of water that is well below the edge of the cup. Simmer slowly, making sure not to boil, and then add beeswax, coconut oil, and honey. Let the beeswax melt slowly—approximately 15 to 20 minutes. Mix with a chopstick, then pour into 1-ounce jars. Add the camphor and peppermint essential oils to each jar before mixture hardens. Seal jar, and let sit for 24 hours. ■

ORGANIC RAW HONEY

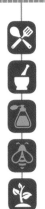

Feverfew

Tanacetum parthenium

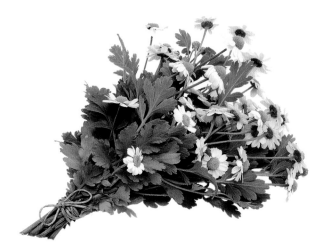

Feverfew, one of the wild chamomiles, is an age-old remedy among country folk for treating migraine headaches, but with its bright, daisy-like blooms, it also makes a cheerful addition to the garden. A member of the daisy or Composite family, Asteraceae, feverfew was originally native to Eastern Europe, particularly the Balkan peninsula, Anatolia, and the Caucasus region. Today it can be found—both cultivated and growing wild—around the world, including in many parts of Europe, North America, Australia, and Chile. The plant particularly prefers scrubby mountainsides, rocky slopes, stone walls, and waste places.

Feverfew's medicinal history goes back at least as far as the ancient Romans, when physician and herbalist Dioscorides recommended it as an anti-inflammatory. The herb's name derives from the Latin *febrifugio,* meaning "fever

DID YOU KNOW?
A short bush with small daisy-like blooms, feverfew may be helpful in preventing migraines and many other common ailments.

reducer." It was once widely used for this purpose, but the plant is no longer seen as effective for fevers. Its specific name, *parthenium,* possibly comes from the folktale that the herb helped save someone who had fallen from the Parthenon, the temple of Athena on the Acropolis.

Feverfew grows into a smallish bush that averages 18 to 24 inches in height, with notched, feathery, citrus-scented yellow-green leaves, and yellow or white flowers that bloom between July and September.

Healing Properties

In addition to easing headaches, feverfew has been used by traditional herbalists to treat arthritis and digestive issues, irregular menstrual periods, psoriasis, nasal allergies, asthma, tinnitus, dizziness, and nausea and vomiting. The herb has also been prescribed for fertility issues in both men and women, to prevent miscarriage, to pep up tired blood, and to treat colds, earache, liver disease, muscular tension, swollen feet, bone disorders, and gas. Its crushed leaves can be placed on the gums to ease toothache or on the skin to kill germs in superficial wounds. A tincture made from feverfew is said to immediately relieve the pain and swelling of insect bites.

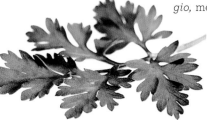

The dried leaves of feverfew are used to make extracts, and the leaves are sometimes eaten fresh.

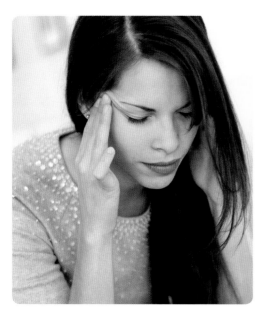

Taken in a capsule or as an infusion or tincture, feverfew may relieve the pain of premenstrual and migraine headaches.

Culinary Uses

While not thought of as a cooking herb, feverfew, with its slightly bitter citrus leaves, has been used as to flavor a number of dishes. The dried flowers can be used to make tea or to as a flavoring in pastries.

History and Lore

» The plant is also known by its synonyms *Chrysanthemum parthenium* and *Pyrethrum parthenium* and is referred to as bachelor's buttons, featherfew, featherfoil, flirtwort, and midsummer daisy.

» In late Anglo-Saxon lore, feverfew was a remedy for the "flying venom" that came from an arrow shot by an elf, a hag, or a god.

» Feverfew can attract harmful snails, slugs, and black flies. Some gardeners place terra-cotta pots on their sides as homes for toads, who will feast on these pests.

» An infusion of the flowers, made with boiling water and allowed to cool, was once used to calm the nerves and treat earaches.

Although there is little scientific evidence to support these many healing claims, the herb's advocates maintain that its curative properties are more than just the "placebo effect." Human studies, on the other hand, do indicate that feverfew can be effective in treating or preventing chronic migraines, but researchers are still not sure what substance in the plant is responsible for this. Some people who stop taking feverfew after prolonged use have experienced withdrawal symptoms.

FOR YOUR HEALTH

Feverfew and Cell Destruction

Feverfew contains the active ingredients parthenolide and tanetin. In studies, the former has been shown to induce apoptosis (programmed cell destruction via biochemical changes in morphology followed by cell death) in some cancer cell lines in vitro. The chemical may also have the potential to target cancer stem cells. These possibilities have yet to be verified in studies on humans, but research is ongoing. Unfortunately, in commercial feverfew preparations, parthenolide content can vary by as much as 40-fold depending on the brand purchased—and studies show that the amount actually found was often far less than the amount printed on the label. ■

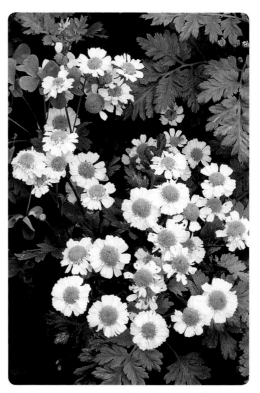

Feverfew is a popular garden plant with many cultivars, ranging from the typical daisy-like blossoms to double-flowered blooms that show off its chrysanthemum heritage.

Feverfew

127

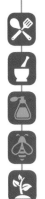

Ginkgo

Ginkgo biloba

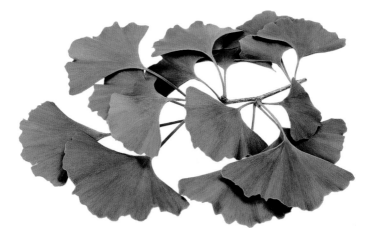

Called a "living fossil," this tree dates back to the dinosaur age and is the lone surviving member of the family Ginkgoaceae. Imprints of its distinctive fan-shaped leaves have been found in shale from the Permian era, roughly 298 to 252 million years ago. At the end of the Permian, the greatest mass extinction in history killed off 90 percent of marine species and 70 percent of terrestrial species—yet not the ginkgo tree, which then ranged throughout both hemispheres.

Ginkgos disappeared from the fossil record at the end of the Pliocene (about 5.333 million to 2.58 million years ago), except for a small area of central China, where the tree continued to thrive. Although it has been cultivated for centuries in Europe and America, the tree has not naturalized. Also known as the maidenhair tree, the ginkgo has been used as a multipurpose remedy for millennia—it was prescribed for treating asthma and bronchitis in 2600 B.C.

The ginkgo is dioecious, but each tree does not reveal its gender until it is about 20 years old. Males produce small pollen cones. Females produce two fruitlike ovules at the end of a stalk; after pollination, either one or both develop into seeds. Despite the stench of the fruit, the peeled seeds, or nuts, are roasted for use in Chinese cuisine.

Trees reach a height of 120 feet or more; young trees have sparse branches, but mature ginkgos sport a broad, towering crown. With its deep roots, it is usually impervious to wind and weather. The tree is also disease and insect resistant, and can sprout aerial roots, making it hardy and adaptable. Due to its longevity—some specimens are more than 2,500 years old—the tree is venerated by a number of Asian faiths.

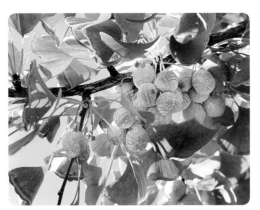

Gingko's fruitlike seedpods are attractive, but the butyric acid they contain makes them smell like rancid butter or vomit.

The Bearers of Hope

Ginkgo trees not only survived a mass extinction event millions of years ago, they also proved resilient in the face of the atomic bomb. After the bombing of the Japanese city Hiroshima in 1945, six mature ginkgo trees growing near the epicenter managed to survive the devastating blast. Charred, scarred, and broken, they all eventually revived, regenerated without major deformities, and remain alive today. Three have actually had temples built around them. The temple tree at Hosshin-ji was saved from demolition in 1994 and has since become an international symbol. Because of their strength and tenacity, ginkgos are known in Japan as the "bearers of hope." ∎

Healing Properties

Ginkgo biloba contains potent antioxidant flavonoids and terpenoids that improve blood flow and is taken as an extract prepared from the leaves. Due to its anti-inflammatory, antifungal, and antiseptic qualities, it has been used in traditional medicine to treat arthritis, bladder ailments, chilblains, skin inflammations, diabetes, digestive disorders, dysentery, edema, headache, liver problems, scabies, seizures, sepsis, and vision problems, and to heal wounds.

In the modern era, the herb's benefits have been the subject of much clinical research. Recent double-blind trials have demonstrated *Ginkgo biloba*'s ability to dilate blood vessels, making it useful in treating conditions related to loss of blood flow to the brain—Alzheimer's disease, memory problems, tinnitus, vertigo, concentration issues, mood disturbances, and hearing disorders. It has also been used to treat glaucoma and macular degeneration, and it has improved the low libidos of some people taking SSRI antidepressants.

Culinary Uses

The roasted seeds, without their fleshy covering, are considered a delicacy in China and Japan. Used in cooking, these low-fat kernels pick up the flavor of other ingredients, similar to soybeans. They can be found in many Asian markets dried or shelled and canned in brine.

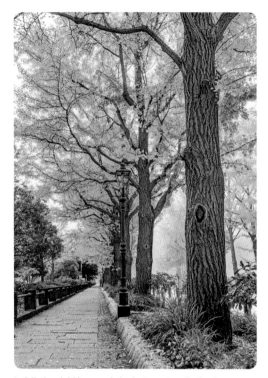

In fall, the vivid leaves of gingko trees turn the landscape a glittering gold. The hardy male ginkgo is now a popular urban plant, beautifying streets and parks in many cities.

History and Lore

» A population of ginkgos in central China was thought to be remnants from the Pliocene, but their genetic uniformity indicates they were probably planted by monks a thousand years ago. Truly wild ginkgos, direct descendants of the ancient ones, possibly grow in China's Qinghair-Tibet Plateau.

» The Chinese have many names for the gingko tree, including *tinxing* (silver almond tree), *baiguoshu* (white nut tree), *yazhangshu* (duck feet tree), *gongsunshu* (Yellow Emperor tree), *fozhijia* (Buddha's fingernail), and *lingyan* (eyes of the cosmic spirit tree).

» Graphic images of the leaf are found in religious and civic artwork throughout Asia, such on a manhole cover in Tokyo, Japan, which depicts ginkgo leaves with a sakura flower (at left).

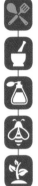

Ginseng

Panax ginseng, P. quinquefolius

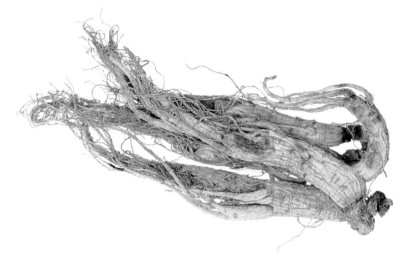

A plant of cooler climates, ginseng is a slow-growing perennial and one of the most popular health supplements in the world. The term *ginseng* can refer to any one of 11 species that belong to the *Panax* genus and the Araliaceae family. Many folk healers utilize Asian ginseng (*Panax ginseng*), or American ginseng (*P. quinquefolius*). Siberian ginseng (*Eleutherococcus senticosus*) is also a popular herbal remedy and is part of the same family, though not in the *Panax* genus.

Originating in China, the ginseng plant once grew wild in many parts of the world. It can

reach 18 inches in height, with stalks bearing with three to five leaflets of 2 to 5 inches in length. The flowers, greenish in hue, are followed by red berries. The pale, fleshy, aromatic root is the part most used by healers. It resembles a small parsnip that forks as it matures.

The name ginseng derives from the Chinese *rénshēn,* combining the words for "man or person" and "plant root," referring to the forked "legs" of the root. The genus name *Panax* comes from the Greek for "all heal."

Healing Properties

Five thousand years ago, Chinese healers in Manchuria valued ginseng for its powers of rejuvenation. Around the same time, the scriptures in the Indian *Rig Veda* lauded the herb for bestowing the strength of the horse, the mule, the goat, the ram, and the bull. Asian herbalists continued to use—and demand—the herb, right up to modern times, when sources worldwide began to diminish. Fortunately, ginseng is now commercially cultivated.

Contemporary herbalists value ginseng because it is considered an adaptogen—a class of healing plants that help the body balance, restore, and

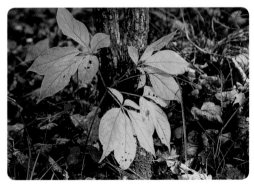

In fall, red berries appear on Asian ginseng *(Panax ginseng)*.

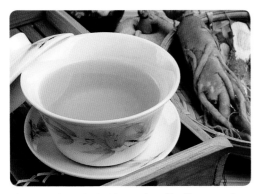

Ginseng tea is credited with a number of healing properties, and it is said to have a soothing effect on the body.

protect itself, especially from stressors. This property is difficult to prove scientifically, however, though some research has shown that Asian ginseng can increase RNA and protein in the muscle tissue of lab animals. In another study, daily doses of Siberian ginseng increased the number of white blood cells—including the number of killer cells that eliminate invading cells and those that have been virally infected. In a double-blind study of 93 volunteers with herpes simplex virus 2 who took ginseng, there was a 50 percent reduction in outbreaks, and if outbreaks did occur, they were less severe and of shorter duration.

The *Panax* species contains ginsenosides, unique compounds with anti-inflammatory effects that are being investigated for potential medicinal use.

Aromatic Qualities

Ginseng, with its strong scent, is one of the most relied-upon botanicals in aromatherapy. It is used to improve mental and physical performance, and can also be employed as an aphrodisiac. American ginseng (yin) offers cooling properties that help with respiratory ailments, while Asian ginseng (yang) helps to improve circulation.

History and Lore

» Chinese emperors not only used the plant for food and medicine, but also had it made into soaps and body lotions.
» Koreans would purify themselves for a week, remaining clean and chaste, before they went to gather the revered plant.
» American frontiersman Daniel Boone dug for the valuable root and sold many tons.

Supply and Demand

By the third century A.D., the demand for medicinal ginseng in China was so great that the Chinese offered silks and other valuables to foreign traders in exchange for it. This demand only increased over the centuries. In 1716, a Jesuit priest in Canada, who knew of the herb's great popularity, began searching for it in French Canada, a region with a climate much like Manchuria, where ginseng originated. The similar plants he found growing outside Montreal came to be known as American ginseng. (Native Americans were already using this herb, called *garantequen,* to treat headaches, fevers, coughs, eye infections, and to poultice wounds.) Botanists soon realized this species was common all over the eastern United States, and so an export trade to China developed and rapidly grew. During the mid-1970s ginseng was again so popular that the wild herb became endangered due to overharvesting. Farmers solved the problem by cultivating ginseng for export. It is currently grown in Wisconsin, Ontario, and British Columbia. Ironically, the American species is now also grown in China ■

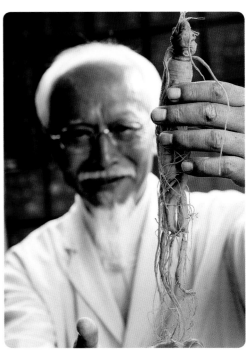

The semi-human shape of the ginseng root made it a powerful symbol of divine harmony to early Asian cultures.

Ginseng

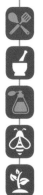

Goldenseal

Hydrastis canadensis

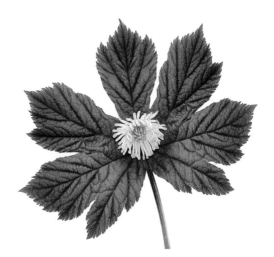

This herb was widely used by Native American healers well before Europeans settled North America. Today, goldenseal reigns as one of America's most popular medicinal herbs, and it continues to gain advocates, who value it for, among other things, its effectiveness as a digestive tonic and an immune booster. More than 150,000 pounds of the herb are consumed in the United States each year.

This low-growing woodland perennial is a member of the buttercup family, Ranunculaceae, and is native to the eastern United States, ranging from northeast South Carolina to lower New

---

DID YOU KNOW?

One of the most popular healing herbs in the United States, goldenseal, a perennial in the buttercup family, is often used as a multipurpose remedy.

York, and from northern Arkansas to the southeast corner of Wisconsin. Due to overharvesting and loss of habitat, the wild herb is now considered endangered, and although it can still be found in Ohio, Indiana, West Virginia, Kentucky, and Illinois, it should never be picked. Most prepared goldenseal products come from commercial cultivation.

The goldenseal plant produces two palmate, hairy leaves with five to seven double-toothed lobes. The single, diminutive flower is a greenish white and ripens into a raspberry-like seed head. The golden yellow root—the medicinal portion of the plant—is dried and administered orally and externally for its anti-inflammatory, astringent, and antimicrobial qualities.

Healing Properties

American Indians used goldenseal for respiratory, digestive, and urinary tract conditions brought on by allergy or infection. The Cherokee made a decoction of the roots to cleanse local inflammations and use as a tonic for general

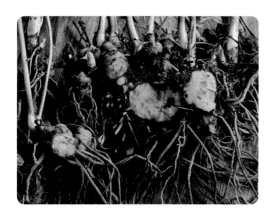

Goldenseal gets it alternate names, orangeroot and yellow puccoon, from the roots' golden color. When sliced, they reveal a bright yellow interior.

debility, indigestion, and to improve appetite. They also mixed the herb with bear grease as an insect repellent. The Iroquois used it to treat whooping cough, diarrhea, liver disease, fever, sour stomach, flatulence, and pneumonia, and combined it with whiskey for heart trouble. They also mixed it with other medicinal roots to make a wash for treating earaches and eye infections.

The European colonists, borrowing cures from the native population, eventually began to use the herb to treat colds and other respiratory infections, hay fever, stomach pain and gastritis, peptic ulcers, colitis, constipation, hemorrhoids, gas, urinary tract problems, liver disorders, fatigue, fever, jaundice, gonorrhea, bleeding after childbirth, vaginal pain, menstrual problems, malaria, and anorexia. It was also applied to the skin to treat rashes, ulcers, acne, itching, eczema, dandruff, ringworm, and cold sores.

Modern studies on the herb have so far validated only some of goldenseal's many healing claims, specifically its antibacterial, anticonvulsive, and choleretic properties. One of the herb's constituents, the alkaloid berberine—responsible for the root's yellow hue, has shown effectiveness against bacteria and fungi. It is known to prevent the bacteria *Escherichia coli (E. coli)*

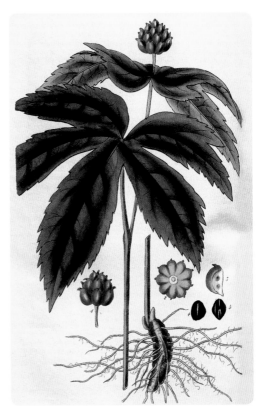

Goldenseal shown in *Curtis's Botanical Magazine* from 1833. In late spring, a single, small, inconspicuous flower blossoms between each pair of the large, palmate leaves of goldenseal. In the summer, a single, red, raspberry-like fruit appears.

from binding to urinary tract walls. Berberine can lower blood pressure, improve an irregular heartbeat, and early research indicates that it can lower blood sugar and "bad" low-density lipoprotein (LDL) cholesterol.

Goldenseal contains calcium, iron, and manganese, and vitamins A, C, E and the B-complex, as well as other nutrients and minerals.

History and Lore

» Goldenseal experienced bursts of popularity in the 1930s and 1970s, and it is much in demand again today.

» This herb contains propolis, a resinous substance gathered by bees from the leaf buds of certain plants; it is used as a "cement" for sealing unwanted open spaces in the hive, keeping out predators, parasites, and disease.

» Contrary to popular myth, goldenseal isn't effective for masking the presence of illegal drugs in the urine.

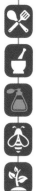

Heartsease

Viola tricolor

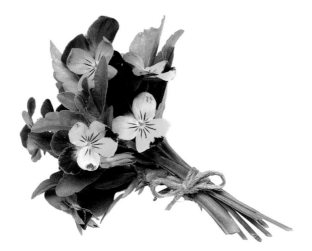

This annual wildflower is the progenitor of the modern-day pansy most gardeners know and love as an early spring bloomer. It is native to Europe, but has naturalized in most of the United States, where it is sometimes called Johnny-jump-up.

The plant's history as an herbal remedy dates as far back as ancient Greece, where Homer recommended the plant to moderate anger; Roman botanist Pliny advised its use for headaches and dizziness.

Heartsease grows to no more than six inches in height, has a clumping tendency, and produces deeply cut leaves and the familiar "small face" pansy blossoms in white, purple, or yellow—or a combination of two or three—with the most color showing on the upper petals. The flowers can bloom throughout the growing season, from spring to fall, especially with regular

DID YOU KNOW?
The wild version of the Johnny-jump-up so familiar to gardeners, heartsease is an age-old herbal remedy often used to make a rejuvenating tonic.

Heartsease displays two basic color patterns: a single color having black "penciling" lines radiating from its center or a combination of white, blue, purple, and yellow with a dark center called a face. The faces can show a wide range of "expressions," from happy to sad.

deadheading. Flowers will droop after dark or just before a rainstorm, keeping the water on the reverse of their delicate petals.

Healing Properties

This plant—often the whole plant—has been used by traditional healers for millennia to treat epilepsy, asthma, respiratory ailments, ulcers, skin diseases, and colds. A common use of heartsease is as a blood cleanser that boosts the metabolism. As an expectorant it is prescribed for bronchitis and whooping cough (pertussis), and its diuretic properties make it useful for treating rheumatism and cystitis. Its blood cleansing properties made it effective against scrofula in children. Chinese herbalists used the plant for almost exactly the same ailments as Europeans did, while North American Indians used it to treat boils and swelling.

As expected from its name, heartsease was also viewed as a love charm or token. In the "language of flowers" its three colors—purple, yellow, and white—stand for "memories, loving thoughts, and souvenirs," the very things that ease the hearts of separated lovers. In truth, the herb might not be able to relieve a lover's woes, but it does have a calming, sedative effect.

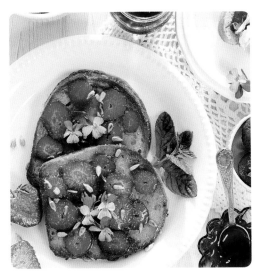

Sprinkle heartsease over french toast and strawberries to add both color and flavor—all *Viola tricolor* blooms are edible.

Chemically, the constituents of heartsease include saponins, mucilage, resins, alkaloids, flavonoids, volatile oil, salicylic acid, and carotenoids. Heartsease is one of the many violas that contains small peptides called cyclotides. Their size and structure lend them high stability, making them ideal for use in drug development.

Many of the cyclotides in *Viola tricolor* are also cytotoxic, meaning they could be useful in treating cancer. The edible flowers also contain beneficial antioxidants.

Culinary Uses

Heartsease leaves can be eaten raw with mixed greens or cooked for addition to soups and light dishes. The flowers are also edible and can be candied as garnish for desserts or added to salads for a touch of color.

History and Lore

» The herb is also known as wild pansy, heart's delight, tickle-my-fancy, Jack-jump-up-and-kiss-me, come-and-cuddle-me, three faces in a hood, or love-in-idleness. The Anglo-Saxon name was *banwort* or *bonewort*.

» The flowers have been used to make yellow, green, and blue-green dyes, while the leaves can be used to make a chemical indicator.

» Heartsease appears in Shakespeare's comedy *A Midsummer Night's Dream;* it is the love-charm picked by Puck, at Oberon's command, that causes a sleeper to become besotted with the first person he or she sees upon waking.

CURIOSITIES

"You Occupy My Thoughts": The Language of Flowers

A long-held tradition in literature and folklore is that different flowers represent various emotions or traits or act as symbols for them in a kind of secret code. This hidden meaning is often based on a flower's appearance or nature. For instance, the mimosa, which closes at even a gentle touch, commonly represents chastity. In *Hamlet,* Shakespeare's poor, mad Ophelia catalogs a host of plants' meanings and even mentions heartsease: "There's pansies, that's for thoughts."

The language of flowers, or floriography, had early advocates in the tulip-mad Turkish court during the early 1700s and was introduced to England by Mary Wortley Montagu in 1717. During the Victorian Age, floriography became a true craze, with courting couples sending each other coded sprays or arrangements or exchanging small "talking bouquets" called tussie-mussies. The trend was also carried out in literature and painting, especially by the Pre-Raphaelites.

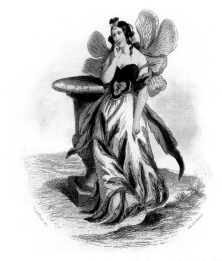

"Pensée" from the book *Fleurs animées,* published in 1846. Heartsease and other pansies—which take their name from the French for "thought"—symbolized "remembrance" in the language of flowers. Heartsease was often given as a reminder of happier times to ease the heartbreak of separation.

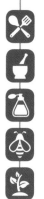

Lemon Balm

Melissa officinalis

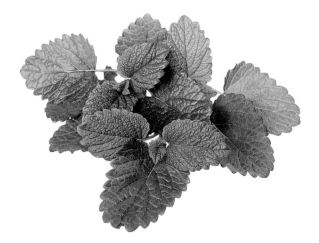

L emon balm, often called the "calming herb," is a versatile perennial that has medical, culinary, and aromatic applications. A member of the mint family, Lamiaceae, it was originally native to south-central Europe and the Mediterranean region. In parts of North America, it escaped cultivation and now grows wild.

The herb goes back to ancient Greece, where it was likely the "honey-leaf" mentioned by Theophrastus, the father of botany, in the third century B.C. Lemon balm remained popular throughout the Middle Ages and could be found in the herb garden of botanist John Gerard in 1596.

DID YOU KNOW?

Considered a "calming" herb, lemon balm produces fresh-scented leaves. Prized for the permanence of their aroma, the leaves are a favorite addition to potpourris and aromatherapy oils.

The plant reaches two to three feet in height, and has erect, clumping stems and heart-shaped, serrated leaves. The delicate white flowers are rich in nectar, attracting the busy pollinators that gave the plant it genus name, *Melissa,* which is Greek for "honeybee." There are many cultivars, some, like 'Quedlinburger Niederliegende', are engineered to be high in essential oils.

Healing Properties

Early natural healers recommended lemon balm, both externally as essential oils or internally as teas, for treating insomnia and anxiety, as well as disorders of the gastric tract, the nervous system, and the liver.

Modern research has discovered that lemon balm possesses impressive levels of antioxidant activity. In studies, high doses of purified lemon balm extracts had a marked effect on laboratory-induced levels of stress in humans, resulting in "significantly increased self-ratings of calmness and reduced self-ratings of alertness." A 300-mg dose also sped up problem-solving skills without any loss of accuracy. A daily dose of herbal tea for 30 days reduced oxidative stress, which can lead to the development of cancer and other

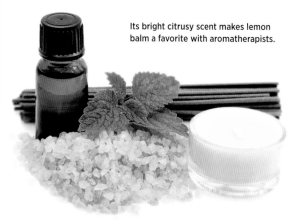

Its bright citrusy scent makes lemon balm a favorite with aromatherapists.

debilitating diseases, in radiology staff members who were exposed to low-level radiation at work.

Lemon balm contains eugenol, which can be used as an antiseptic and anesthetic; tannins, which act as astringents, and terpenes, which are biosynthetic building blocks and the primary constituents of essential oils.

Easy Lemon Balm Projects

Soothing lemon balm can be used so many ways— to make herbal tea, an herbal bath sachet, even a healing lip balm. Here are a few simple projects:

- Make an infused oil by filling a heatproof glass jar a quarter full of dried, crumbled leaves, then pouring in light olive oil. Cap and store in a dark place for six weeks. Make a compound oil by adding dried calendula flowers.
- To create a healing lip balm, combine three parts lemon balm oil to one part beeswax and one half to one part solid butter. Add one or two drops of essential oil (such as peppermint or tea tree) per tablespoon of ingredients, blend well, and transfer to a small tin or jar.
- Fill a small gauze bag with lemon balm leaves and rose petals and hang from the spigot as you draw a bath.
- For a delicious spread to put on muffins or cornbread, mix a pinch of lemon balm into a half stick of butter and add a drizzle of honey.
- Make a refreshing summer drink by filling a pitcher with fresh lemon balm leaves and slices of fresh lemon and cucumber and then adding water. Refrigerate for several hours. ∎

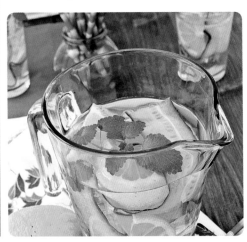

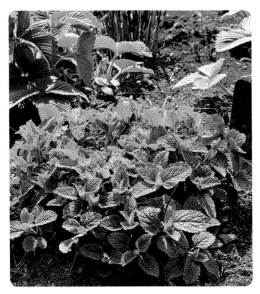

Lemon balm is an easy-to-grow and attractive addition to a kitchen garden. Cut back the plants after they flower, and they will keep producing fresh batches of aromatic foliage.

Culinary Uses

Lemon balm's light citrus flavor makes it a natural in the kitchen. The herb is used as a flavoring for ice cream, in fruit dishes and candies, and in both hot tea and iced tea. It is the key ingredient in lemon balm pesto, and it also works well with fish or poultry dishes. Its taste combines especially well with its mint family cousin spearmint.

Aromatic Qualities

Aromatherapists call this herb melissa, valuing both its sweet scent and its potent healing capabilities. They use it for treating headaches, depression, and stress, but it has also had success as a calming agent in patients with dementia.

History and Lore

» When the leaves are crushed and rubbed on the skin, they act as a mosquito repellent.

» Lemon balm might be a better, more healthwise, preservative for sausages than the butylated hydroxy anisole that is currently used.

» Lemon balm is the chief ingredient in carmelite water, an alcoholic extract which combines the herb with lemon peel, nutmeg, and angelica root. It was originally made by 12th-century French nuns and monks and used as a toilet water and tonic to ward off nervous headaches and fever. It is still sold in German pharmacies.

Lemon Balm

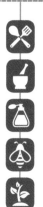

Lemon Verbena

Aloysia citrodora

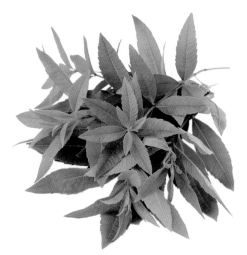

This herb of the New World was once considered a sacred healing plant and was frequently woven into wreaths for celebrants to wear at festivals and weddings. It was originally native to western South America, and, after the Spanish brought the plant to Europe, it became an important raw material for perfumes. It was introduced to England in 1784 and was soon a favorite for use in teas, desserts, and meat dishes.

Also called lemon beebrush, this deciduous shrub is a member of the Verbenaceae family and makes an attractive garden addition, often reaching six feet or more in height. The glossy, lance-shaped leaves release their citrusy fragrance whenever they are touched, and the clustering, small white or pale purple flowers form on panicles.

Its genus name, *Aloysia*, was meant to honor Maria Louisa, Princess of Parma, in 1819.

> **DID YOU KNOW?**
> With its heady citrus scent and flavor, lemon verbena has a place in the kitchen pantry, as well as the medicine cabinet.

Healing Properties

Lemon verbena, with its anti-inflammatory, antispasmodic, and antioxidant benefits, was once used by natural healers to treat a variety of ailments, but it has become undervalued in recent years. It was known for its sedative effect and ability to soothe stomach pains, but also for treating joint pain, sleep disorders, asthma, colds and fevers, hemorrhoids, varicose veins, skin ailments, and chills. Today it is prescribed as a digestive tonic, a mild expectorant, a tension reducer, and as relief for arthritis pain.

Culinary Uses

Lemon verbena leaves can be used to enhance both meat dishes and desserts. They add lemony tang to fish dishes, salads, and stir-fried vegetables. The syrup is delicious over ice cream or mixed into a cocktail, for instance, a gin and tonic, gin fizz, or daiquiri. In summer, the leaves can be infused in water with mint to create a refreshing drink. In cooler weather, a half cup of leaves steeped in boiling water make a relaxing tisane. Lemon verbena can even be blended with garlic,

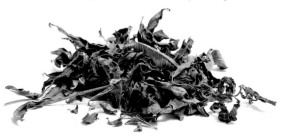

Dried lemon verbena leaves. The leaves, whether fresh or dried, emit a powerful citrus odor, hence the Latin specific name *citrodora,* which means "lemon-scented."

The Clean Scent of Lemon: Keeping Pests and Odors at Bay

Lemon verbena's potent lemon scent makes an excellent insect repellent. In the past, stablemen hung bunches of the herb over stall doors to keep flies and midges away and scattered it on stable floors so the horses would trample it and release the scent. Today, the leaves can be tucked behind books or placed on kitchen shelves to discourage silverfish that feed on paper and starch.

To freshen the bath, hang a posy of leaves on your tub faucet; to refresh your home, add a few sprigs to your vacuum cleaner bag. Or make a zesty, lemony room freshener by adding a quarter cup clove and cinnamon pieces, a quarter cup dried coriander seeds, and a quarter cup thinly sliced lemon rind to one cup dried lemon verbena leaves. Combine these in a bowl with a teaspoon each of clove oil and lemon oil. Place in a covered jar and shake daily for three days. Then place room freshener in small bowls around your house. Return mixture to covered jar at night. ■

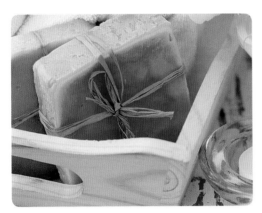

Used in handmade soaps, lemon verbena imparts a crisp, refreshing scent. In aromatherapy, it is said to lift the spirits.

pine nuts (or walnuts), olive oil, and Parmesan cheese to make a pesto that's perfect over roasted vegetables like asparagus or green beans.

To gain the freshest flavor, preserve lemon verbena leaves by processing two cups of leaves with one-half to one cup sugar in a food processor until they form a paste. Freeze the paste in a thin layer in zip bags. To serve, break off whatever amount is required and sprinkle over tea, fruits, and desserts, or mix into meat marinades or rubs.

Aromatic Qualities

This plant is often considered the "queen of lemon-scented herbs." It was valued by the perfume industry for hundreds of years, but the oil extraction process eventually grew too expensive. Today, the herb is found in potpourris and air fresheners, while the essential oil is used in aromatherapy for nervous and digestive problems and to sharpen concentration. Dried lemon verbena leaves will retain their odor for many years.

History and Lore

» In *Gone with the Wind,* lemon verbena is mentioned as the favorite plant of Scarlet O'Hara's mother, Ellen.

» In the practice of the magical arts, lemon verbena is ruled by the planet Mars and represents dreams, happiness, and harmony. It is said to prevent nightmares, aid true love, and can be added to other magical herbs to increase their strength.

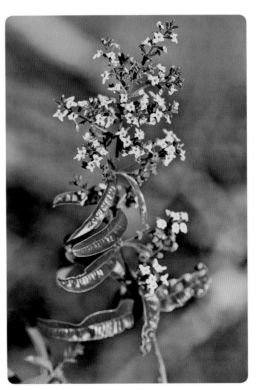

In late spring or early summer, sprays of white to pale purple flowers rise above the long, glossy leaves of the plant.

Lemon Verbena

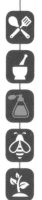

Milk Thistle

Silybum marianum

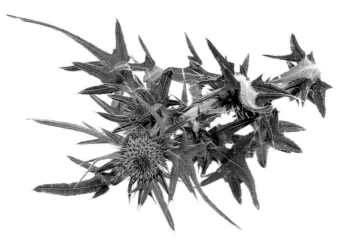

Milk thistle is a striking, prickly member of the daisy family, Asteraceae. It is often considered a garden invader, but don't weed it out too quickly—the dried seed heads attract finches, and its roots and stems can be cooked. The common name comes from the milky white fluid that is produced from the crushed leaves. Other names include *cardus marianus,* blessed milk thistle, Marian thistle, Saint Mary's thistle, Mediterranean milk thistle, variegated thistle, and Scotch thistle.

Native to Mediterranean Europe and Asia, this annual or biennial plant is now found worldwide. For more than two thousand years, milk thistle has been used to treat liver ailments—a folk remedy now validated by modern clinical studies.

DID YOU KNOW?

Used medicinally for more than two millennia, milk thistle is now recognized for its ability to protect the liver

It is commercially cultivated for pharmaceutical use in Austria (Waldviertel), Germany, Hungary, Poland, China, and Argentina.

The plant can reach an impressive ten feet in height, and, like most thistles, has red to purple flowers. It also produces pale green leaves covered with fine, woolly hairs. The leaves have sharp prickles on the margins and white streaks along their veins. The "milk" in the plant's name may refer to these white streaks, as well as the plant's milky sap.

Healing Properties

In addition to its beneficial effects on the liver, milk thistle was considered a cure for baldness from the days of ancient Greece and Rome to the Middle Ages. Greek Theophrastus called it *pternix,* while Roman Pliny called it *silybum.* For many centuries, herbalists prescribed it for headaches, canker sores, vertigo, jaundice, and the plague. In the modern era, the herb again came into its own as a liver treatment after studies done in Germany in the 1960s.

The seed shells contain a powerful flavonoid complex called silymarin, and in 40 years of intensive research, more than 400 studies have confirmed that this extract can both prevent and

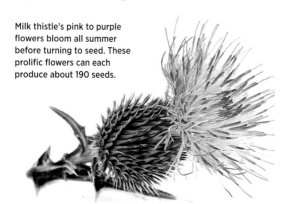

Milk thistle's pink to purple flowers bloom all summer before turning to seed. These prolific flowers can each produce about 190 seeds.

140

repair liver damage. This makes it invaluable for treating ailments such as cirrhosis, hepatitis, gallstones, fatty liver, and even poisoning. (Milk thistle is still used as an antidote to poisoning by amanitas mushrooms, including death cap and destroying angel.)

In one key study, workers who had been exposed to the harmful vapors of toluene and/ or xylene for five to twenty years were given 80 percent silymarin. All showed significant improvement in liver function and platelet counts compared to a control group taking a placebo. Silymarin was also found to reduce drug-induced liver damage in patients taking several psychotropic drugs used for treating schizophrenia and bipolar disorder. In 2010, the medical journal *Cancer* reported that a double-blind placebo study of 50 children indicated that milk thistle could treat liver damage caused

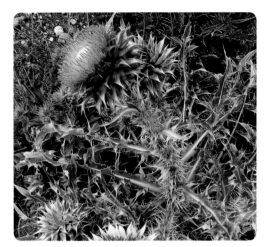

Classified as a noxious weed in many places, milk thistle thrives in waste places with dry and rocky soil. It will also form dense stands in pastures and rangelands.

by chemotherapy. Silymarin might be useful in treating primary biliary cirrhosis of the liver and could also be effective as an antidepressant—a selective serotonin reuptake inhibitor (SSRI)—in the treatment of obsessive-compulsive disorder.

Culinary Uses

In spite of the spines, milk thistle is edible. The roots are eaten raw, boiled and buttered, or parboiled and roasted. In the spring, tender young shoots can be cut down to the root and their "wool" rubbed off, and then served boiled and buttered. The stems can be peeled, soaked overnight to remove bitterness, and then stewed. The leaves make a tasty spinach substitute once they are trimmed of prickles and boiled. They can also be added to salads.

History and Lore

» The milk thistle's spines keep most livestock from browsing on the leaves. A good thing, because the potassium nitrate found in the plant can be toxic to cud-chewing ruminants like cattle and sheep.

» The thistle in an ancient Celtic symbol and, according to the language of flowers, it stands for nobility of character.

» Thistles feature in the works of many writers, including poets Ted Hughes and Hugh McDiarmid, and fiction authors Leo Tolstoy and A. A. Milne—in *Winnie the Pooh*, thistles were Eeyore the donkey's favorite food.

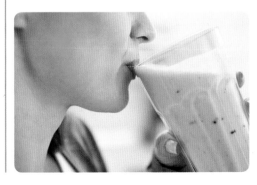

Mugwort

Artemisia vulgaris

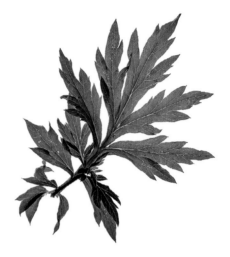

A common perennial plant, which can be found growing in lowly hedgerows and country lanes, mugwort was once a valued household necessity—as both a trusted healing herb and a protector of the home that could ward off evil. A member of the daisy family, Asteraceae, mugwort was originally native to Europe, Asia, and North Africa.

The "mug" in its name possibly derives from the herb's use as a flavoring for beer before the introduction of hops. It is still used in some parts of England to flavor home-brew. "Mug" might also come from the Anglo-Saxon word *moughte,* for "maggot" or "moth," because from the time of early Roman botanist Dioscorides, the herb has been used to repel moths. Its reputation as a healing herb goes back that far as well.

DID YOU KNOW?

For centuries, the stems and leaves of the humbly named mugwort have been used in herbal medicine. The plant has also been used as a beer additive and flavoring and a smudging herb.

Mugwort reaches three feet or more in height, and its pointed, frilled leaves are smooth and dark green on the upper surface, while the undersides are covered with whitish down. The red or pale yellow flowers are small and arranged in long, terminal panicles. The light brown root is about eight inches long, covered with short, tough rootlets. It tastes sweet but acrid.

Healing Properties

Both the leaves and the root of the plant are used medicinally, in teas or tinctures. The main constituents are a volatile oil, an acrid resin, and tannin. Natural healers have used mugwort for female reproductive problems, to stimulate digestion, and as a mild sedative. The herb was also used to treat bronchitis, colds, and kidney ailments. The leaf tea induces sweating, and promotes appetite and liver function. The Japanese used the downy leaves to prepare moxas, a traditional cure for rheumatism, while the Chinese burned the herb as part of moxibustion heat therapy—heating certain acupuncture points with rolled moxa—to stimulate the *qi* and ensure general health.

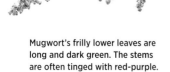

Mugwort's frilly lower leaves are long and dark green. The stems are often tinged with red-purple.

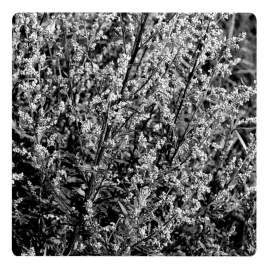

Mugwort is a tall herbaceous plant with small white to red flowers radiating from its erect stems. The leaves and roots are the parts most often used for medicinal purposes.

Oddly, for a time-honored medicinal herb that has been used by both Asian- and European-based healers, there have been very few clinical studies on mugwort's health benefits. Conversely, studies have been conducted on the plant's allergenic properties—its pollen affects roughly 15 percent of hay fever sufferers in Europe.

Culinary Uses

Mugwort is not only used as a savory seasoning for rich dishes—meats, poultry, and game—it can make them easier to digest. Because the herb's flavor is intense, it should be used sparingly. Mugwort is also occasionally employed as one of the green herbs with which geese are stuffed during roasting.

CURIOSITIES

The Magic of Mugwort

Mugwort was a favorite of village wise women and practitioners of Wicca for centuries, and it is also one of nine sacred herbs, representing purity, used in shamanistic rituals. It is the plant of Midgard (the human domain in the nine worlds of Norse mythology) used to begin and end ceremonies; it is burned like incense to sanctify a space and remove all negative influences and energies. Native American also burned bundles of the herb as "smudge" to purify the spiritual and physical aspects of the environment. ■

CULTURAL CONNECTIONS

The Genus of Moonlight

Artemisia, the genus of mugwort, tarragon, and wormwood, among others, takes its name from Artemis, the Greek goddess of the hunt and the moon—who was known as Diana by the Romans. She was said to have given the *Artemisias* to Chiron, the centaur, to care for. It's also possible the genus was so named because most of its plants have pale, silver-gray coloring, resembling the light of the moon. ■

History and Lore

» In the Middle Ages, mugwort was known as *Cingulum Sancti Johannis* because it was believed that John the Baptist wore a girdle of the herbs in the wilderness.

» Mugwort could supposedly preserve the traveler from fatigue, sunstroke, wild beasts, and evil spirits.

» In Holland and Germany, gathering the herb on St. John's Eve—June 23—offered protection against disease and misfortune.

» In Cornwall, during the days of World War II rationing, the dried leaves were used as an economical substitute for black tea.

» Many species of Lepidoptera feed on the mugwort, including the common emerald, bordered pug, scalloped hazel, and mouse moths.

» The plant is also known as felon herb, cranewort, Artemis herb, naughty man, old man, old Uncle Henry, muggons, and sailor's tobacco (because it was smoked when sailors ran out of regular tobacco while at sea).

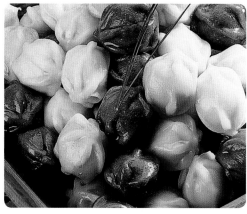

Korean cooks use mugwort to make *tteok,* a steamed rice cake.

SENIOR HEALTH SOLUTIONS

Baby boomers can benefit from alternative health remedies.

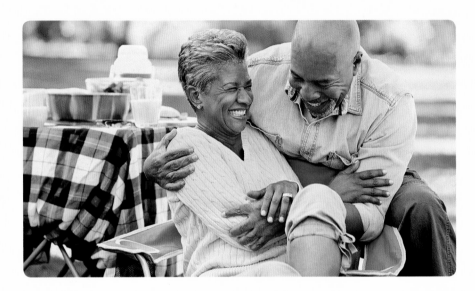

Now that the baby boomers, the generation born directly after World War II, have started entering their "golden years," they will need to address the many health problems associated with aging.

Many boomers have doubtless already investigated herbal alternatives to modern medicine—after all this is the generation that gave us hippies and the counter-culture and spurred the New Age movement. In any case, here are some common medical problems that seniors face—and suggestions for herbal remedies.

Herbs to Investigate

» For *arthritis*, time-tested treatments include alfalfa, feverfew, ginger, nettle, cayenne, turmeric, and burdock root.
» To combat *chronic fatigue syndrome*, try burdock root, dandelion, ginger, gold-enseal, ginkgo, valerian, licorice, milk thistle, or St. John's wort.
» Try St. John's wort, lemon balm, pepper-mint, ginger, ginkgo, Siberian ginseng, or valerian for *depression*.
» To control *digestive issues* and main-tain the gastrointestinal tract, especially the colon, try German chamomile, milk thistle, ginger, or psyllium.
» Try dong quai for *erectile dysfunction*.
» To maintain a strong and *healthy heart,* try rosemary, turmeric, borage seed, nettle, ginger root, valerian root, ginkgo,

or green tea, which may improve pulmonary function and circulation.

» For *kidney ailments,* useful diuretics include dandelion, nettle, and parsley.

» Dong quai relieves the symptoms of *menopause,* including vaginal dryness, depression, and hot flashes. Aloe vera with slippery elm also works for vaginal dryness. To acquire natural estrogens, take anise, fennel, licorice (seven-day limit), or sage. For loss of libido, take ginseng, and for insomnia try chamomile, catnip, hops, lemon balm, passionflower, or valerian root.

» Take dandelion greens, safflower, nettle, or watercress to strengthen bones and avoid *osteoporosis.*

» For *prostate problems,* try Chinese ginseng, parsley, cayenne, saw palmetto, or turmeric with nettle.

» Combat the tension and anxiety of *stress* with ginkgo, chamomile, milk thistle, catnip, hops, passionflower, St. John's wort, or valerian.

Contraindications

It is always a good idea to discuss any program of herbal supplementation with your physician. Even an herb you've been taking for decades with no side effects might now be contraindicated, either because it conflicts with a current prescription medication or it could augment it to a dangerous extent. For instance, taking an herb that thins the blood, like ginkgo—typically used to enhance memory—while on blood thinners such as warfarin (Coumadin), can lead to excess bleeding. On the other hand, alfalfa can encourage clotting, and it should also be avoided.

Herbal Immunity Boosters

To stay healthy and also to combat serious ailments like cancer and heart disease, it pays for all of us, but especially seniors, to pump up our immune systems. Many plants are proven immunity boosters, such as members of the *Allium* genus. Grow or shop for herbs and spices, such as those shown below, that are rich in antioxidant and anti-inflammatory properties. ■

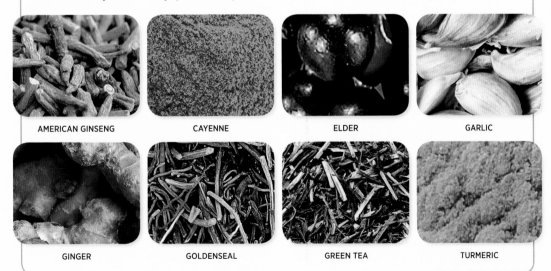

AMERICAN GINSENG   CAYENNE   ELDER   GARLIC

GINGER   GOLDENSEAL   GREEN TEA   TURMERIC

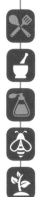

Mullein

Verbascum thapsus

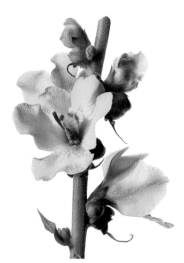

With a towering, central stalk of bright yellow blossoms, this familiar biennial herb grows wild in fields and vacant lots, but it can also be cultivated in the garden. Great or common mullein (*Verbascum thapsus*) is a member of the figwort family, Scrophulariaceae, and is the species most often used in herbal medicine. It originated in Europe and Asia and prefers temperate or subtropical climates. Mullein eventually naturalized in North America, where the Indians discovered its value for treating skin and respiratory ailments.

The plant's fuzzy, pale green leaves form a dense rosette at ground level the first year; the next year, the plant produces a sturdy, central

DID YOU KNOW?
An herbalist's delight, mullein, with its imposing spikes of golden blossoms, has strong anti-inflammatory, antispasmodic, antiviral, and antibiotic properties.

stem that reaches four to eight feet in height and then yellow blooms that circle the spike. The buds typically open at random—not in progression as with foxgloves—and feature five symmetrical petals. They range in color from yellow, orange, and reddish brown to pink, purple, blue, and white. The sap- and nectar-rich flowers soon become a magnet for pollinating insects.

The name *mullein* possibly comes from either of two Latin words: *mollis*, meaning "soft," referring to the downy leaves, or *mulandrum*, from *melanders*, meaning "leprosy," a disease the plant was used to treat. Or possibly the name is based on a French word of Celtic origins, *moleine*, meaning "yellow." The genus *Verbascum* derives from the word *barbascum*, "with beard," again recalling the hairy leaves. The species name *thapsus* came from the mullein's resemblance to the European genus of flowers *Thaspium*, named after an ancient city in Tunisia.

Healing Properties

This plant has a long history as a reliable, multipurpose herbal remedy. A poultice of mullein was prescribed by the Roman physician Dioscorides for hemorrhoids, and recommended by Roman

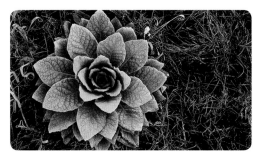

In its first year, mullein leaves form a stalkless basal rosette.

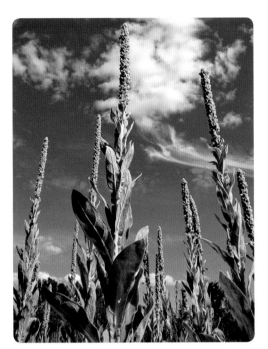

From June through September, mullein's huge flower spikes can be found growing in sunny open ground like fields, roadsides, streamsides, gardens, and forest clearings.

possess expectorant qualities and are effective for treating coughs, bronchitis, tuberculosis, pneumonia, colds, flu, fever, allergies, tonsillitis, and sore throats. The infused oil is known to banish earaches or ear infections.

Modern science concurs that mullein offers a number of medicinal benefits. In 2010, in an article that discussed using mullein to treat tuberculosis, the Cork Institute of Technology in Ireland reported: "Extracts of the mullein leaf have also been shown in laboratory studies to possess antitumor, antiviral, antifungal, and—most interestingly for the purpose of this paper—antibacterial properties." The plant also displays anti-inflammatory and antispasmodic properties. Mullein tea is both a sedative and diuretic and provides vitamins B2, B5, B12, and D, choline, hesperidin, PABA, sulfur, magnesium, mucilage, saponins, and other active substances.

botanist Pliny—as well as by healers in the Middle Ages—for treating arthritis.

Herbalists in Europe used a conserve made of the flowers to treat ringworm, while distilled water of the flowers was an effective cure for burns. The flowers have been used in traditional Austrian medicine, taken internally as tea or used externally as an ointment. Mullein was also added to a bath or a compress for ailments of the respiratory tract, skin, veins, the gastrointestinal tract, and the locomotor system. The leaves

History and Lore

» Mullein has a host of evocative folk names, including Our Lady's flannel, blanket herb, velvet plant, rag paper, wild ice leaf, clown's lungwort, Bullock's lungwort, Aaron's rod, Jupiter's staff, Jacob's staff, Peter's staff, shepherd's staff, beggar's stalk, Adam's flannel, beggar's blanket, Cuddy's lungs, feltwort, fluffweed, hare's beard, old man's flannel, and hag's taper. It was also called, candlewick plant, torches, or candelaria because dried flower stalks were dipped in tallow to make torches.

» The lore of ancient Greece relates that the warrior Ulysses took mullein to protect himself from the wiles of the sorceress Circe.

FOR YOUR HEALTH

Mullein Facial Splash

Most dermatologists agree that skin ages as a result of inflammation. It is possible, though, to rejuvenate aging skin and soothe acne and irritations by applying a refreshing facial splash that offers the anti-inflammatory properties of mullein.

Combine one cup of hot distilled water with two tablespoons dried mullein or seven or eight fresh mullein leaves. Add the petals from two or three roses and allow to steep for 20 minutes. When cool, blend in 8 to 12 drops of rose essential oil. Keep in the refrigerator. ■

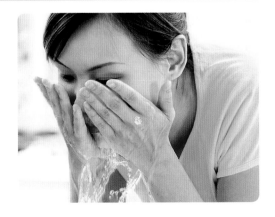

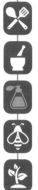

Nasturtium

Tropaeolum majus, T. minus

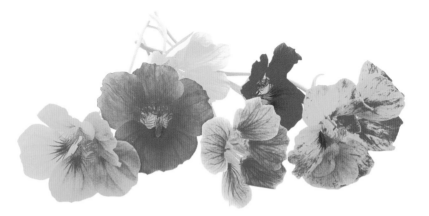

The old gardener's adage, "Be nasty to nasturtiums" is not far off the mark—this attractive mounding plant prefers lean soil. Too much nitrogen-rich fertilizer will yield healthy green leaves, but not a flower in sight. Nasturtiums were found growing the in rocky soil of Peru by European explorers in the 1600s. The early Mesoamericans used nasturtiums to treat urinary and kidney infections and for their antibiotic effect. European healers quickly adopted this versatile South American plant and soon no cottage garden was complete without it. Within

DID YOU KNOW?

With its intense colors, nasturtium makes a cheerful addition to a summer garden. All of its parts are edible and rich in vitamin C.

two centuries, it had naturalized in the temperate regions of North America and Europe.

The name comes from the Latin *nas* and *tortum,* or "nose twist," referring to a common reaction to the taste of the spicy leaves.

Garden nasturtiums descend from two species: *Tropaeolum majus* forms a trailing vine that can be trained to climb, while *T. minus* is bushy and does well in window boxes and containers. Members of the Tropaeolaceae family, the plants are perennial from zones USDA 9–11 but are treated as annuals in cooler regions. The bluish green leaves resemble water lily pads and form dense mounds from which the vivid flowers peek out. The flowers come in nearly every warm shade of the color spectrum, as well as a creamy white. Arrange nasturtiums so that they spill over the top of a wall, edge a border, or climb a trellis in a patio pot.

Healing Properties

Nasturtiums contain high levels of vitamin C, and in 19th-century Europe, they were used to combat a severe outbreak of scurvy. Natural healers also used the leaves to treat colds and the flu, regulate menstruation, purify the blood, repel insects, and to treat skin conditions, including acne.

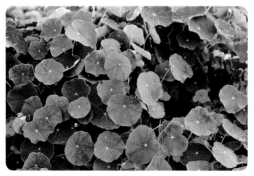

Showy nasturtium is popular in borders, herb gardens, window boxes, and hanging baskets. With its nearly circular leaves, nasturtium is charming even when it is not in bloom.

Stuffed Nasturtium Salad

Taking full advantage of the bright colors of nasturtium, this formally prepared salad is pleasing to the eye and the taste buds.

Ingredients
- 8 nasturtium flowers
- 2 cloves garlic, crushed
- ¼ teaspoon black pepper
- 4 ounces cream cheese
- 1 head Boston lettuce
- ½ head radicchio
- 3 large tomatoes chopped
- handful of black olives
- 4 or 5 chives, finely sliced
- white wine vinegar
- olive oil

Directions
Blend cream cheese, garlic, and pepper together, and stuff flowers with mixture. Set on whole lettuce leaves and arrange other ingredients around them. Mix oil and vinegar, ideally three parts to one, and add a pinch of chili powder, cayenne, or paprika. Shake well, and pour over salad. Serves four. ∎

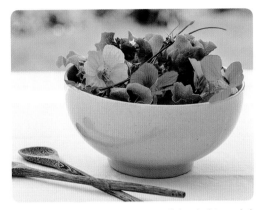

Add a shot of bright color and a boost of vitamin C to a salad by sprinkling on a handful of edible nasturtiums and borage.

dry, and store in zip bags. Cooks use them in stir-fries, with pasta, and even stuff the flowers. The young buds are also pickled as a caper substitute, but they contain high levels of oxalic acid and should be eaten sparingly.

Nasturtiums not only makes a tasty addition to your recipes, they also stimulate the appetite and aid digestion and metabolism.

History and Lore:
» If you grow different colors of nasturtium in the same garden, they will cross pollinate, and you might get some surprising results.
» Nasturtiums are prone to aphid infestations and are sometimes used as a trap crop in vegetable gardens. A blast of water usually rids the plant of the pests.

Today, researchers know that nasturtiums possess antibiotic and antiseptic qualities as well as diuretic and mild laxative properties. In addition to supplying ten times as much vitamin C as lettuce, the plant contains vitamins A and D and the minerals iron, sulfur, and manganese. It offers healthful flavonoids, carotenoids, and amino acids.

Culinary Uses

When the nasturtium was first introduced to England, it was called Indian cress due to its resemblance to watercress. In 19th-century France, it was used as an accessible vegetable during times of famine. During World War II, the seeds were ground up and used as a pepper substitute.

The plant's tangy, peppery taste is found in the flower, buds, and leaves, which are all delicious in salads. Harvest them early in the day—heat-stressed plants taste the strongest—then wash,

Nasturtiums of Many Colors

Nasturtium is a garden classic. Popular cultivars include 'Apricot Twist', with red and orange flowers; 'Empress of India', with scarlet blossoms with blue-green leaves; 'Jewel of Africa mix' with red, cream, yellow and pink flowers and variegated leaves; 'Moonlight', with pale yellow flowers; 'Night and Day', with white and deep red flowers; 'Peach Melba', with cream flowers with raspberry pink throat. In the 'Tall Trailing' mix the vines grow 8 to 10 feet long, while with 'Tip Top Alaska' mix they grow just 10 inches long. ∎

Nasturtium

149

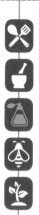

Nettle

Urtica dioica

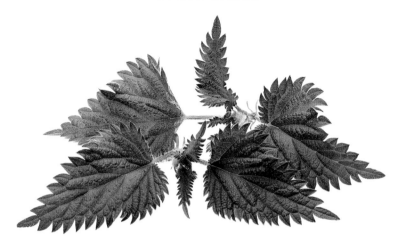

Also known as common nettle and stinging nettle, this perennial plant is a member of the family Uticaceae. Despite its off-putting name, this native of Europe, Asia, Africa, and North America, has been used in a variety of ways over the years, especially for its medicinal and food value and as a source of industrial fiber.

The plant, which can reach seven feet in height, bears opposite serrated leaves on a wiry stem. The greenish or brownish flowers are tiny and form dense clusters. Underground, the roots, rhizomes, and stolons are a bright

DID YOU KNOW?
Known for its toothed, hairy leaves and for its sting, nettle is a highly useful medicinal and culinary plant.

yellow. The nettle does more than prick its victims—in five of the six subspecies, the hairs on the stem and leaves, called trichomes, act like hypodermic needles, actually injecting histamines and other chemicals into the skin. No surprise the plant earned the folk names burn nettle, burn weed, and burn hazel.

Nettles yield a bast—or skin—fiber similar to linen, which has been used for more than two millennia to make fabric. At one point during World War I, German uniforms were woven from nettles due to a cotton shortage. The root is used as a yellow dye, while the leaves produce a yellow-green dye.

Healing Properties

Known as *stiðe* to the Anglo-Saxons, nettles were one of plants invoked in the pagan Nine Herbs Charm used to treat poisoning and infection and recorded in the tenth century. The plant was known for its anti-inflammatory qualities, but was also considered an expectorant, decongestant, astringent, diuretic, antiallergenic, tonic, herpetic, and antihistamine.

Flogging with nettles was a folk remedy for arthritis—the warmth flooding the irritated skin would ease joint pain. In Europe, the nettle was

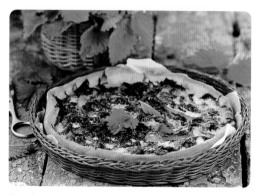
Try using nettles in place of spinach for a tasty and nutritious quiche. Be sure to gather young nettles early in the year.

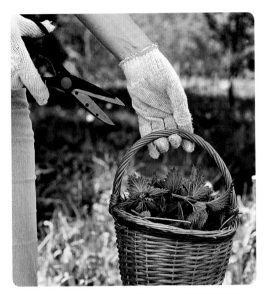

When gathering nettle, be sure to wear protective gloves—the plant is known for the sting of its toothed, hairy leaves.

also employed against kidney and urinary tract disorders, flu, and hemorrhage, as well as to aid the digestive tract, the locomotor system, the skin, and the cardiovascular system. It was used as a blood purifier and, in powdered form, to staunch wounds. The juice rubbed onto the scalp was said to induce hair growth.

In modern times, in extensive human clinical trials, the root extract was shown to improve urine flow in patients with benign prostatic hyperplasia compared to a placebo group. Currently testing is underway to explore the herb's use in helping with glycemic control in type-2 diabetes sufferers. The herb contains beneficial flavonoids, histamine, and serotonin.

Culinary Uses

Nettles, with their rich, earthy flavor—like a blend of spinach and cucumber—have long been used as a food source by many cultures. In the mountain villages of Nepal, as well as in parts of Scandinavia, stinging nettle soup is a staple—inexpensive, warming, and nutritious. Nettle tea is known as an immunity booster, and the plants do contain impressive amounts of iron, calcium, potassium, and vitamins A and C. In spite of this, however, the stinging spines intimidate many cooks. Yet, once the leaves are detached from the stems and boiled until wilted, they lose their sting and can then be substituted for young

spinach or chard as a vegetable, or used in soups, stews, pastas, and egg dishes.

If harvesting nettles for the pot—early spring is the ideal time to snip tender upper leaves—wear heavy leather gloves and long sleeves. Soak leaves in warm water for ten minutes to remove most of the sting, then transfer to a pot, barely cover with water, and blanch for ten minutes.

History and Lore

» Nettles thrive around abandoned dwellings, possibly because human and animal waste elevate levels of phosphate and nitrogen in the soil.

» In Dorset, England, an annual World Nettle Eating Championship draws thousands of people to watch competitors consume raw nettles.

» The Tibetan saint Milarepa was purported to have lived on nothing but nettles during decades of meditation.

» Hardy nettles are able to quickly reestablish themselves after brush fires.

CURIOSITIES

Butterfly and Moth Buffet

Many gardeners have started leaning toward xeriscaping—creating gardens that conserve water and protect the environment by encouraging native plants that sustain animal and insect life. Nettles work great in such gardens and are critical to many Lepidoptera. They are the exclusive food source of the larvae of the peacock butterfly and the small tortoiseshell, and are also consumed by the larvae of some moths—angle shades, buff ermine, dot moth, the flame, the Gothic, grey chi, grey pug, lesser broad-bordered yellow underwing, mouse moth, setaceous Hebrew character, and small angle shade. The larval ghost moth has been known to eat the roots of the nettle. ■

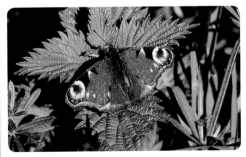

A peacock butterfly *(Aglais io)* rests on nettle leaves.

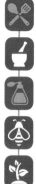

Passionflower

Passiflora incarnata

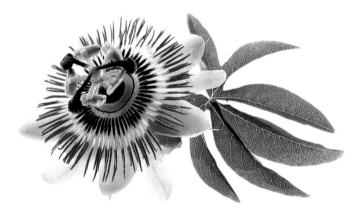

MEDICINAL HERBS

I f only for the beauty of its exquisite blossoms, passionflower would be welcomed into most gardens. But the plant, also known as purple passionflower, is also a time-tested sedative that has been used to treat anxiety and insomnia. This perennial native of the Americas had its origins in Peru—where the Spanish discovered it in 1569—and it can now also be found growing throughout the American southeast and Europe. For all its elegance, passionflower has a weedy habit and can often be seen massed in ditches and vacant lots.

This member of the Passifloraceae family is a hardy climbing vine with three-lobed, finely serrated leaves and a sturdy woody stem that can reach a length of 30 feet or more. The flowers consist of five white petals and five sepals that range in color from magenta to blue;

A different species than the well-known passionfruit (*Passiflora edulis*), the fleshy fruit of *P. incarnata* is known as maypop and is about the size of a hen's egg.

DID YOU KNOW?
An evergreen climber, passionflower produces stunningly unusual blooms. Its leaves and roots are used medicinally to treat anxiety and other mood disorders.

blooms begin in July and continue until the first frost. The egg-shaped berry may be yellow or purple.

Healing Properties

Passionflower has been employed as a sedative and antispasmodic as far back as the days of the Aztecs in Central America. European herbalists added the flowers to numerous pharmaceutical mixtures to treat nerve disorders, heart palpitations, epilepsy, anxiety, and high blood pressure.

Today passionflower is often recommended for treating anxiety, stress, and insomnia. Scientists believe the plant produces this calming effect by increasing levels of a chemical called gamma aminobutyric acid (GABA) in the brain—GABA has the ability to lower the activity of certain brain cells. Passionflower is much gentler than the sedative herb valerian, although it is sometimes combined with valerian, lemon balm, or kava kava to treat anxiety. Passionflower has the added benefit of calming twitching muscles and tension without affecting respiratory rate or mental acuity the way many prescriptions sedatives do. It is also nonaddictive.

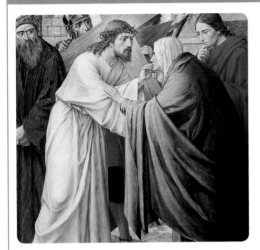

Christ carries the cross to his crucifixion in the Stations of the Cross series in Our Lady of St Peter's Church, Ghent, Belgium.

Symbols of Christ

Since they were first discovered by the Spanish, the passionflowers have been associated with Christian symbolism. In 1608, Spanish Jesuits presented drawings and samples of the plant to Pope Paul V. Because the plant bears five anthers, scholar Giacomo Bosio called it *la flor de las cinco llagas*—the flower of the five wounds—referring to the wounds of Christ. The plant likely got its common name because its corona resembles the crown of thorns worn by Jesus during the crucifixion (known as "the Passion"). The five petals and five sepals are said to represent the ten faithful apostles (omitting Judas Iscariot and Peter), and the three stigmas, the nails of the crucifixion, while the sharp tips of the leaves replicate the Roman centurion's spear. ■

A number of studies have been done, with and without placebo groups, and one nonplacebo result was that the herb had a similar effect to the prescription antianxiety drug Serax. In conjunction with other herbs, passionflower can help relax patients before surgery and has been effective for treating a psychiatric condition known as "adjustment disorder with anxious mood." It can relieve symptoms of narcotic drug withdrawal when used in combination with the medication clonidine

Herbalists also consider this plant useful for treating nervous stomach, burns, hemorrhoids, asthma, heart problems, high blood pressure, seizures, fibromyalgia, and other conditions. Passionflower is available via infusion, teas, liquid extracts, and tinctures. The stems, leaves, and flowers of the plant have all been used for healing purposes.

History and Lore

» Some common names include wild passion vine, purple passionflower, true passionflower, wild apricot, and maypop—for the way they just "popped" out of the ground.
» In Tennessee, Native Americans named the plant *ocoee*, as in the river and valley of the same name. Passionflower is now the Tennessee State Wildflower.
» The small fruits can be used to make jelly, but they are most useful as a food source for several species of butterfly and their larvae.

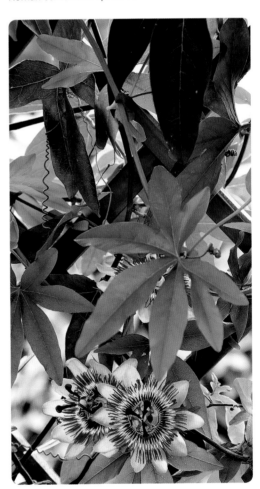

Passionflower is a vigorous climbing vine that works well in a backyard garden, twining its stunning flowers around a trellis.

Passionflower

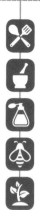

Rose Hips

Rosa spp.

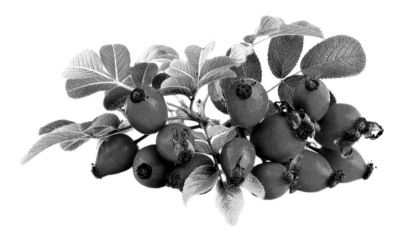

Rose hips, the bright red-orange fruit of the rose blossom, have been providing humans with a nutritious food supplement since the Stone Age. The rose plant itself goes back 35 million years according to fossil records. Rose hips, also known as rose haw or rose hep, have been employed by herbal healers since before Roman times.

Roses are woody shrubs with thorny stems and serrated, oval leaves. The flowers are generally showy and can have single or multiple rows of velvety petals. The hips start to form in late spring or early summer, after the flower has been successfully pollinated, and they ripen in late

DID YOU KNOW?

The fruits of the rose plant, vitamin C–rich rose hips can be harvested from many species of roses.

summer through to autumn. Rose hips are decorative in the garden, but can also be cut on the stem to use in dried or fresh flower arrangements. If left to overwinter, they bring birds into the garden to feed.

While domestic roses produce larger hips, they do not have the same flavor or medicinal value as those produced by wild roses, which typically have only five petals. For harvesting rose hips, try growing the dog rose *(Rosa canina)*, which bears a white to pink, heavily fragrant flower, or the Japanese or beach rose *(R. rugosa)*, which bears a white or rose-colored flower and grows large hips. (In some states in America, this plant is considered invasive.) In Chinese traditional medicine, the China rose *(R. chinensis)* has long been used. The cinnamon rose *(R. majalis)* is also a good choice for rose hips.

Healing Properties

Over the centuries, natural healers have utilized rose hips to treat colds, kidney disorders, wounds, and skin problems—acne, scars, burns—and to boost overall immunity.

Rose hips are known to have antiviral, antibacterial, and anti-inflammatory properties; recent studies in Germany and Denmark have shown them to be useful in treating arthritis and

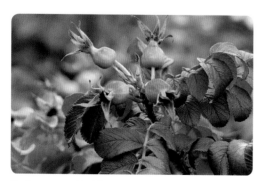

Most roses are prized for the beauty of their flowers, but a few species are grown for the ornamental value of their hips.

osteoarthritis, improving patient mobility by more than 25 percent. They contain a variety of antioxidants—carotenoids, flavonoids, polyphenols, leucoanthocyanins, and catechins—making them a possible preventative against cancer and cardiovascular disease. A simple, healthful tea can be made by steeping a tablespoon of crushed, dried hips in a cup of boiling water, then straining and drinking.

Culinary Uses

In addition to their amazing healing qualities, rose hips are an edible "superfood" loaded with A and B-complex vitamins, and, in some cases 50 times more vitamin C than oranges. They also contain calcium, silica, iron, and phosphorus. The fleshy outer shell—a sweet and tart combination of apple, plum, and rose petal—can be peeled away from the seeds. Rose hip seeds irritate the bowel and should be avoided. Rose hips can be purchased dried and deseeded. They are used to make jams, syrups, relishes, or teas, or added to desserts and sauces. Powdered hips add complex flavor to black bean soup or chili.

Most health food stores carry dried rose hips. For home harvesting, hips are sweetest after one frost, but pick them quickly or you risk brown spots. To dry, slice open, scoop out seeds with a knife tip, and spread the hips in a flat basket. Change their position frequently. When dried—it will take up to ten days—store in a glass lidded jar.

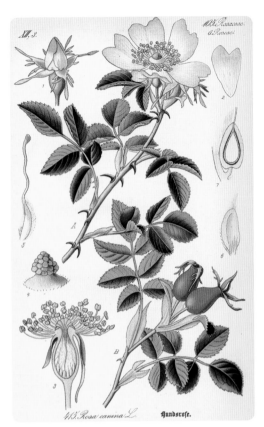

A 1885 botanical illustration of the dog rose *(Rosa canina)*, a hardy climber that is found in meadows, fields, beaches, and woods. It has long been valued for its rich vitamin C content.

Aromatic Qualities

Many modern rose cultivars are heavily scented, but roses have been valued for their sweet smell for millennia. Dried rose hips have a mild fruity odor, making them popular in potpourri mixtures.

History and Lore

» Rose hip soup, *nyponsoppa,* is especially popular in Sweden. *Rhodomel,* a type of mead, is also made with rose hips.

» The traditional Hungarian drink *palinka,* also popular in Romania, is made from rose hips. They are also the main ingredient in Cockta, Slovenia's sweet, fruity national soft drink.

» When shipments of citrus fruits could not reach England during World War II, parents were encouraged to make syrup from wild rose hips so that their children could receive sufficient amounts of vitamin C.

» The astringent qualities of rose hip oil makes it a valuable addition to cosmetic preparations.

A Brief History of Roses

The cultivation of roses began around five thousand years ago, possibly in China. During the Roman Empire, roses were grown extensively in the Middle East for celebratory confetti, medicine, and perfume. Since then, roses have gone in and out of style. In 15th-century England, two warring factions each adopted a rose as their standard, the white of York and the red of Lancaster, resulting in the "War of the Roses." In the 17th century, a high-water mark for the plant, French nobles considered rose bushes legal tender. Cultivated roses—including repeat bloomers—were introduced to Europe from China in the late 18th century, resulting in yet another craze. These became the source of most modern-day roses. ∎

HEALING TISANES

Brew your own healthful and delicious herbal teas.

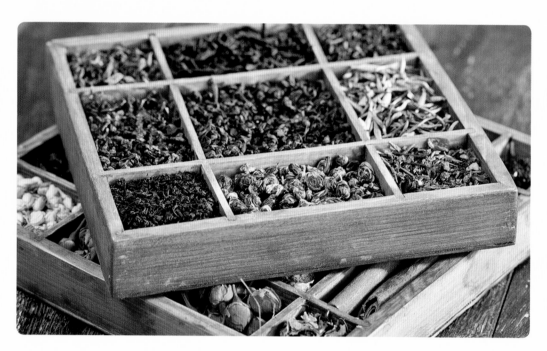

Long before Asian black tea, *Camillia sinensis,* became available worldwide as a hot libation, many people in Europe, Africa, and the Americas were already drinking dried plants steeped in hot water. Furthermore, a majority of these teas were made from health-wise, beneficial herbs—and over the passing centuries their popularity has never quite diminished. Perhaps nothing is more comforting than "taking one's medicine" in the form of a soothing hot beverage in fall or winter—or a refreshing iced drink during the warmer months.

What Is a Tisane?

Herbalists generally refer to herbal tea as a tisane. Most herbal tisanes contain antioxidants and nutrients. Some are specifically classified as medicinal—such as "detox teas"—while others are considered culinary, primarily taken for pleasure.

There are two methods of turning herbs into tisanes: infusion and decoction.

» **Infusion** involves pouring boiling or hot water over plant matter—dried leaves or berries, for example—and allowing the mixture to steep before straining out the solids. The term *infusion* usually applies to herbal teas or tisanes, but it can also be used in relation to black teas. This method works best with tisanes made from leaves, flowers, or seeds.

» Decoction involves placing the dried ingredients in a non-aluminum pot or saucepan, and then bringing the water to a boil until two thirds have evaporated. The mixture is then strained and served. Decoctions release more flavor and oil from the herbs than infusions and are often used to prepare the tougher parts of plants, such as the stems. Decoction is preferred when preparing bark, root, fruit, or berry tisanes.

Brewing a Healthy Cup

Brewing times vary from herb to herb, with some steeping for just 2 minutes, while others as long as 15. Quantity is just as variable, from just a pinch of plant material per cup of water to several tablespoons. Ask your health food supplier for suggestions, or experiment until you discover the level of intensity you prefer. And never use aluminum pans to brew herbs: the metal could react and create toxicity in the tea.

A Tea Chest of Herbs

Tisanes, or herbal teas, can be made from a vast array of herbs. Tisanes are broadly categorized by the part of the plant used for brewing: leaf, flower, bark, root/stem, fruit, or seed/spice. Some tisanes, however, are a combination, including the mixed parts of a single plant or parts from several different herbs brewed into one flavorful drink. Below are the main categories of tisanes—and some examples of delicious and beneficial herbs to keep in your herbal tea chest. ■

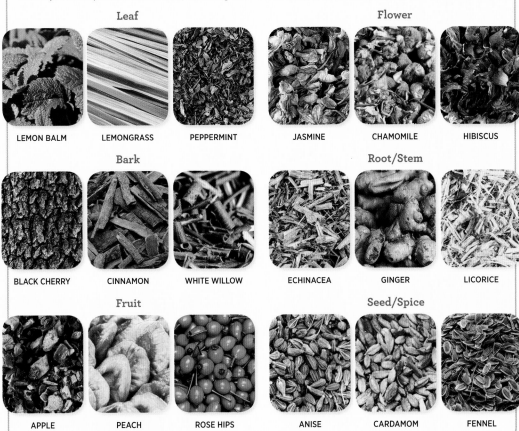

Leaf
LEMON BALM LEMONGRASS PEPPERMINT

Flower
JASMINE CHAMOMILE HIBISCUS

Bark
BLACK CHERRY CINNAMON WHITE WILLOW

Root/Stem
ECHINACEA GINGER LICORICE

Fruit
APPLE PEACH ROSE HIPS

Seed/Spice
ANISE CARDAMOM FENNEL

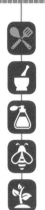

St. John's Wort

Hypericum perforatum

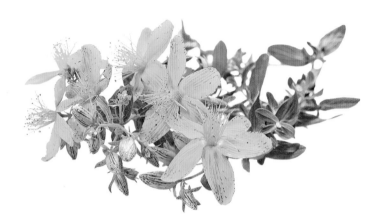

T his is another of the medicinal herbs of antiquity, in this case, an apothecary's trusted ally for treating depression. Today, St. John's wort is possibly the most studied of all medicinal herbs. A member of the Hypericaceae family, it was originally indigenous to Europe, but can now also be found in most temperate regions including Turkey, Ukraine, Russia, the Middle East, India, and China. It has naturalized in North America—and elsewhere—and is considered invasive in some regions. It is often called common or perforate St. John's wort to distinguish it from the more than 370 other species in the genus.

This bushy perennial, with its creeping rhizomes, typically reaches two or three feet in height. It has opposite, oblong, yellow-green leaves and produces small, bright yellow flowers that

DID YOU KNOW?

St. John's Wort, a yellow-flowering perennial herb indigenous to Europe, is known for its long history of medicinal use.

feature five petals and three clusters of elongated stamens.

Its genus name *Hypericum* is Latin for "over an apparition," reflecting the belief the plant should be gathered to make evil spirits flee away. The species name, *perforatum*, refers to the black dots on the underside of the leaves, tiny oil glands that resemble punctures. The plant is associated with St. John the Baptist—its blooms were traditionally gathered on St. John's Day, June 24, and made into an anointing oil called the "Blood of Christ."

Healing Properties

Depression is not a modern ailment—the early Greeks recognized melancholia as an illness, believing it stemmed from an imbalance of the four bodily fluids, or humors. (The humors dictated personality types: sanguine—hopeful, carefree; phlegmatic—thoughtful, patient; melancholic—serious, despondent; choleric—restless, easily angered.) Hippocrates described the symptoms of melancholy as "all fears and despondencies, lasting a long time." The Greeks used St. John's wort to treat melancholy as well as insanity. Later, European and Slavic healers would mention the herb in their writings.

Petite colorful berries, which turn from yellow to a pale red, follow St. John's wort's midsummer-to-fall flowering.

MEDICINAL HERBS

A Noxious Invader?

Unfortunately, for all its beneficial properties—and in spite of the fact that it is grown commercially in parts of southeast Europe—St. John's wort is considered a noxious weed by more than 20 countries. There are already introduced populations in North and South America New Zealand, Australia, India, and South Africa. When introduced to pasturage, it can replace native forage vegetation, as well as imperil existing ecosystems and habitats. It often makes once-productive land no longer viable. When consumed by livestock, the plant can cause photosensitization, central nervous system depression, spontaneous abortion, and even death. A number of herbicides are effective against it, however, and in the American West, three beetles, *Chrysolina quadrigemina*, *Chrysolina hyperici*, and *Agrilus hyperici*, have been used as biocontrol agents. ∎

Modern scientific studies have shown that the extract actually does affect the brain in a manner similar to a mild antidepressant. Those people who can function in their lives but still suffer from dysthymia—long-term depression—are good candidates for St. John's wort therapy.

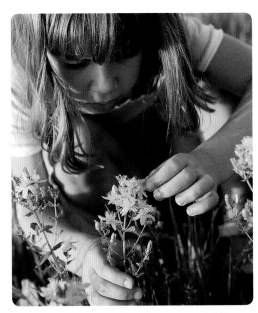

The cheery yellow flowers of St. John's wort may brighten many fields, meadows, and other sunny locations, but it can crowd out native species and forage on pasturelands.

St. John's wort can be administered as a hot or cold tea, as a liquid extract, in capsules, or in another concentrated form of the herb.

St. John's wort has anti-inflammatory and antiviral has properties and is also known to help digestion, support the thyroid, and gently balance the neurotransmitters GABA, norepinephrine, serotonin, and dopamine. One major constituent of the plant is a chemical called hyperforin, which researchers feel might be useful in the treatment of alcoholism. Additional studies on dosage, safety, and efficacy are still required. Extracts of the herb are sometimes used as a topical remedy for wounds, abrasions, burns, and muscle pain. The flowers are rich in hypericin, a flavonoid that improves venous-wall strength, making them useful in treating swollen veins, bruising, or injury to the skin or muscles.

St. John's wort can cause photosensitivity in some individuals. Discontinue use if this occurs.

Aromatic Qualities

St. John's wort has a rich, sweet scent. It is popular in aromatherapy for treating neuralgia, sciatica, and fibrositis, as well as sprains and burns. Combined with calendula oil, it us used to treat bruises. The essential oil is infused from the yellow blossoms, yet it shows a characteristic red color, caused by the presence of hypericin. Unlike the herbal extract, the infused oil does not work on depression.

History and Lore

» The plant has also been known as Tipton's weed, rosin rose, goatweed, chase-devil, and Klamath weed.

» During the Crusades, the herb was used to staunch battle wounds

» The herb is associated with the energies of Midsummer's eve. It was also worn to ward off fevers and colds, to cure melancholy, or to attract love.

» In rural England, householders tied the herb into bunches and hung them in windows to prevent lightning strikes.

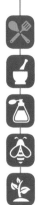

Valerian

Valeriana officinalis

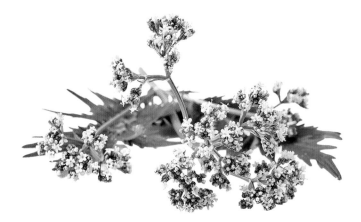

Valerian is a time-honored medicinal herb that has been used as a mood elevator and to induce sleep for more than two thousand years.

Native to Europe and Asia, this tall, flowering perennial has also been introduced in North America. It is a member of the Valerianaceae family—of roughly 200 species—and is typically found thriving in grasslands, damp meadows and along streams.

The mature plant can reach five feet in height and produces fernlike serrated leaves and small white or pinkish blossoms that form terminal clusters. They will continue to bloom from June through September. The plant's name possibly

DID YOU KNOW?

Sweetly scented valerian, a perennial flowering plant, is valued for its sedative qualities and has been used as a sleeping aid for centuries.

derived from the Latin word *valere,* meaning "to be strong and healthy."

Healing Properties

The use of valerian root as a medicinal herb goes back at least to ancient Greece and Rome; Hippocrates wrote of its therapeutic uses, Galen prescribed it for insomnia in the second century, and both Indian and Chinese healers mention it in texts. During the Renaissance it was a treatment for anxiety, headache, and palpitations. In the mid-19th century it was held in dislike, believed to be a stimulant that caused the very conditions earlier healers felt it cured. Its popularity rose again in the 20th century, especially during World War II, when it proved effective at relieving the stress caused by air raids.

Unlike some prescription medications, valerian does not result in a hung-over or drugged feeling. It has also been employed to treat gastrointestinal spasms, epileptic seizures, and attention deficit hyperactivity disorder. There is no conclusive evidence, however, that it is effective in these instances.

For medicinal use, valerian roots, which contain essential oil, are chopped up and made into a tea or extract. Supplements are also available in tablets, capsules, and tinctures.

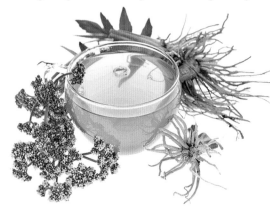

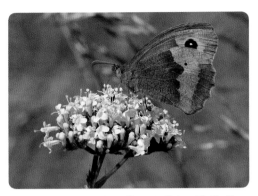

The pleasant scent of valerian flowers will attract butterflies like the meadow brown (*Maniola jurtina*) to your garden.

It's a different story in terms of its effects on insomnia. According to the Mayo Clinic, "several small or short-term studies indicate that valerian . . . may reduce the amount of time it takes to fall asleep and help you sleep better." The correct dosage is still somewhat unclear, however, although the herb does seem to work better after it is taken regularly for a few weeks. It is not safe for women who are pregnant or breastfeeding or those with liver disease.

Medicinal preparations of the herb are made from its roots, rhizomes, and stolons—horizontal stems, which yield a yellowish green to brown oil. The roots are administered as a tincture or a tea and the dried extracts or plant materials can be made into tablets. There is no scientific consensus on what the active ingredients of the herb are; it is likely that valerian's calmative effects are the result of interactions between several constituents acting synergistically rather than one specific compound.

CURIOSITIES

The Pied Piper's Secret

According to the well-known folk tale, the town of Hamelin was infested with rats and needed someone to drive them away. So they hired a rat-catcher called the Pied Piper, and when he played his pipes, the rats all followed him from the town. Legend insists it was not his music, though, but valerian stuffed in his pockets—which rats and cats both love—that lured them away. When the townspeople refused to "pay the piper," he then lured their children away, though it is not clear which herb he used to perform that feat. ∎

Aromatic Qualities

The flowers are sweetly scented, but the stems, leaves, and the dried root have an unpleasant odor that has been compared to dirty socks or stinky cheese. In spite of this, valerian was used in the preparation of perfumes for many years. It is possible it is still part of some scent manufacturer's secret recipe.

History and Lore

» Valerian is also known as setwall, garden heliotrope, and all-heal in English, *Valerianae radix* in Latin, *Baldrianwurzel* in German, and *phu* in Greek. The word *phew*, meaning "to express disgust at an unpleasant odor," possibly derived from the latter usage.

» In medieval Sweden, the herb was often placed in the wedding clothes of the groom to ward off the "envy" of the elves.

» This plant is a favorite with the larvae of some species of Lepidoptera, including the grey pug.

» Valerian is sometimes used to flavor foods and drinks such as root beer.

» Valerian is a frequent ingredient in love and harmony spells and potions.

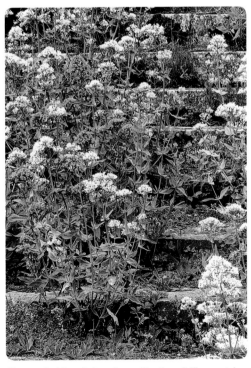

Clusters of white valerian, along with other wildflowers, take over the damp stone of an abandoned outdoor stairway.

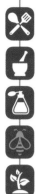

Wormwood

Artemisia absinthium

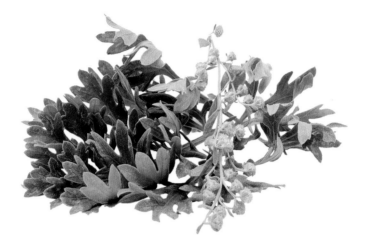

Healers have relied upon this grand, showy example of the silvery *Artemisia* genus to stimulate the appetite since the days of ancient Egypt. The plant is native to the temperate regions of Eurasia and North Africa, and it has since naturalized in several regions, including North America and the Kashmir Valley in India. Wormwood is not a fussy plant and will grow on rough, arid ground, on rocky slopes, and at the edges of lanes and fields.

A member of the Asteraceae family, wormwood is a perennial herb with fibrous roots and a grooved stem that can reach three feet in height. The feathery leaves grow in a spiral around the stem, showing gray-green above and white below, and are covered with a fine fuzz. The pale yellow, tube-shaped flowers form tight clusters on branched panicles.

It is available as an essential oil, but many products labeled "wormwood" are really a related species, *Artemisia annua,* which is often known as sweet wormwood or sweet annie.

Healing Properties

Considering its name, it is not hard to guess that wormwood was once regularly prescribed as an anthelmintic—a substance used to rid the body of pinworms, roundworms, and other parasites.

Wormwood was often employed to stimulate digestion, the way that modern-day bitters are taken before a meal. This is because a bitter taste triggers the production of bile from the gall bladder and other intestinal glands—a process called the cholagogue effect—which then aids in the digestion of food. So those prone to indigestion or with insufficient stomach acid often benefited from a dose of this herb. Some people discovered, however, that wormwood could cause diarrhea: its bile-stimulating properties also made the intestines empty quickly.

The herb now has a somewhat uncertain future as a medicinal plant. Wormwood contains the same psychoactive constituent, thujone, as tansy. This compound has been shown to cause convulsions and kidney failure when ingested in large amounts. The herb, therefore, must be consumed with extreme caution, taken in small amounts for a only short time, and only after consultation with a physician.

Culinary Uses

In the Middle Ages, wormwood was used to spice mead. The bitter substance in the herb, called absinthin, was also used to flavor beer and distilled alcohol. A once-popular anise-flavored French liquor called absinthe was made from a number of herbs, including the flowers and leaves of grand wormwood. Wormwood also lent its flavor and its name to vermouth: The German word for wormwood is *wermuth*, which is the source of the modern word *vermouth*.

Aromatic Qualities

The scent of wormwood has been described as intense, pungent, and herbaceous, similar to cedarleaf. The dried leaves and flowers are steam-distilled to make the oil, which is used in minute amounts as a top note in aromatic accords—men's perfumes.

History and Lore

» *Artemisia absinthium* was commonly burned as a protective offering by the early Persians.
» A tract of open land in West London called Wormwood Scrubs was the former site of a famous dueling ground; it now houses Hammersmith Hospital, Linford Christie Stadium, and HM Prison Wormwood Scrubs.

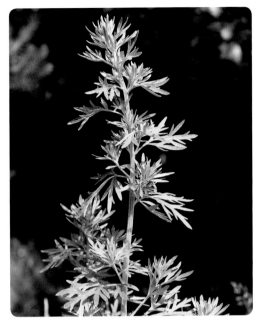

Wormwood has naturalized in North America, and you can now find these tall, feathery perennials growing in the wild on arid ground, often at the edges of trails and fields.

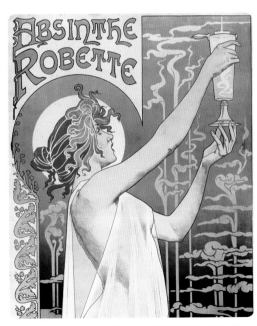

An advertising poster for Absinthe Robette from 1896, when absinthe was all the rage in Europe and the Unites States.

Return of the Green Fairy

In the late 19th and early 20th centuries, many artists, writers, and musicians in Paris and elsewhere—such as painter Henri de Toulouse-Lautrec and author Oscar Wilde—made absinthe their drink of choice, claiming it stimulated their creativity. This "liquid muse" became known as the Green Fairy due to absinthe's natural emerald hue. The drink was typically prepared with water and a sugar cube held above the glass by a special spoon.

Social conservatives soon labeled this drink of bohemians and nonconformists "dangerously addictive" and further claimed it "makes you crazy and criminal." This accusation was due in part to the presence of the compound thujone, which was believed to induce seizures and hallucinations, and which was discovered by scientists studying absinthe. As a result, by 1915, the drink had been banned in the United States and most European countries. Studies have recently determined that absinthe contains only minute levels of thujone and is no more harmful than other alcoholic beverages, and so production began again in the 1990s. There are now more than 200 brands being produced in a dozen countries. ∎

Wormwood

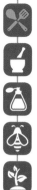

Yarrow

Achillea millefolium

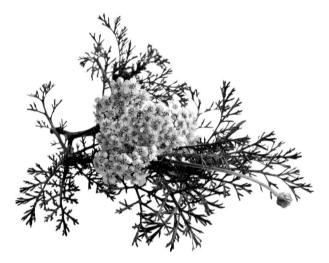

Yarrow, or common yarrow, has a long history as a well-regarded healing herb in both the Old World and the New World. This perennial denizen of grasslands and open forests can range from sea level to impressive altitudes of 11,000 feet. A member of the daisy family, Asteraceae, it is native to the temperate Northern Hemisphere—Europe, Asia, and North America. In the United States, both native and introduced yarrow species can be found.

Yarrow can reach three feet in height; its featherlike, hairy leaves are evenly distributed and grow spirally on the erect stem. (Yarrow's

DID YOU KNOW?

Yarrow is an attractive plant that makes an appealing ornamental, but all of its parts—roots, flowers, stems, and leaves—are also used medicinally.

species name, *millefolium*, is Latin for "a thousand leaves.") It produces flowering inflorescences with four to nine bracts that contain tiny ray and disk blossoms in white, pink, or yellow. Some common names include nosebleed plant, old man's pepper, devil's nettle, milfoil, and soldier's woundwort.

Yarrow is useful for combating soil erosion, due to its resistance to drought. Before the arrival of ryegrass monocultures, permanent pasture typically contained yarrow in the grazing mixture. With the plant's deep roots, yarrow's leaves would become rich in minerals, helping to prevent mineral deficiencies in the ruminants that fed upon it.

Healing Properties

During the Crusades, yarrow was known as *herbal militaris*, or "knight's milfoil," because it could staunch the flow of blood from battle wounds. It was also used for treating heavy menstrual flow and bleeding ulcers, and as a compress could ease bleeding hemorrhoids. It is part of the Ayurvedic tradition of India, while Chinese physicians value its ability to affect the spleen, liver, kidney, and bladder meridians, as well as energy channels.

A honeybee alights on a yarrow plant. Yarrow's tiny disk blossoms look like clusters of miniature daisies.

Science has acknowledged yarrow's medicinal capabilities, reporting that the herb displays antiseptic action against bacteria and is an antispasmodic. It also contains pain-killing salicylic acid (similar to the active ingredient in aspirin) and a volatile oil with anti-inflammatory properties. Studies show that yarrow taken in tincture or tea form can relieve painful gynecological conditions such as cramps and endometriosis, as well as stomach problems—like wormwood, yarrow's bitter constituents stimulate the production of digestion-enhancing bile.

Its decongestant properties make it effective against sinus infections, loose coughs, and nasal allergies, and it promotes sweating during colds, flu, and fevers. Yarrow can intensify the action of any other herbs taken with it.

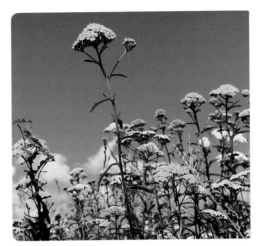

Tall stands of yarrow, with airy foliage and pastel blooms of pink, white, and yellow, flower in grasslands and open forests from May through June.

Aromatic Qualities

The plant's aroma—woody and herbaceous—has been compared to that of the chrysanthemum. The flowers are steam distilled to produce an essential oil, which is used in aromatherapy to treat low spirits or mood swings. The scent is considered grounding, opening, restorative, revitalizing, and strengthening to the spirit. It helps to balance the intellectual and creative forces. Today, the oil is produced mainly in Germany, Hungary, and France.

History and Lore

» According to Homer's *Iliad,* the legendary Greek warrior Achilles used yarrow to heal his comrade's wounds.

» In New Mexico and southern Colorado, the herb is called *plumajillo* (Spanish for "little feather") for the shape and texture of its leaves.

» Chinese herbalists believe yarrow represents the perfect balance between yin and yang; they use the dried stalks as randomizing agents in *I Ching* divination.

CULTURAL CONNECTIONS

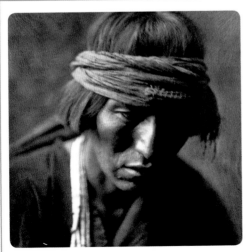

Hastobiga, a Navaho medicine man, photographed in 1904. The western variety of yarrow (*A. millefolium* var. *occidentalis*) is a standard herb in the Navajo pharmacopeia, with both medicinal and ceremonial uses.

Native American "Life Medicine"

In many Indian tribes across North America, common yarrow—and its American varieties—was of great value to shamans and medicine men. The Navajo of the Southwest considered it "life medicine," using it as a tonic to restore vitality. They also chewed it for toothaches and made infusions for earaches. To the Miwok of California, it was a painkiller and headache remedy. Plains Indians, like the Pawnee, also used it for pain relief. The Chippewa inhaled the steamed leaves for headaches, and they also chewed the root, and then applied the saliva to their skin as a stimulant. The Cherokee used a tea to reduce fever and encourage restful sleep. The Zuni used the *A. occidentalis* variety, chewing the blossoms and roots and then applying the juice before firewalking. They also pulverized the plants to make poultices for burns. ■

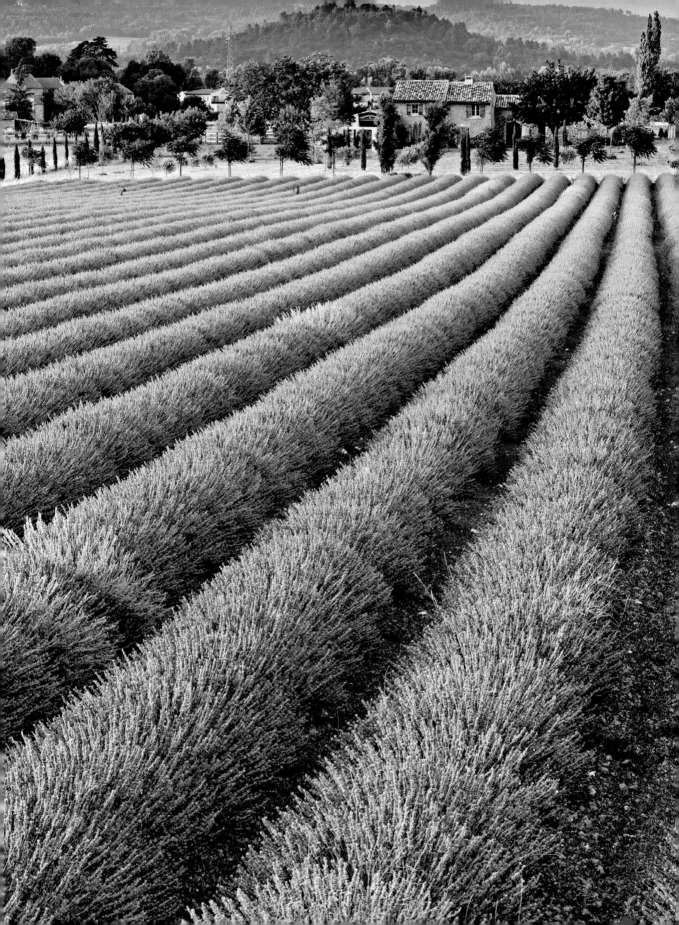

AROMATIC HERBS

Opposite: **Lavender**

Scents of Ritual and Romance

THE ALLURE OF AROMATIC HERBS

The aromatic herbs are the stuff of legends. Their fragrant essences are the source of the sultry perfumes of seduction, like jasmine; the carefully guarded embalming secrets of the ancients, like lavender; and the hallowed incense used for worship and sacrifice, like spikenard of Biblical fame.

Aromatic herbs were less visible in day-to-day life than the culinary or medicinal herbs, but these plants still played a vital part in many early cultures. Fragrant herbs were employed in the garden or field to ensure a steady supply of pollinators or to keep predators away from a vital crop. Some scented herbs were even cultivated to lure pests to consume their leaves over those of a more valued plant. Other herbs were used to repel the fleas, flies, midges, and mosquitoes that often plagued humans and their domesticated animals and pets.

Sprigs of lavender with scented candle and bath salts

Throughout history, they have held a revered place in religious ceremonies—acrid incense accompanied animal sacrifices or funeral rites; sweetly scented herbs offered a benediction at weddings or baptisms; and the cloying, heady fumes from swaying censers filled the air during the Catholic or Orthodox mass—the very word *perfume* was Latin for "through smoke." Native American shamans employed bundles of smoldering herbs to "smudge," or purify, the air before certain ceremonies, a practice echoed by mystics in far away Europe, Asia, and Africa.

During the Middle Ages, "strewing herbs" were scattered around the floors of both castles and humble cottages to welcome guests by creating a pleasant scent when stepped upon. Some herbs also kept away invasive creatures like ants, roaches, silverfish, or scorpions. From the Georgian period on, the notion

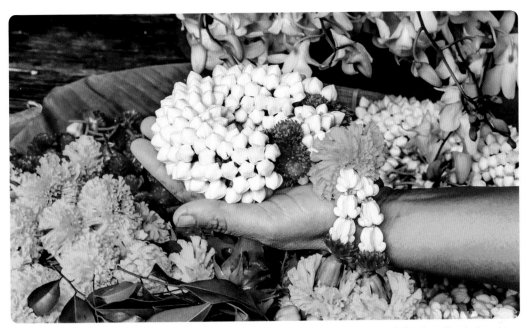

A Thai florist displays a completed jasmine garland, which is meant as a holiday gift or religious offering. For millennia, humans have picked flowers and captured the essences of fragrant herbs to use in ceremonies and to scent their homes and their bodies.

of freshening the home with aromatic herbs became an established trend, until the Victorian era, when potpourris, sachets, pomander balls, and scented pillows could be found in nearly every room of the house.

HEADY PERFUMES

Since the time of the pharaohs, people have used the essential oils of aromatic herbs to create provocative perfumes, dabbing them on both their hair and bodies and their clothing. This habit of using strong scents was especially critical to courtship and procreation during the Middle Ages, when Europeans felt that bathing in water was dangerous. During the Renaissance, the production of perfume

> **"When nothing else subsists from the past . . . the smell and taste of things remain."**
>
> —*Marcel Proust*

became a major industry. Eventually four main scent families were established: *floral*—including fresh flowers and sweet spices; *oriental*—vanilla, orange blossom, sweet spices, and amber; *woody*—sandalwood, vetiver grass, and patchouli; and *fresh*—citrus, marine, grass, lavender, and other aromatic herbs.

AROMATHERAPY

In the late 20th century, an aspect of natural medicine gained increasing popularity, one that traditional herbalists had been utilizing for millennia. This practice came to be known as aromatherapy: inhaling, ingesting or applying the essential oils of aromatic herbs to heal the body, aid relaxation, and restore the spirits.

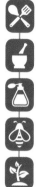

Bee Balm

Monarda didyma, M. fistulosa, M. citriodora

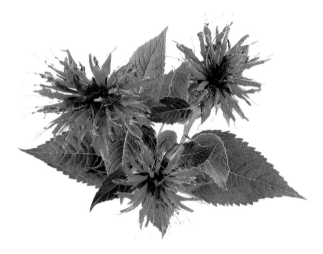

With its potent scent, tall, ornamental bee balm attracts all manner of pollinators besides its winged namesake, and it is also a staple of Native American medicine. It is a member of the mint family, Lamiaceae, and native to the eastern United States. It now ranges from Ontario and British Columbia to Georgia and Mexico and is found in parts of Europe and Asia. It typically grows in clearings, thickets, and the edges of woodlands.

Other common names include horsemint and bergamot, the latter inspired by the scent of the leaves, which smell like bergamot orange. Bee balm grows to a height of two feet or more, and its square, grooved stem, typical of all mints, displays paired, toothed leaves that are roughly textured on both sides. Its showy, tubular, nectar-rich flowers form whorls of 20 to 50 at the top of

DID YOU KNOW?

Bee balms are several species of brilliantly colored midsummer bloomers that scent the air with an earthy mint aroma.

the stem and are supported by leafy bracts. The root system consists of short, slender rhizomes.

Several species of bee balm are used medicinally, with the crushed leaves exuding a fragrant essential oil. *M. didyma,* with the highest concentration, has airy blossoms of bright carmine red. Wild bergamot or purple bee balm *(M. fistulosa)* is a tall perennial with narrow lavender flowers. It is also called Oswego tea. It got this name after the American colonists dumped a shipment of tea into Boston Harbor to protest British taxes and then discovered an alternative hot beverage made from the young leaves of wild bergamot; it was called Oswego tea after the Oswego Indians of western New York. Lemon bergamot or lemon mint *(M. citriodora)* has edible purple-pink flowers that are used in desserts and salads and lemon-scented leaves that flavor teas and liquors.

Aromatic Qualities

Bee balm's distinctive aroma, with hints of mint, oregano, and thyme, is found in both the leaf and flower, making it a favorite for potpourris or sachets. The plant blossoms from June to July, which is when the leaves and blooming flowers should be

With its intense red bloom, *Monarda didyma,* also called crimson bee balm, scarlet bee balm, and scarlet monarda, is especially attractive to hummingbirds.

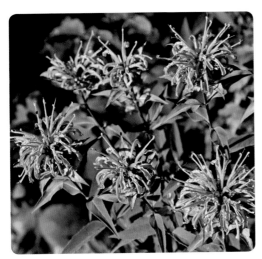
Wild bee balms, such as *Monarda fistulosa,* have wispier petals than garden varieties and bloom in shades of pale purple.

gathered for drying. At home, the plants should be dried inside a paper bag and hung in a well-ventilated area.

In aromatherapy, the essential oil is used as a calmative, antidepressant, and anxiety reducer.

Healing Properties

Even before Europeans discovered the New World, Native Americans were using bee balm extensively as a medicinal plant; they even identified four separate varieties that had different odors. Wild bee balm was used as a sweat inducer in ceremonial sweat lodges, it was made into hair pomade, and used to heal skin and mouth infections—due to its high levels of the antiseptic compound known as thymol.

Colonists applied the herb as the Indians did and also steamed the entire monarda plant and breathed in the vapor to unblock swollen sinuses. The Shakers, members of a 19th-century religious sect, believed that bee balm was effective against colds and sore throats.

In alternative medicine, the herb's leaves and flowers are employed to relieve gas and induce sweating, and as a diuretic, a stimulant, and an antiseptic. An infusion is taken internally to treat colds, headaches, and gastric disorders, to reduce low fevers, and to relieve menstrual pain and insomnia. Steam inhalation of the herb is effective for sore throats and bronchial irritation. Externally, it can be applied to skin eruptions and infections.

History and Lore

» Bee balm should not be confused with *Mentha citrata,* an herb called bergamot mint, or *Citrus bergamia,* the bergamot orange tree, whose fruit is the source of the flavor in Earl Grey tea.

» According to folklore, carrying bee balm in your wallet will attract money, and rubbing the leaves onto bills before spending them will ensure their return.

IN THE KITCHEN

Sparkling Berry Punch

This punch, brightened with the addition of citrusy bee balm, is perfect for lawn parties and other summer gatherings.

Ingredients
- 1 cup sugar or stevia
- 1 cup lemon juice
- 1 cup young bee balm leaves
- 1 cup strawberries/raspberries, mixed
- ½ cup chopped mint leaves
- 2 cups cranberry juice
- 1 large can of pineapple juice, chilled
- 2-liter bottle of lemon-lime soda

Directions
Heat sugar and lemon juice in a pan until sugar is dissolved. Add bee balm and berries and simmer for 15 minutes, while stirring to soften berries. Strain leaves and berries, stir in mint and cranberry juice, and chill for one day. Add pineapple juice and soda just prior to serving in a punch bowl. Float fresh strawberries or raspberries or an ice ring with frozen berries in the bowl. ■

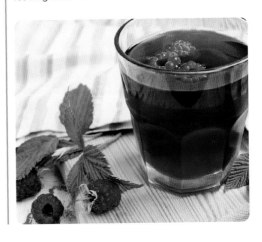

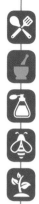

Bergamot Orange

Citrus bergamia

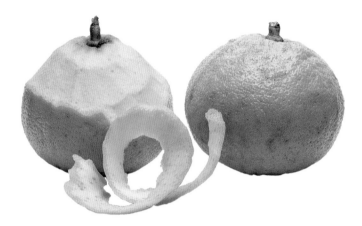

AROMATIC HERBS

The bergamot orange tree bears an aromatic fruit that is used as a perfume component, an ingredient in skin-care products, and a flavoring for food. The tree was originally native to Southeast Asia, but since the 16th century, it has been found in the Mediterranean region. Venetian traders were most likely the first to bring bergamot oranges to Italy, possibly obtained from Arab traders. Calabria, a region in southern Italy, is the major commercial supplier. In the south of France and the West African Côte d'Ivoire, it is cultivated for its essential oil, while in Antalya, Turkey, it is grown for marmalade.

DID YOU KNOW?

The leaves and peel of bergamot orange release a highly fragrant citrus-scented oil that is prized in the perfume industry.

The bergamot orange tree is a member of the Rutaceae—rue or citrus—family, and it is likely a hybrid between sweet lime or sweet lemon (*Citrus limetta*) and bitter orange (*C. aurantium*). It is a relatively small tree that blossoms in the winter. The fruit is the size of an orange, but is closer to the color of a lemon.

Aromatic Qualities

Bergamot orange peel is widely used in the manufacture of perfume. It is known for its ability to combine with a variety of other scents to create distinct complementary fragrances. It is estimated that one third of men's perfumes and roughly half of women's contain the essential oil. One hundred bergamot oranges will produce only three ounces of the oil. Because the adulteration of the oil with cheaper products, such as rosewood or bergamot mint, has been a problem in the past, Italian authorities tightly control the production of bergamot orange oil, testing it for purity and issuing certificates.

The aromatic roots of bergamot orange are thought to mask the scent of the roots of other nearby plants from agricultural pests, and so the trees are sometimes used as companion plantings in vegetable gardens.

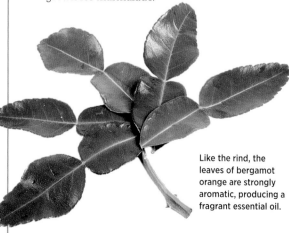

Like the rind, the leaves of bergamot orange are strongly aromatic, producing a fragrant essential oil.

The Pride of Cologne

Eau de Cologne, or "water of Cologne," has over time become the generic term for any scent that has a concentration of essential oil less than that of perfume or toilet water (usually 2 to 5 percent). It was originally, however, the name of a specific fragrance created by Italian perfume maker Giovanni Maria Farina. His creation used a delicious blend of citrus oils, including a significant amount of bergamot orange—which was mentioned as a perfume ingredient in the Farina Archive from 1714. Farina wrote to his brother: "I have found a fragrance that reminds me of an Italian spring morning, of mountain daffodils and orange blossoms after the rain." He named the scent after his new hometown, Cologne, Germany, and delivered it to nearly all the royal houses of Europe. There is a statue of Farina, who became

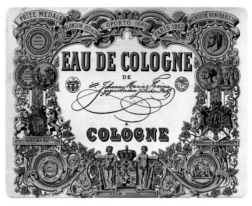

A label from an 1858 version of Farina's Eau de Cologne

known as Johann Maria Farina in Germany, on the Town Hall of the city he helped make famous. His shop, which opened in 1709, is still in business as the world's oldest fragrance factory. ■

Culinary Uses

The actual pulp of the sour fruit is considered inedible, bit the essence extracted from the scented peel is a popular flavoring. It is the

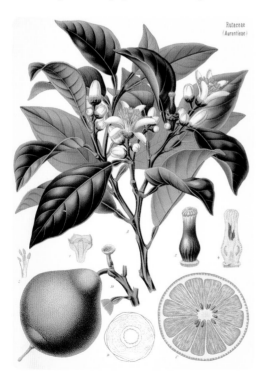

An illustration of bergamot orange from *Köhler's Medicinal Plants,* published by Franz Eugen Köhler in 1887

"secret" ingredient behind the tangy citrus taste of Earl Grey and Lady Grey teas and is used in the making of the confection called Turkish Delight. Italians use it to make marmalade and a digestive liqueur called Liquore de Bergamotto. In Sweden and Norway, bergamot orange flavors a smokeless tobacco product called *snus* and it is used in regular snuff blends as well. The juice can be added to marmalades and vinaigrettes.

Healing Properties

For many years, an extract from bergamot oil, called psoralen, was used as an ingredient in tanning accelerators and sunscreens. As of 1959, this extract was known to be photocarcinogenic—causing cancer after exposure to light—but was not banned from sunscreens until 1965.

Today, psoralen plus UVA—ultraviolet light—is used in a therapy called PUVA, to treat serious skin disorders like eczema, psoriasis, graft-versus-host disease, vitiligo, mycosis fungoides, and cutaneous T-cell lymphoma.

History and Lore

» During World War II, bergamot orange oil could not be exported from Fascist Italy to the Allied countries, so substitutes from Brazil and Mexico made from sweet lime and other citrus fruits were used.

Bergamot Orange

173

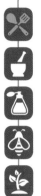

Cretan Dittany

Origanum dictamnus

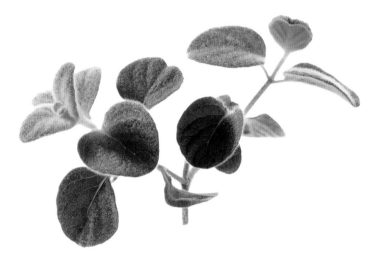

Cretan dittany, also known as dittany-of-Crete and hop marjoram, is an aromatic ground cover that was one of the best-known healing agents of antiquity, beginning with the Minoans. This native of the Grecian island of Crete grows wild on rough mountainsides and in rocky gorges. It is also often found in temperate zones, and does especially well in water-conserving xeriscapes because it prefers acid soil on dry, wooded slopes.

The small, creeping bush, which reaches only a about a foot in height, is a perennial member of the mint family, Lamiaceae. It is easily identified by the whitish, woolly hairs on the surface

DID YOU KNOW?

Cretan dittany is a drought-tolerant bush with a fragrant scent that attracts bees, butterflies, and birds.

of its arching stems and oval, gray-green leaves, which make them look like velvet. The tiny, drooping, rose-colored flowers grow in tufts and are surrounded by numerous, overlapping purple-pink bracts.

Cretan dittany benefits the environment—its flowers attract and feed hummingbirds, butterflies, skippers, bees, and other insects, and its roots prevent erosion, holding the soil in place on the steep slopes where it grows. The name is believed to come from Dicte, the mountain in Crete where Zeus is said to have been born.

Aromatic Qualities

Cretan dittany is greatly prized for its aroma. It is gathered while blooming during the summer months, and it is exported for use in pharmaceuticals, perfume making, beauty products, and to flavor liquors such as vermouth and absinthe, and the liqueur Benedictine. Cultivation in Crete is currently centered in Embaros, south of Heraklion, and its surrounding villages.

Sadly, the wild, naturally growing dittany of Crete is classed as "rare" and since 1997 has

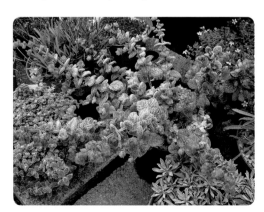

With its love of dry environments, Cretan dittany is perfect for a xeriscape garden, which is planned to conserve water.

been listed on the International Union for the Conservation of Nature's Red List for endangered species.

The plant's main aromatic constituents are thymol, an antiseptic also found in thyme; carvacrol, an antibacterial also found in oregano; minty-citrus phellandrene, found in fennel; and cymene, found in cumin and thyme. The scent of dittany is pungent, reminiscent of oregano, thyme, and marjoram.

Healing Properties

Dittany has a long history as a healing agent for various kinds of digestive issues, or, as a Cretan grandmother might say, it is "very strong and good for the stomach." Greek physician Hippocrates prescribed it for many ailments, including arthritis, digestive issues, to induce menstruation, and as a poultice for wounds. In his book *The History of Animals,* Aristotle relates that when wild goats on Crete were wounded by a hunter's arrow, they went in search of dittany, which could supposedly eject the arrow. *Origanum dictamnus* is also mentioned in the writings of Homer, Euripides, Virgil, Theophrastus, Plutarch, Dioscorides, and Galinos. Charlemagne catalogued it as one of the herbs on his agricultural farms.

Although medicinal use of this herb has waned recently, herbalists still recommend dittany as a poultice for wounds or as a tea to treat headaches, digestive problems, neuralgia, and to relieve periodic pain.

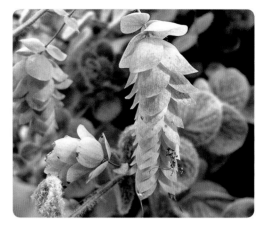

The fragrant flowers of Cretan dittany form papery pink bracts that make excellent dried flowers for potpourris.

History and Lore

» In Virgil's *Aeneid,* the goddess Venus heals the wounded Aeneas with a stalk of "dittany from Cretan Ida." In art, the goddess Artemis is often shown wearing a crown of dittany.

» Occultists believe that incense made of dittany, vanilla, benzoin, and sandalwood aids astral projection—the separation of the consciousness from the physical body.

» In the Cretan dialect the plant is called *erontas,* or "love," and is considered an aphrodisiac. The men who harvest it commercially are called *erondades,* or "love seekers." Legend claims that many ardent young men died while trying to pluck the blossoms from remote mountainsides as a gift for their sweethearts.

Madam Blavatsky's Magical Herb

Occultists regularly use dittany in the art of divination and for healing and protection. Madam Helena Blavatsky, a famous practitioner, considered dittany to be one of the most powerful of all "magical" plants. Blavatsky, a Ukrainian who lived in the 19th century, founded the Theosophical Society and promoted a system of beliefs called Theosophy—"the archaic Wisdom-Religion, the esoteric doctrine once known in every ancient country having claims to civilization." Blavatsky's philosophy eventually had an effect on the Buddhist modernism and Hindu reform movements. She is also considered a herald of the 20th-century New Age Movement. ∎

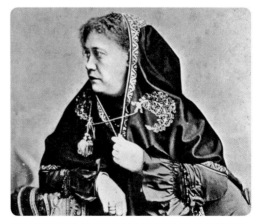

Helena Blavatsky, the foremost occultist of the 19th century, credited "magical herbs" for many of her mystical insights.

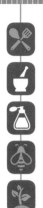

Eucalyptus

Eucalyptus globulus

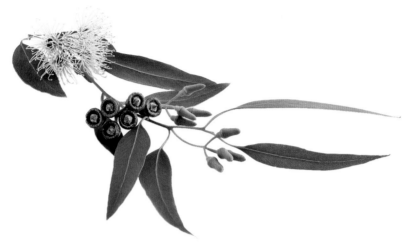

The eucalyptus is part of a diverse genus of flowering trees and shrubs of the myrtle family, Myrtaceae. There are more than 700 species of eucalyptus, which originated in Australia and Tasmania, where at least 691 species grow, dominating the tree flora. They can also now be found in most subtropical regions of the world.

The species vary greatly—some are the size of ornamental shrubs, while others grow to be giants. The source of most medicinal eucalyptus is *Eucalyptus globulus,* called the blue gum or Australian fever tree, which can reach 230 feet in height. The large leaves of this attractive tree are a shiny dark green, while the blue-gray bark peels back to reveal the cream-colored inner bark. Australia's famous blue forests

DID YOU KNOW?

The eucalyptus species known as the blue gum supplies the richly scented oil prized for its therapeutic, aromatic, and flavoring properties.

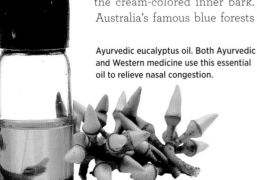

Ayurvedic eucalyptus oil. Both Ayurvedic and Western medicine use this essential oil to relieve nasal congestion.

are actually named for the haze created by the trees' essential oils rising above the canopy.

Aromatic Qualities

The active ingredient in this plant is called cineole, an anti-inflammatory that is responsible for its camphor-like, slightly pungent aroma. The scent is said to increase brain-wave activity and counteract physical and mental fatigue. Travelers are advised to carry eucalyptus with them on long car trips, and students should inhale the scent to help them study. Researchers at International Flavors and Fragrances, a research and development corporation in New Jersey, found that sniffing eucalyptus increases energy. In aromatherapy, the oil is used to help resolve disagreements, clear the air, and ease interpersonal conflicts.

Healing Properties

Medicinally, eucalyptus is antibacterial and antiviral, a deodorant, and an expectorant that clears mucous from the lungs. It is also used as a liniment to relieve rheumatism, arthritis and other types of joint pain. The oil is made from the fresh leaves and branch tops of the eucalyptus plant. Eucalyptus leaves contain tannins, which

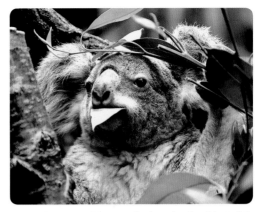

Leaves of many eucalyptus species form the diet of Australia's indigenous koala bears; sadly, deforestation has seriously impacted populations of these sweet-faced marsupials.

CULTURAL CONNECTIONS

Combating Malaria

When the eucalyptus tree was introduced to Europe at the Paris Exposition of 1867, the director of the botanical gardens in Melbourne had an ulterior motive. He believed that its essential oil might be a low-cost replacement for an antiseptic, expectorant called cajeput oil, which is distilled from the tree *Melaleuca leucadendra*. It turned out he was correct. The French government then began planting the fast-growing eucalyptus in Algeria, where malaria was a widespread problem. They believed that the aromatic trees could counteract the unhealthy air, or miasma, thought to cause malaria. The trees did lower the incidence of malaria, but this was not due to their essential oil. It was because the water-hungry eucalyptus transformed the Algerian marshes into dry land, eliminating the wet habitat of the malaria-carrying *Anopheles* mosquitoes. ■

researchers think may help reduce inflammation, along with flavonoids or plant-based antioxidants, and volatile oils.

In traditional Aboriginal medicine, the plant was employed to heal wounds and treat fungal infections, and eucalyptus tea was known to reduce fevers. After the exploration of Australia began, it wasn't long before this plant's healing abilities were recognized by other cultures—it was soon integrated into Chinese, Ayurvedic, and Greek and European medicine. In the 19th century, it was commonly employed to disinfect urinary catheters—and research later confirmed that the oil contains antibacterial properties.

Today, eucalyptus essential oil is used in over-the-counter preparations to treat coughs, colds, and flu. Herbalists recommend using the fresh leaves in teas and gargles to ease sore throats and treat bronchitis and sinusitis. A vaporous eucalyptus ointment is often used as a chest rub on ailing children. The oil is also included in creams and ointments meant to ease backaches and muscle and joint pain.

Because the oil is rich in cineole, which kills the bacteria that can cause bad breath, many mouthwashes contain eucalyptus, along with other oils. There is also some evidence that eucalyptus may help prevent plaque and gingivitis.

History and Lore

» The wood is commonly used for lumber, firewood, paper pulpwood, and fencing. A large, long, resonating Aborigine instrument, called a didgeridoo, is also often made from this wood.
» All parts of the tree can be used to manufacture dyes for silks and woolens, in colors ranging from yellows, oranges, and greens through to deep rust and chocolate.
» Eucalyptus forests are excellent for reducing carbon dioxide emissions: one tree absorbs 660 pounds (300 kilograms) a year.

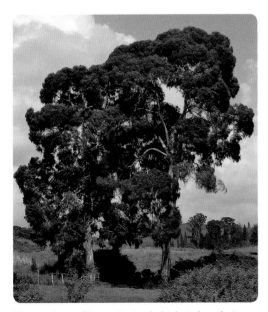

Blue gum is one of the most extensively planted eucalyptus trees. It leaves are distilled to extract the fragrant essential oil.

Eucalyptus

AROMATHERAPY

Relax, restore, and rejuvenate with healing oils.

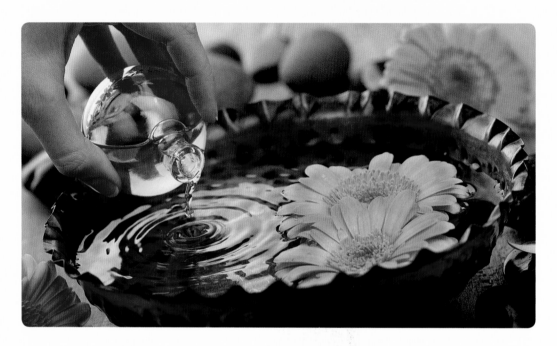

Aromatherapy, also called essential oil therapy, is a form of natural healing that incorporates the aromatic oils of various botanicals, or beneficial herbs. Practiced by herbalists for centuries, this approach has recently become more widespread, especially in health-conscious segments of the population.

Historians believe that early humans, maybe as far back as 7000 B.C. and perhaps by accident, discovered that heated animal fat absorbed the scent of aromatic plants. They used these fragrant oils as perfume, hair dressing pomades, skin protectors, and insect repellents. They also used them for massage and rituals—and for medicinal purposes.

Aromatic healing was an accepted part of Chinese, Indian, Egyptian, Greek, and Roman culture, and, over time, healers realized that scented oils could also affect mood and emotions. This was possibly because the nose is the quickest route to the blood-brain barrier, making the sense of smell extremely powerful; humans can distinguish roughly ten thousand different scents. With their ability to heal the body and lift the spirits, essential oils became one of the cornerstones of alternative medicine.

French perfumer and chemist René-Maurice Gattefossé first used the word *aromatherapie* in his 1937 book of the same name to distinguish the medicinal use of essential oils from their use in perfumery.

Treating the Whole Person

The aim of aromatherapy is simple: to treat ailments and influence mental states in a natural, noninvasive manner that affects the whole person, not just the symptoms or disease—and further triggers the body's ability to heal and maintain itself. Fortunately, many of the essential oils used in aromatherapy are far less expensive, more accessible, and have fewer side effects and risks than synthetic or chemically produced drugs.

Something in the Air

Once you determine your health goal, you will know which aromatherapy application to use: using it topically; taking it internally, or inhaling the aroma. Oil can be massaged into the skin; or ingested as tea or used as a gargle. The oil can be dispersed in the air with a diffuser or inhaled from a steam vaporizer. Adding essential oil to your bath serves a dual purpose: you will breathe in the healing scent while absorbing the oil into your skin.

Making Sense of Scents

Whether you want to freshen your living space, lift your mood, or promote healing, you can use aromatherapy at home. Many herbs can be blended to achieve multiple benefits, such a clarifying mix of peppermint and rosemary. Here are some favorite herbs and spices, and what their scents do. ■

Soothe Stress and Anxiety

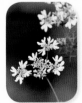 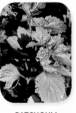

| BEE BALM | LAVENDER | VANILLA |

Boost Memory and Cognitive Function

 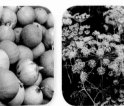 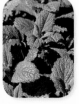

| BASIL | CLARY SAGE | JUNIPER BERRY |

Relieve Fatigue and Elevate Energy

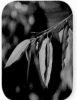 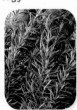

| EUCALYPTUS | PEPPERMINT | ROSEMARY |

Promote Calmness and Comfort

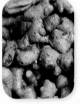 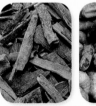 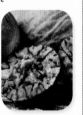

| CINNAMON | GINGER | NUTMEG |

Evoke Sensuality and Romance

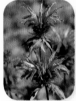 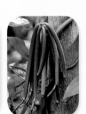 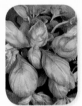

| CORIANDER | JASMINE | PATCHOULI |

Lift Spirits and Mood

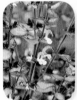 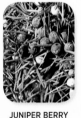

| BERGAMOT ORANGE | FENNEL | LEMON BALM |

Aromatherapy

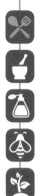

Hyssop

Hyssopus officinalis

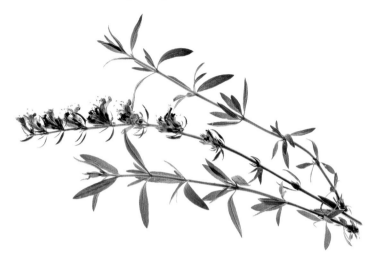

Hyssop's history as an aromatic and medicinal herb goes back to Biblical times. The plant originated in central Asia but has naturalized in most temperate regions of the world. The common and genus name is from the Greek *azob,* or the Hebrew *ezob,* meaning "holy herb," because hyssop was once used to cleanse sacred places.

Hyssop, an evergreen, semi-woody herb, is a member of the mint family, Lamiaceae. It grows to three feet high, and has straight, square stems and slender,

---

DID YOU KNOW?

A versatile perennial herb, hyssop is the source of a fragrant essential oil with a clean and aromatic scent. With its purple bloom, it also makes itself at home in gardens.

---

oblong-shaped leaves. Pollinators flock to the warm, woodsy scent of the bluish purple flowers that form whorls at the top of the stem as summer approaches.

Aromatic Qualities

All the visible parts of the hyssop plant are highly aromatic, offering a sweet, camphor-like scent. Perfume makers value hyssop's essential oil even more so than oil of lavender, and it is used to produce eau de cologne. It is also employed in the manufacture of alcoholic beverages and is one of the "secret" ingredients in the French liqueur Chartreuse. Bees are drawn to the plant, and the nectar gives their honey a wonderful scent. Hyssop was employed in medieval times as a strewing herb, used to refresh the atmosphere in cottages and castles both.

The essential oil of hyssop is extracted from the leaves and small blue flowers, primarily from plants grown in Germany and Provence. In aromatherapy, the oil is used as a tonic that encourages the secretion of hormones, for massage, and to promote overall organic health. Spiritually, it is also believed to stimulate a stronger connection to people and increase the sense of harmony and oneness if shared within a group.

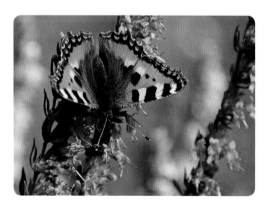

A small tortoiseshell butterfly *(Aglais urticae)* visits a slender purple spike of hyssop. This perennial is a must-have for anyone planting a butterfly or hummingbird garden.

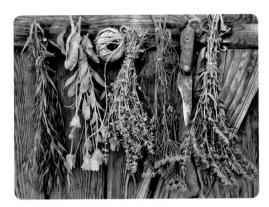

Hyssop leaves and blooms (far right) bundled to air-dry with tarragon, calendula, thyme, and dill. As a kitchen herb, hyssop is used to make broths, decoctions, and, occasionally, salads. The dried leaves can be made into a beneficial tea.

Healing Properties

Over the centuries, natural healers have valued hyssop's qualities—as an antispasmodic, antidepressant, antiseptic, expectorant, diuretic, and aid to circulation. It has also been used for the treatment of female reproductive complaints, diarrhea, colds, fevers, sore throat, and influenza. The herb's astringent properties make hyssop helpful for treating skin ailments such as eczema or dermatitis.

For relief from colds or flu, hyssop is usually administered as a warm infusion, often mixed with horehound. Hyssop tea is beneficial to weak stomachs, while the tops of the herb are sometimes boiled in soup as a treatment for asthma.

History and Lore

» Hyssop mixed with frankincense and mastic creates a rich incense that has been employed since the ancient Minoan kingdom of Crete.

» The herb is mentioned at least ten times in the Bible, often in conjunction with cleansing and purification. Some scholars believe the hyssop referred to in some places is actually the caper plant (*Capparis spinosa*), which grows throughout the Holy Land.

» Hebrew holy men would make brooms out of hyssop stalks to "sweep" negative spirits out of temples. Early Christians used hyssop during baptisms; it was later considered it a symbol of forgiven sins.

» Hyssop is a bee magnet—so much so that it is said that beekeepers once rubbed it over their hives to encourage bees to stay.

Governed by Water

According to early British herbalist Nicholas Culpeper, hyssop is governed by the Zodiac water sign Cancer and should therefore be effective against anything involving fluids. Culpeper documented several uses for the herb in treating "rheum," what healers of the Middle Ages called the mucouslike fluids that collect in the throat or lungs, or around joints. It turns out hyssop, as a simple syrup, is beneficial for treating wet, hacking coughs. When applied as heat therapy, it is useful for treating arthritis inflammation and muscle aches. To make a hot compress, add a handful of dried hyssop to one pint of very hot water, soak a washcloth in the mixture, apply immediately to injury or inflamed joint, and wrap inside a warmed towel for 15 minutes. ■

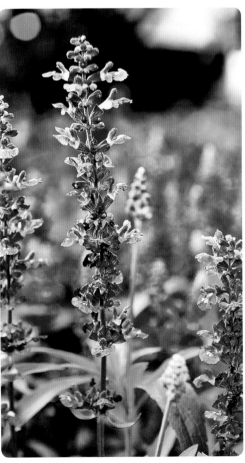

Plant hyssop as a low hedge along a walkway or massed in a garden border to scent the air with its sweet fragrance.

Hyssop

181

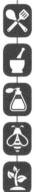

Jasmine

Jasminum spp.

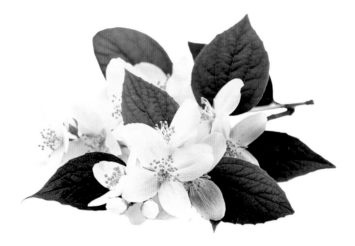

Evoking the music of a fountain playing in an exotic moonlit garden, the heady scent of night-blooming jasmine has been synonymous with romance and desire since the beginning of recorded history. Even the source of its common name is poetic, *yasmin* means "heavenly felicity" in Persian and "fragrant flower" in Arabic.

Jasmine is a member of the olive family, Oleaceae, and there are roughly 200 species of this evergreen shrub, some annual, some perennial. The plant is a woody climber that can reach more than 40 feet in length, with green, pinnate leaves and white, star-shaped flowers that grow in clusters. Jasmine was most likely native to Persia (Iran) or India, but around 1000 B.C. it

> **DID YOU KNOW?**
> A genus of tropical and subtropical shrubs and vines, jasmine has an illustrious history, and it is often cultivated for the fragrance of its heavenly scented flowers.

found its way to Egypt, then naturalized in Turkey and Greece. Today, it grows in many tropical or warm temperate regions. In the United States, *Jasminum officinale* is hardy as far north as Washington, D. C.

Jasmine is sometimes called the queen of flowers and, indeed, it was a favorite of royalty. It was found in the gardens of the Sung Dynasty emperors of China (A.D. 960 to 1279), and planted at the residences of the kings of Afghanistan, Nepal, and Persia in the 1400s. During the 1600s, the Moors introduced the flower to Spain, from where it spread to France and Italy.

Aromatic Qualities

Jasmine has a distinctive, rich, warm floral fragrance that is sweetly exotic, with a fruity-tea undertone. As early as the 1200s, the Chinese were using jasmine to scent their green tea. Jasmine is also found in many of the most exclusive scents—Spanish jasmine *(J. grandiflorum)*, which has been grown in France for centuries, is a key part of the perfume industry that has become so associated with that country.

Jasmine's principle constituent is jasmone, which is used commercially in perfumes and cosmetics. In aromatherapy, the essential oil,

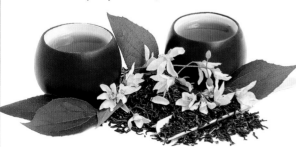

The flowers of Arabian jasmine *(J. sambac)* are blended with tea—usually green—to create the highly fragrant jasmine tea.

Capturing Scent with Enfleurage

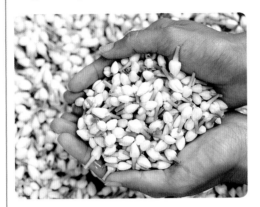

Jasmine is known as the Mistress of the Night and Moonlight of the Grove because late evening is when the flowers produce the most oil and when their heady scent is at its peak. It is also the best time to gather the blossoms for the manufacture of perfume. To capture the essence of this delicate floral botanical, perfumers have long used the enfleurage method. In this process, the flowers are first laid on a layer of odorless fat. Subsequent layers of flowers make sure the fat—now called pomade—is saturated with fragrance. The pomade is then soaked in alcohol, the fat is separated, and the alcohol is allowed to evaporate, leaving the fragrant and valuable "absolute" behind. Unlike other floral scents that have been re-created chemically, jasmine cannot be duplicated. ■

as well as jasmine-infused candles and incense, are used as an antidepressant, to relax the nerves, to combat addiction, and to relieve muscle spasms and cramping.

Healing Properties

The early Chinese, Arabians, and Indians all valued jasmine for its medicinal effects. In China, the root was used to treat headache, insomnia and dislocated joints. In India, the leaves and flowers were used to make a putty, which was eaten with rice to cure scabies and other skin irritations. In Borneo, young jasmine leaves were boiled and the infusion taken to treat gallstones.

Jasmine is considered an astringent, an antibacterial, an antiviral, and a cooling and bitter herb. Jasmine oil makes a beneficial treatment for sensitive or mature skin. In India, jasmine flowers infused into sesame oil are applied to abscesses and sores. A similar ointment can be made by adding two drops of jasmine essential oil to one ounce of vegetable oil.

Studies at Toho University School of Medicine in Tokyo indicate that it also enhances mental alertness and stimulates brain waves. In another study, jasmine helped computer operators reduce the number of mistakes they made by one-third.

History and Lore

» The only continents that do not have any native species of jasmine are Antarctica and North America.

» To the Chinese, the flower represents feminine kindness, grace and delicacy, and attracts both wealth and romance. To the Thai people, it symbolizes motherhood, and, in India, it is called *jui* and is used in Hindu ceremonies.

» In Hawaii, Arabian jasmine is called *pikake*—pronounced pea-cock-y—and the flowers are fashioned into fragrant leis.

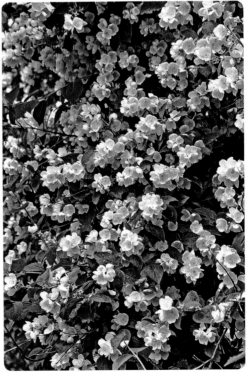

Jasmine is a woody shrub with cascades of heavily scented flowers. Some species will bloom from spring until fall.

Jasmine

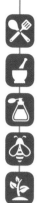

Lavender

Lavandula angustifolia

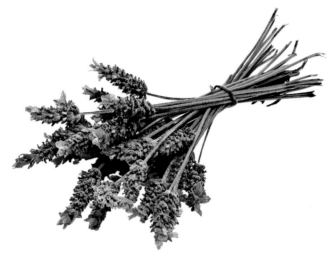

If basil is the king of herbs, then lavender might well be the queen. The applications for this stately herb transcend categories. For more than two millennia, lavender has been a source of perfumes, incense, sachets, cut flowers, dried bouquets, potpourris, room fresheners, medicines, insect repellents, culinary flavorings, and adornments. It ultimately provides a vital cash crop to the south of France, England, the United States, and elsewhere.

The ancient Egyptians applied it as a perfume and also dipped shrouds in it for use in mummification. The Greeks called it *nardus* or *nard*—from

DID YOU KNOW?

Lavender, with its famously soapy scent, is a flowering mint that is cultivated as an ornamental and culinary herb. It also commercially grown for its much sought-after essential oils.

the Syrian city of Naarda—and prescribed it for insomnia, backaches, and even insanity. It became so valuable, Roman merchants sold a pound of nard flowers for the equivalent of a farm laborer's monthly wage. Romans used it for scenting bath water, hence its name, *Lavandula*, from *lavare*, meaning "to wash." In the Middle Ages, it was a strewing herb, used to disinfect and deodorize homes. During the Great Plague of London in the 17th century, fearful citizens wore sprigs of lavender or gloves scented with the oil to guard against infection. Because fleas carried the plague bacillus and lavender repels fleas, it is possible that the herb actually did prevent many people from contracting the deadly disease.

This perennial member of the mint family, Lamiaceae, lends itself to mass plantings in large gardens or borders. It likely originated in the Mediterranean, the Middle East, and India, but today is found throughout Europe, Australia, New Zealand, and both North and South America.

Depending on species—there are 39—the height, leaf shape, and color can vary, but the best-known, English lavender (*L. angustifolia*), is a shrubby plant that reaches from three feet

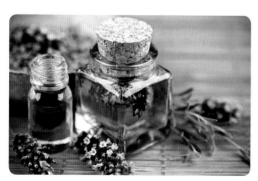

The classic, clean scent of lavender oil is used extensively in scented products, such as bath oil, colognes, and soap.

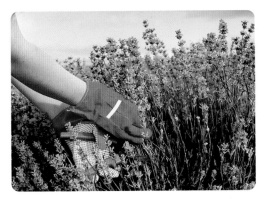

In summer, collect the strong stems of blooming lavender to use in fresh bouquets and flower arrangements or dry them in bunches to use all year round in potpourri and sachets.

In aromatherapy, lavender oil is said to soothe headaches, migraines, and motion sickness when massaged into the temples. It is also used as an aid to sleep and relaxation.

Culinary Uses

Like other members of the mint family, lavender has been used as a seasoning for centuries, lending a floral, elegant taste to salads, soups, and meat and seafood recipes. It is often an ingredient in herbes de Provence and is also used to flavor cheeses, sparkling summer drinks, and omelets, as well as cakes, pastries, and ice creams. The dried flowers are preferred for cooking.

Healing Properties

Natural healers have relied on lavender for its properties as an anti-inflammatory and an antiseptic. An infusion of the herb can soothe and heal sunburn, small cuts, and insect bites or stings. It works on many inflammatory conditions, including acne, and can be taken internally to ease heartburn and indigestion.

to six feet in height, with dusty blue-green foliage and pinkish purple flowers that form spikes atop strong, leafless stems. Other popular species include French lavender, either *L. stoechas* or *L. dentate,* and Spanish lavender, referred to as *L. stoechas, L. lanata* or *L. dentate.*

Aromatic Qualities

Lavender, like the wine grapes of Provence, picks up many scent characteristics from the soil—earthy, floral, fruity, clean, and dry. The essential oil is used to create scented bath and body products, soaps, candles, perfumes, incense, household cleansers, and laundry detergent.

While lavender attracts bees and other pollinators, a tray of dried lavender flowers set in a window can discourage small, crawling invaders, especially in the south of France, where scorpions and insects insist on coming indoors.

History and Lore

» According to legend, Cleopatra used lavender to seduce both Julius Caesar and Mark Antony.
» The Shakers—a strict, celibate sect of the Quakers—grew lavender and were the first to offer commercial, lavender-based products for sale in North America.
» Mystics believe the odor of lavender contributes to a long life and a greater acceptance and understanding of old age.

IN THE GARDEN

Lavender by the Yard

The recent trend toward xeriscaping—creating a garden of hardy plants that require little water and form a habitat for wildlife—has led to many homeowners replacing their water-hungry front lawns with swaths of lavender. When in bloom, this herb creates as much of a unified effect as an all-green lawn, except that the plantings are taller and a pleasing mix of purple hues. The herb's distinctive scent and its benefits for endangered bees are two more reasons for turning your yard into a mini patch of Provence—not to mention the vibrant view every time you gaze out your windows. ■

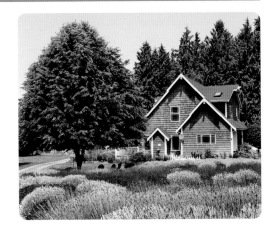

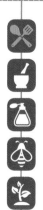

Patchouli

Pogostemon cablin

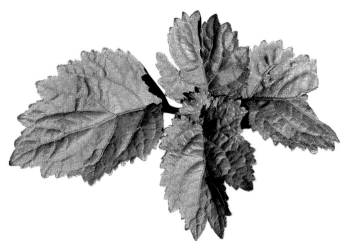

If one aroma could be said to capture an era, it might well be patchouli—"the scent of the 1960s." This was the Age of Aquarius, the era of the counterculture, of hippies, Woodstock, and suburban teens who aspired to be groovy . . . and there was something about the acrid, musky, slightly minty scent of patchouli that made every girl feel like a gypsy queen and every guy swagger like a rock star. Today, its distinctive essence remains a favorite with artists, performers, and other creative types. The herb is also one of those versatile cure-alls valued by healers for centuries, making it one of the most popular oils on the market.

DID YOU KNOW?

The scent of patchouli, forever associated with the hippie culture of the 1960s, comes from the essential oil obtained from the leaves of the *Pogostemon cablin*.

Patchouli is a perennial herb of the mint family, Lamiaceae, and is native to Southeast Asia, growing wild in Sumatra and Java, even at elevations between 3,000 and 6,000 feet. The bushy plant features erect stems that reach two or three feet in height, with soft, hairy, ovoid leaves and small, pale, pinkish white flowers. The name derives from the Tamil words *patchai,* or "green" and *ellai,* or "leaf." In addition to *Pogostemon cablin,* other species cultivated for their essential oils are *P. commosum, P. hortensis, P. heyneasus,* and *P. plectranthoides.*

Aromatic Qualities

Patchouli has a dusty, resinous aroma, and legend insists that its popularity with hippies and bohemians started because its strong scent was able to obscure the odor of marijuana.

The oil has been used for centuries as a fixative in perfumes, and, in recent times, in incense and insect repellent. Patchouli both repels and kills insects, and it was used in Asia to protect fabric from moth damage. In the 19th century, silks imported from India bore the distinctive smell, and so French imitators infused it into their fabrics as well. Today, it lends its scent to paper

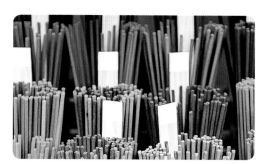

Sticks of incense for sale. Patchouli incense, made from the essential oils of the plant, gives off an earthy, exotic fragrance.

towels, laundry detergent, and air fresheners. Two major aromatic components of the essential oil are patchoulol and norpatchoulenol.

In aromatherapy, patchouli is considered a useful balancer, relaxing yet stimulating, restoring an immunity system weakened by overwork and anxiety. It also harmonizes the three principal forces within the body—the creative at the navel, the heart center, and transcendental wisdom at the crown. Patchouli oil can relieve the strain of excessive mental activity, restoring the balance between the intellect and sensuality.

This oil blends well with the essential oils of bergamot, clary sage, geranium, lavender, and myrrh. When wearing patchouli, keep in mind that the scent is intense, and some people dislike it, so apply it with restraint if you don't want to smell like a Greenwich Village hippie shop.

Healing Properties

Patchouli oil has been used for centuries by herbal healers in the Far East—Malaysia, China and Japan—primarily to treat skin conditions such as dermatitis, eczema, acne, and dandruff. It is also employed as an antidepressant—the oil stimulates the release of the pleasure hormones serotonin and dopamine, relieving sadness and anxiety; an anti-inflammatory; an antiseptic; a diuretic; and a deodorant. Its astringent properties strengthen the hold of the gums and prevent

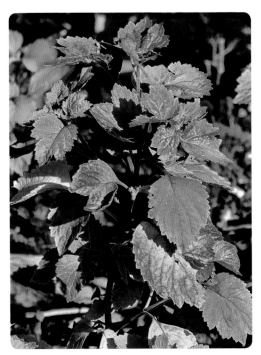

Patchouli has the square stem of most mints. Its flowers are fragrant, but it is the leaves that produce the essential oil.

sagging skin. It boosts the immune system and can rejuvenate cells, making it excellent for wound care and the reduction of scarring. It aids production of red blood cells, thus increasing energy, and improves circulation, oxygenating organs and cells and speeding up metabolism.

History and Lore

» Patchouli possessed such an aura of opulence and luxury in 19th-century Europe that it was used to scent the linen chests of Queen Victoria.

» In 1985, the Mattel toy company used patchouli oil in the plastic of action figure Stinkor, part of the Masters of the Universe line.

» The herb is said to be a bringer of prosperity and abundance. To attract wealth, place patchouli leaves in purses and wallets or scatter them around the base of green candles.

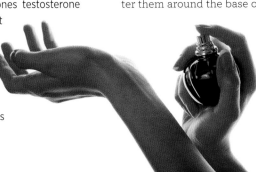

Patchouli oil has many uses in perfumery. Although it is worn as a stand-alone scent, when blended with other oils, it adds musky depth. It is also used as a base note and fixative.

POLLINATORS AND PESTS

Encourage beneficial insects; discourage destructive invaders.

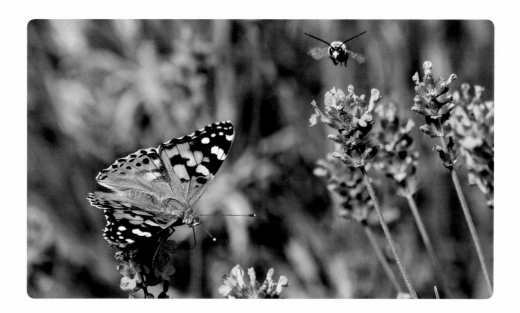

By using plants and herbs that encourage beneficial pollinators and discourage harmful insects, you can help determine whether your garden flourishes or fades away. Still other garden herbs can protect you and your pets from nuisance insects like fleas, midges, and mosquitoes.

Attracting Pollinators

Making your garden attractive to pollinators is both wise and worthwhile. After all, what is more soothing than the hum of busy honeybees or the sight of a swallow-tail alighting on a flower? Make sure your herb garden welcomes these insects with plenty of nectar-filled and pollen-rich blossoms. Nectar furnishes sugar for energy, and pollen supplies proteins and fats. Avoid pesticides and use native plantings. Place clumps of herbs in sheltered areas, chose blossoms of different colors and shapes, and time flowering of plants to span spring, summer, and fall.

Herbs that beneficial insects cannot resist include bee balm, basil, echinacea, elder, hyssop, lavender, marjoram, milk thistle, rosemary, and sage. Passionflower is a food source for butterfly larvae, while yarrow attracts predatory wasps that use insect pests as food for their larvae.

Repelling Garden Pests

Modern gardeners are increasingly aware of the environmental and health risks posed by chemical insecticides. Fortunately, there are many garden herbs that keep insects away, either from themselves or from other plants. Marigolds, for example, lure pests—including earworms, rabbits, maggots, whiteflies, potato beetles, and slugs—away from desirable plants. Essential oils can even be diluted and sprayed in the garden to target invaders.

Based on the world's shortest poem, *Fleas* by Ogden Nash, "Adam had 'em," fleas and other insects that plague humans and domestic animals have been around since the dawn of time. Early humans discovered that certain herbs could be applied to the skin to discourage these biting pests: citronella oil repels ants, fleas, gnats, and mosquitoes; feverfew contains pyrethrin, a natural insect repellent; pennyroyal works against ants and fleas; tansy repels flies and fleas; and patchouli essential oil inhibits bed bugs, ants, fleas, lice, and other crawling creatures. Even pinecones can be used to repel mosquitoes, fleas, and ticks.

Plant a Nuisance-Free Garden

Keep garden pests at bay by carefully planning a garden that includes nature's own insect repellents.

- **Alliums:** Chives act as a trap plant for aphids and control Japanese beetles. Onions and garlic repel ants, aphids, flea beetles, ticks, and mosquitoes. Leeks repel carrot flies.
- **Basil:** Repels flies and mosquitoes.
- **Borage:** Repels tomato worms and, planted with strawberries, will attract bees.
- **Coriander and fennel:** Controls aphids, slugs, snails, and spider mites.
- **Lavender flowers:** Attract numerous bees, but its essential oil, when strengthened with other oils, will repel mosquitoes.
- **Mints:** Catnip controls aphids, earworms, and squash bugs, and cucumber, Japanese, and flea beetles. Peppermint controls ants, aphids, cabbage loopers and grubs, flies, cucumber beetles, flea beetles, squash bugs, whiteflies, and mites. Spearmint controls bee mites.
- **Nasturtium:** Lures aphids, flea beetles, and black flies from desirable plants, like tomatoes. Also repels potato and cucumber beetles.
- **Nettle:** Controls black flies.
- **Oregano:** Repels whiteflies.
- **Sage:** Repels cabbage moths and loopers, flea beetles, carrot flies, and a number of harmful flying insects.
- **Tansy:** Planted with cucumbers and squash, or with roses and certain berries, repels ants, harmful beetles, and squash bugs.
- **Thyme:** Controls cabbage loopers, flea beetles, and whiteflies.
- **Wormwood:** Boughs between rows of onions and carrots will deter flies; deters cabbage moths and fruit tree moths.

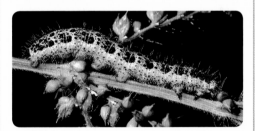

The larvae of *Pieris brassicae,* the cabbage butterfly, can skeletonize their host plants, especially cabbage species.

You can also use essential oils to deter pests.

- **Peppermint oil:** Repels ants, aphids, bean beetles, flies, lice, moths, beetles, spiders, and squash bugs.
- **Patchouli essential oil:** Repels gnats, snails, weevils, and woolly aphids.
- **Sandalwood oil:** Keeps weevils and aphids at bay, and repels mosquitoes.
- **Rosemary essential oil:** Repels carrot flies. ■

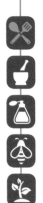

Rue

Ruta graveolens

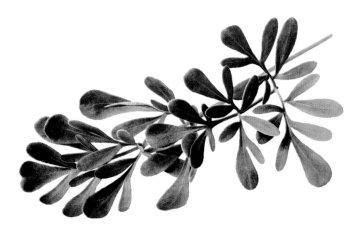

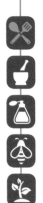

Rue, also known as common rue, herb of grace, country man's treacle, or herbygrass, is another venerable plant that has seen its glory days fade. It was popular from ancient Rome through to the Middle Ages as a seasoning, an aromatic plant, and a protective herb in medicine and magic. Today, it is chiefly grown as an ornamental landscape plant for its attractive bluish leaves, its sunny yellow flowers, earthy aroma, and its tolerance for dry soil conditions.

Native to the Balkan Peninsula or the Mediterranean, rue is now naturalized almost worldwide. This woody-stemmed plant grows to about three feet in height and produces velvety trefoil leaves and clusters of small yellow flowers that develop

DID YOU KNOW?
Yellow rue contains an aromatic volatile oil, which is not always pleasant to all noses, in glands distributed over the entire plant.

into fruit. The leaves, stems and the dried fruit are all used by herbalists.

Aromatic Qualities

Despite rue's somewhat bitter flavor, its scent is pungent and soothing. In the past, it has been used as both a strewing herb on the floors of medieval homes and as an insect repellent. More recently, it has been used in the manufacture of perfumes and cosmetics.

In aromatherapy, rue is directed toward muscle spasms, the central nervous system, heart circulation, epilepsy, diarrhea, hepatitis, pleurisy, and the arteries, and used to release sorrow, regret, and pain. Some practitioners advise against applying rue oil because it can irritate the skin and mucous membranes. It is beneficial in the garden, however, attracting numerous pollinators, and feeding the caterpillars of some subspecies of the butterflies *Papilio machaon* and *P. xuthus*. It makes a good companion plant for roses, along with lavender or geranium, but don't plant rue near cabbage.

Culinary Uses

Rue eventually fell out of favor with cooks, but in ancient Rome the seeds were ground and used as a spice. Both the berries and the seeds are found

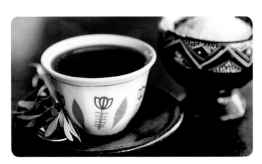

Ethiopian coffee is traditionally served with a sprig of rue.

Rue Sends Its Regrets

The bitter taste of rue has led the herb to symbolize "regret" in literature and poetry. Shakespeare's doomed Ophelia intones, "There's rue for you, and rue for me," while in *Richard II,* the herb marks the spot where the queen wept when hearing of the capture of the king. In *The Winter's Tale,* Perdita gives rue to her disguised father, advising him, "For you there's rosemary and rue; these keep, Seeming and savor all winter long." The angel Michael gives it to Adam to clear his sight in John Milton's *Paradise Lost,* and when the protagonist of Jonathan Swift's *Gulliver's Travels* returns from his adventures to live among humans again, he stuffs rue in his nose to block out their foul smell. ■

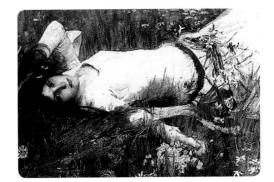

Ophelia by John William Waterhouse (1889). In Hamlet, Ophelia collects an assortment of flowers, handing out the blossoms most suited to various characters. She saves some rue for herself, wearing it as a symbol of regret and grief.

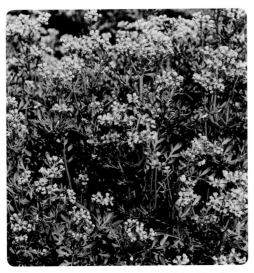

In midsummer, rue blooms in clusters of bright yellow flowers amid foliage that has a strong, pungent scent when bruised.

in recipes from *Apicius de re Coquinaria,* and they are still a part of Ethiopian cuisine. Rue is also an important flavoring in Middle Eastern and Mediterranean cooking. In Northern Italy and Croatia, rue lends a special taste to the liquor called *grappa* or *raki.* When a sprig of the herb appears in the bottle, it is known as *grappa alla ruta.*

Medical science now cautions that eating rue can be toxic to humans in moderate-to-large quantities, although some cooks still use very small amounts. In spite of the plant's reputation for bitterness, young leaves are tasty. Older leaves can be salted to remove the bitterness.

Healing Properties

Rue was once believed to enhance creativity and eyesight, and both Michelangelo and Leonardo da Vinci reputedly ate regular servings of the leaves. Rue had the power to promote the onset of menstruation and stimulates uterine contractions, and, since the time of the Romans, it was sometimes employed to induce abortions. The herb does contain pilocarpine, which induces abortion in horses.

Modern-day healers use rue for treating insomnia, headaches, nervousness, abdominal cramps, and renal troubles. The plant has sedative qualities and rue oil is a commonly used homeopathic medicine for treatment of joint pain and eczema and psoriasis. Rue possibly possesses antiviral properties when combined with certain other herbs. In Brazil, rue is mixed with caramelized sugar and honey to use as an herbal cough syrup.

History and Lore

» Even though the legendary basilisk's breath could crack stone and wilt plants, it had no effect on rue. Weasels bitten by the beast were said to eat rue to counteract the poison.

» In a deck of playing cards, the symbol for the clubs suit is said to be the trefoil leaves of rue.

» At one time, a brush of rue was used to sprinkle holy water during a Roman Catholic High Mass, resulting in one of the herb's common names, herb of grace.

» Rue is the national herb of Lithuania. Often referred to in folk songs, it is associated with young girls, maidenhood, and virginity. It is also popular in the folk music and poetry of Ukraine.

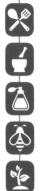

Spikenard

Nardostachys jatamansi

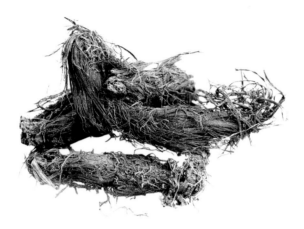

Spikenard, also known as nard, nardin, and muskroot, is a time-honored aromatic that was used to create incense and perfume as well as in the medicinal and culinary arts throughout Asia and Europe. The Egyptians so valued spikenard's anointing oils, they kept them in treasuries along with blue lotus, frankincense, and myrrh, and they guarded them as closely as they would gold.

A native of the Himalayan regions of Nepal, China, and India, this perennial plant is a member of the Valerian family, Valerianaceae. The common name comes from the Latin *spica* and *nardi,* meaning "grain" and "ointment." Spikenard can reach three feet in height and produces green, lanceolate leaves, and pink, bell-shaped flowers that form dense terminal clusters atop sturdy stems. The plant's underground rhizomes are dried and crushed, and then steam-distilled to make a thick, amber essential oil that is highly fragrant.

Aromatic Qualities

The spikenard rhizome possesses a woody, musky, sweet-spicy scent and has been used for millennia as a source of perfume and incense. It was the main ingredient of the Roman perfume *nardinum,* a word derived from the Hebrew *nerd.*

DID YOU KNOW?
Known as nard in the Bible, spikenard has long been valued for the rich, musk scent of its essential oils.

Spikenard was part of the Hebrew *Ketoret,* or consecrated incense offering, made at a special incense altar in the First and Second Temples in Jerusalem.

In the New Testament Book of John, after Jesus arrives in Bethany, Mary, the sister of Lazurus, anoints his feet with a whole pint of nard, causing Judas to grumble that the valuable unguent might better have been sold and the moneys given to the poor. In the Book of Mark, an unnamed woman breaks open an alabaster jar of nard and lets it wash over Jesus' head.

In Homer's *Iliad,* the herb was used by Achilles to perfume the body of Patroklos. In his *Natural History,* Pliny lists 12 species of "nard," including lavender, tuberous valerian, and the true spikenard of today, *Nardostachys jatamansi.*

Although its popularity as a medicinal plant has waned, spikenard is still used in aromatherapy to create a deep state of mediation, increase sensuality, and heighten awareness of touch. Occultists believe the scent of spikenard carries a very high vibration, which enables a deep connection to the spiritual self, and encourages emotional reconciliation and forgiveness, especially prior to death. They call it the "herb of the student," in part because it increases mental clarity.

Easing the Queasy Stomach

Spikenard's mildly sedative qualities means that an external application of the herb in a carrier oil can calm an unsettled, nervous, or churning stomach. Rubbing spikenard oil onto the stomach in a clockwise motion can ease heartburn or nausea. Inhaling the scent from a diffuser can also reduce the tension that creates nervous indigestion. Alternately, one drop of the oil can be ingested at the end of a meal. The oil is useful as a laxative, as well, again by massaging it in a clockwise motion around the lower abdomen. This method can also relieve menstrual cramping. ■

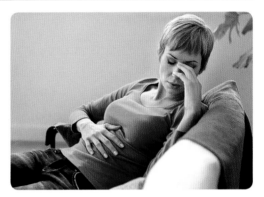

Massage the abdomen with spikenard oil in a clockwise direction to ease menstrual cramps or to alleviate nausea.

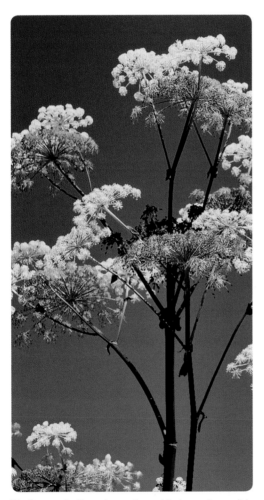

The flowers of spikenard range from white to rose to purplish, growing in dense, lacy clusters. It is not the flowers, however that are used to produce spikenard's amber-colored essential oil. The plant's rhizomes are extremely aromatic, and when they are uprooted, their warm scent will fill the air.

Culinary Uses

The ancient Romans were fond of ground spikenard root as a spice. It is frequently listed as an ingredient in the recipes collected in the cookery manuscript *Apicius* from the late fourth or early fifth century A.D., though it recommends using it in small amounts only. It was a popular seasoning during the medieval period in both European and Arabic cultures. In Europe, it was mixed with other herbs to flavor *hypocras,* a sweet, spicy wine drink, and, starting in the 17th century, the herb was used to prepare a strong beer called stingo.

Healing Properties

Spikenard was part of ancient Greek medicine and Ayurvedic tradition and has been used for thousands of years to treat insomnia, birthing difficulties, migraine headaches, tension headaches, and skin complaints. It has powers of rejuvenation when applied to the face as a wrinkle cream, smoothing out and rehydrating mature skin, and it can also cool and calm inflammations due to allergic reactions.

History and Lore

» The coat of arms of Argentina-born Pope Francis includes a spikenard flower in reference to St. Joseph, the patron saint of the Universal Church, who is depicted in Hispanic iconography holding spikenard.

» American spikenard, *Aralia racemosa,* is a rhizomatous, shrubby perennial of the ginseng family, and no relation to Indian spikenard.

Spikenard

193

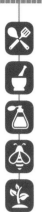

Sweet Woodruff

Galium odoratum

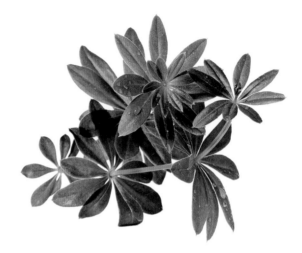

This attractive, fragrant, mat-forming herb is a member of the Rubiaceae family and has a history as an aromatic, medicinal, and culinary herb. Sweet woodruff loves the shade and will thrive in herb or rock gardens, naturalized areas, shady borders, or as ground cover or an edging plant. The plants rarely reach more than a foot in height and produce whorled, dark green, lanceolate leaves and tiny, white, star-shaped blossoms in April and May. These flowers are hermaphroditic, meaning that they can pollinate themselves, although they do also attract bees and butterflies.

DID YOU KNOW?

As its name suggests, sweet woodruff is valued as a pleasant aromatic herb, whose dried leaves give off a fresh scent.

The herb's common name comes from an Old English term meaning "wood that unravels," possibly in reference to the creeping habit of the roots. Now known as *Galium odoratum*, its former scientific name, *Asperula odorata,* comes from the Latin word *asper,* or "rough," referring to the texture of the leaves.

During the Middle Ages, the herb lent its sweet aroma to church interiors on holy days and to the linen stores, floors, and mattresses of stately homes. The leaves were brought indoors to act as air fresheners, and they were scattered on the floors of sick rooms and root cellars to keep the air from growing dank. Sweet woodruff's leaves were also used to produce a pale brown dye, while the roots were used to produce a reddish dye similar to madder.

Aromatic Qualities

Sweet woodruff has been valued for centuries for its aromatic qualities. Although the fresh foliage has little scent, when the leaves are dried and crushed, they emit the odor of freshly mown hay or peach blossoms. This scent arises from the chemical compound coumarin, which has a powerful affect on the brain. Not surprisingly, the plant has been used commercially in perfumes.

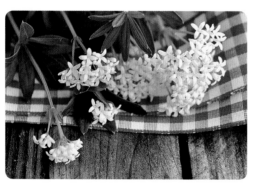

Sweet woodruff is sometimes called wild baby's breath because of its delicate white flowers. The specific epithet *odoratum* describes sweet woodruff's aromatic leaves.

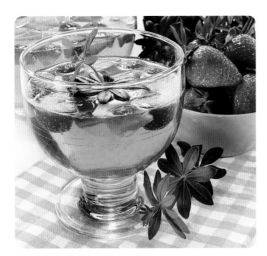

The arrival of summer, especially in Germany, has long been marked by the drinking of May wine. Sweet woodruff is the herbal base for a mix of sparkling wines. Strawberries, which are in season at the same time, are often floated in the drink.

Sweet woodruff is also ideal for adding to linen closets and bed linens. When dried, its aroma intensifies, and the scent can last for years. To make sachets or potpourris, it's best to harvest the plants right after they bloom. The branches should be tied into bunches and hung in a warm, dark place to dry.

This plant has a history as an insect repellent; its active ingredient, coumarin, also wards off moths and kills fleas. Muslins bags of the dried herb can be placed in drawers, closets, pantries, and cellars, or the dried leaves can be sprinkled directly on windowsills and doorsills.

Culinary Uses

The herb's taste was said to remind some people of vanilla, and the leaves were used to flavor teas and cold fruit drinks, as well as to prepare May wine, a warm-weather punch made from white wine flavored with woodruff and fruit. The Food and Drug Administration no longer considers it safe to ingest sweet woodruff, however, unless it is taken in an alcoholic beverage.

Healing Properties

This herb has been prescribed by healers as a sedative and to treat liver problems such as jaundice. As a tea, it was used to treat stomach disorders, while a poultice made from the crushed leaves eased headaches and promoted the healing of wounds, varicose veins, and hemorrhoids.

Celebrate Summer with May Wine

In the ancient Celtic calendar, May 1—called May Day or Beltain—is regarded as the first day of summer. This return to life and fertility is celebrated by dancing around the Maypole, eating oatcakes, and drinking May wine.

Ingredients
- ½ cup dried sweet woodruff leaves
- 1 bottle Riesling white wine
- 1 bottle of German sparkling white wine or champagne
- ¾ cup chopped strawberries
- pinch of fresh sweet woodruff for garnish

Directions

Infuse the dried herbs in the white wine bottle for an hour, then strain. Poured infused wine into a large pitcher, and slowly add sparkling wine. Add strawberries and a large pinch of sweet woodruff and stir slightly. Serve with oatcakes, shortbread, vegetable quiche, or smoked salmon. ■

History and Lore

» In Germany the herb is referred to as *Waldmeister* meaning "master of the woods."
» Other names for sweet woodruff are herb walter, kiss-me-quick, Our Lady's lace, sweet scented bedstraw, and wood rove
» Pillows scented with sweet woodruff sachets were said to ward of nightmares.
» The powdered leaves of sweet woodruff were once mixed with fancy snuffs because their scent lasted so long.

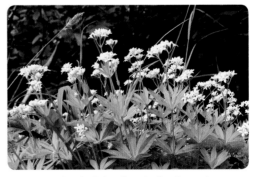

With its graceful whorled spokes of pointed green leaves framing clusters of white flowers, sweet woodruff makes an attractive ground cover for shady areas with moist soil.

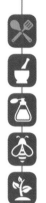

Tansy

Tanacetum vulgare

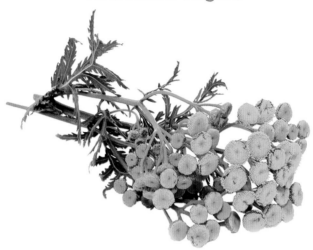

Tansy is an is upright herb with a crown of bright yellow clustering flowers. It is a member of the Asteraceae family and is also known as common tansy, bitter buttons, cow bitter, mugwort, and golden buttons. It grows to a height of three feet and produces pinnate, lance-shaped leaves that are uniformly toothed. Its button-shaped flowers sit atop erect, reddish stems.

Native to Europe and Asia—and of possible Asian origin—the plant was likely first cultivated as a medicinal herb by the Greeks. In the eighth century, it grew in the herb gardens of

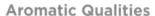

DID YOU KNOW?

With buttons of bright flowers, tansy makes a lively garden display, and its camphor scent also makes it an organic insect repellent.

Charlemagne and at the Abbey of Saint Gall in present-day Switzerland, now a UNESCO World Heritage Site. At that time, it was used to treat worms, digestive issues, rheumatism, fevers, sores, and to cause the eruption of measles. In the Middle Ages, high doses were administered to induce abortions, while lower doses were thought to encourage conception. During the Catholic Lenten season, tansy was served with meals to replicate the bitter herbs eaten by the Israelites. By the 16th century, the British considered tansy "necessary for a garden."

Aromatic Qualities

The oddly agreeable scent of tansy is similar to that of camphor, with some hints of rosemary. It is used as an ingredient in some expensive perfumes. It was also long used in embalming; it would be packed into coffins and wrapped in winding sheets to ward off worms.

Its medicinal benefits may be in question, but tansy still offers a major boon to humans—it is a powerful insect repellent. At one time, farmers

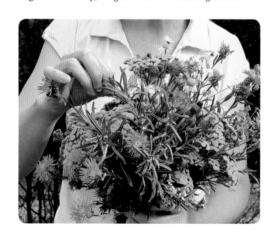

Although once part of the herbalist's pharmacopoeia, tansy is no longer considered safe, and it is best to limit its use to decorative fresh-cut bouquets or dried-flower arrangements.

planted tansy in valuable orchards to keep away aphids and other destructive insects. In England, tansy was hung in windows to keep out flies and placed in bedding to repel moths and fleas.

Culinary Uses

Even though Europeans used tansy as a seasoning from the Middle Ages on, we now know that the leaves and flowers can be dangerous if consumed in large quantities. The herb's volatile oil contains toxic compounds, including thujone, and ingesting too much tansy can cause convulsions and liver and brain damage. The flower extract is still used as a flavor corrective by the liquor industry.

Healing Properties

Tansy had a centuries-long run as a medicinal herb and was valued by herbal healers of many nations. During the Middle Ages, a bitter tea made with the flowers was used to treat parasitic worm infestations. In the 15th century, Christians regularly ate tansy cakes during the Lenten season because it was believed that the heavy diet of fish during that season could cause

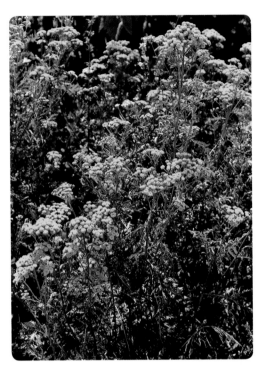

Tansy in bloom makes for a cheerful sight. It can also help keep flies, ants, rodents, and other pests out of your garden. Be careful with this hardy grower, though; in many places, tansy is considered a noxious or invasive weed.

intestinal worms. Tansy was also used for treating migraine, neuralgia, and rheumatism.

Recent research has shown, however, that due to the presence of thujone, this herb can be dangerous to ingest in any but the smallest quantities.

Tansy has also been used to repel human pests like flies, midges, and mosquitoes, and a 2008 Swedish study showed that tansy oil had a 64 percent effectiveness rate at repelling ticks.

As a companion planting, it has many uses—tansy can repel the Colorado potato beetle, sometimes reducing the population by as much as 60 percent, and it keeps destructive pests away from cucumbers and squash, as well as roses and some berries.

History and Lore

» Nineteenth-century Irish folklore insisted that bathing in a solution of tansy and salts would cure joint pain.

» Some beekeepers use dried tansy as fuel in their smokers.

» During the English Restoration, a "tansy" was a sweet omelet flavored with tansy juice.

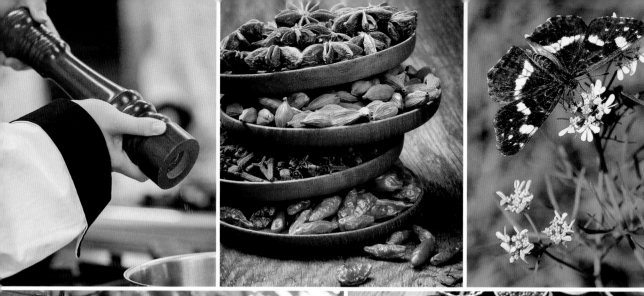

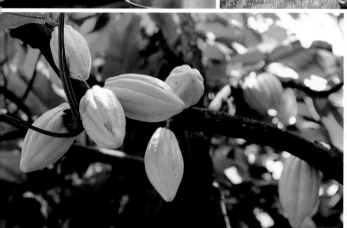

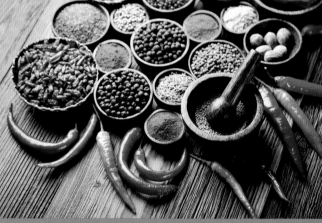

SPICES

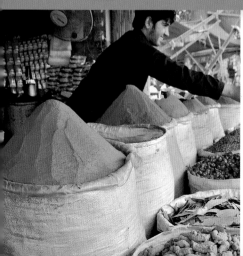

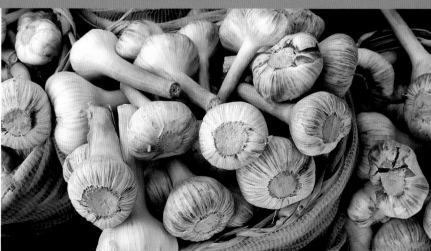

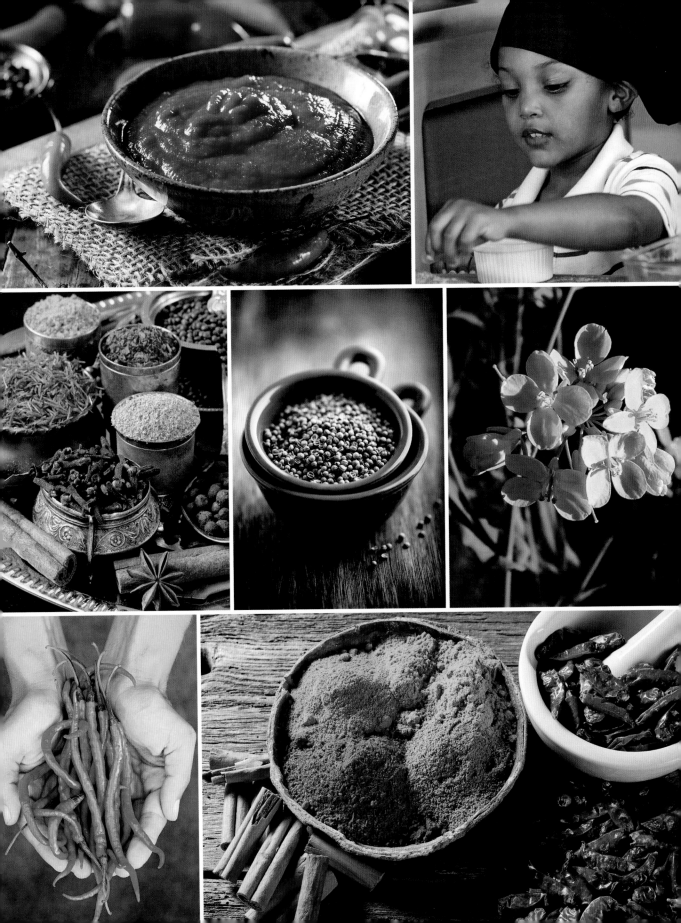

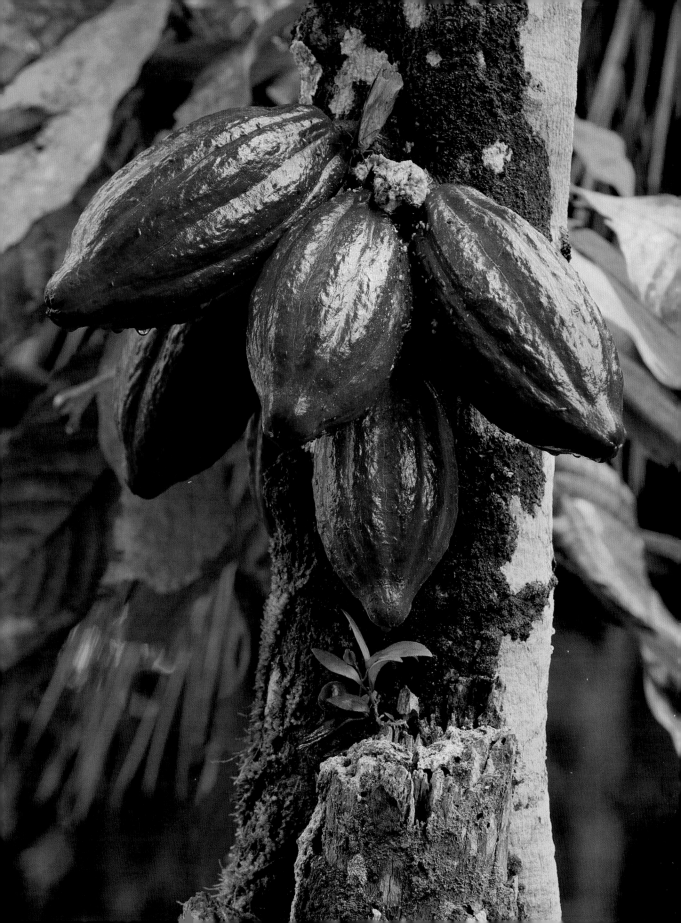

CHAPTER FOUR

SWEET SPICES

Opposite: Cacao tree

Tastes of Warmth and Comfort

ELEVATING DESSERTS WITH DELECTABLE FLAVORS

The sweet spices are the culinary province of French and Austrian pastry chefs, of Scandinavian and German bakers, of moms at Thanksgiving, and of grandmothers at Christmas. Conversely, they are often the surprise kick that makes the savory dishes of Mexico, the Mediterranean, the Middle East, India, and Asia so memorable.

These complex, flavorful spices naturally lend themselves to the preparation of desserts, candies, and other confections. And from Biblical times through to the Renaissance, they remained carefully guarded treasures in the strongholds of emperors, kings, and nobles—common folk could simply not afford such luxuries.

LIFE WITHOUT CHOCOLATE?

It's hard to credit, but two of the planet's favorite flavors—chocolate and vanilla—were unknown to the Old World until explorers unlocked the culinary secrets of the Americas in the 1500s. Although Christopher Columbus had been seeking spice routes, the Spanish conquistadors who followed were unabashedly seeking gold. Yet, they stumbled across something nearly as valuable—unknown, delectable spices, including vanilla, cacao, and allspice, as well as piquant cayenne pepper—around which agricultural empires grew and over which wars were fought.

As travel to the Far East—a long arduous journey by caravan or ship—became safer, and with the opening of the New World, traders introduced a whole range of novel flavors to the Old. Sweet spices once only spoken of with yearning, were now within the reach of many. Soon, even humble families could afford to purchase a nutmeg for grating on eggnog or a few sticks of cinnamon.

According to archeological findings, some of the earliest

Cinnamon sticks with (from left to right) vanilla beans, cloves, and nutmeg

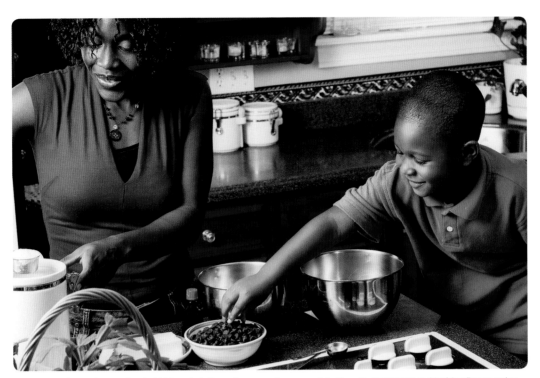

Sweet spices have a long and varied history, but, these days, we often appreciate them for their warm and inviting flavors, using spiced baked goods to commemorate happy events. Sharing their preparation (and the results) is part of the spirit of celebration.

sweet spices used by humans include aniseed, which predates ancient Egypt and was used in cooking, medicine, and perfumery; cinnamon, a seasoning used by early Egyptians for embalming and by Moses as an anointing oil; sesame seeds, flavoring food for five thousand years; carob, which survived the most recent ice age, has been grown around the Mediterranean for more than four thousand years; cardamom, used by the pharaohs to cleanse their teeth; star anise, a decorative dessert spice for three millennia; and fragrant ginger, a "gift from the gods" that has served as a garnish, medicine, and aphrodisiac since 1000 B.C.

> ## "All you need is love. But a little chocolate now and then doesn't hurt."
>
> —*Charles M. Schulz*

SWEET MEDICINE

For all their tasty delights, these sweet spices were not just frivolities to be used for desserts—they were valuable additions to the healer's art in the early cultures of the Egyptians, Israelites, Greeks, Romans, Chinese, Japanese, Aztecs, Incas, and Native Americans. Among the most prized of the sweet medicinal spices were cinnamon, a warming expectorant used to loosen congestion; cloves, high in antioxidants and good for easing gas and bloating; aniseed, used by Romans to relieve heartburn after lavish feasts; and ginger, an effective cure for nausea, indigestion, respiratory ailments, and colds.

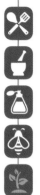

Allspice
Pimenta dioica

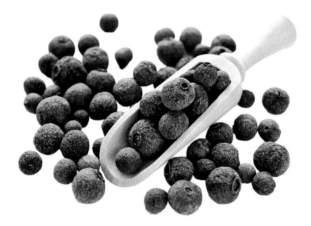

E nglish cooks of the early 1600s named this versatile seasoning allspice because its taste is a blend of cinnamon, nutmeg, and cloves with a hint of juniper and peppercorn. Allspice is also called Jamaica pepper, myrtle pepper, *kurundu, pimienta, pimento,* English pepper, and newspice. It comes from the dried, unripened fruit of the *Pimenta dioica,* a slow-growing evergreen tree. A native of the rain forests of the Greater Antilles, southern Mexico, and Honduras, the tree is now cultivated in many warm regions of the world. Jamaica currently exports the majority of allspice for consumption.

DID YOU KNOW?

The berry-like fruit of the evergreen allspice tree has a complex flavor that tastes like a rich blend of many spices.

A member of the Myrtaceae, or myrtle family, the allspice is a medium-sized tree that reaches from 20 to 40 feet in height. It is similar in appearance to the bay laurel tree, and its glossy, aromatic leaves can be used in the same manner as those of bay leaves. The allspice tree produces small white flowers, which in turn produce rough, reddish brown berries that are slightly larger than peppercorns and contain two seeds. The berries are harvested when they reach full size—but before they ripen and lose their flavor.

This is the only spice grown exclusively in the Western Hemisphere. More than two thousand years ago, the Maya employed it as an embalming agent, and they and other Mesoamerican and South American tribes also used it to flavor chocolate. Columbus came across it growing in Jamaica and, never having seen *Piper nigrum,* thought he was bringing back real pepper to Spain. There it got the name *pimienta,* Spanish for "pepper." The native Arawaks of the Caribbean used allspice to cure meat and the preserved result was called *boucan* in their language. Settlers who cured meat the same way were called *boucaneers,* which later became the word *buccaneer*—a synonym for pirate.

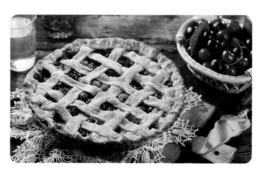

Spiced Cherry Pie. Warm spices like allspice and cinnamon lend flavorful depth to stone fruit pie recipes, turning a summertime favorite into a perfect fall or winter dessert.

Culinary Uses

Allspice is a hallmark of Caribbean cooking, used to make Jamaican jerk seasoning, mole sauce, and pickles, as well as a West Indian liqueur called *pimento dram*. In Middle Eastern cooking, it flavors meat pies and stews. The Poles call it *kubaba* and use it in soups and pickling. It makes a tangy seasoning for beef, pork, lamb, game, soups, and stews, as well as beets, cabbage, carrots, grains, onions, pumpkin, spinach, squash, sweet potatoes, tomatoes, and turnips. It is also included in commercial sausage and curry powders, as well as many barbecue sauce recipes. The famous French liqueurs Benedictine and Chartreuse also contain allspice.

In America, allspice is almost always used in desserts—pumpkin pie, stone fruit pies, applesauce, fruit compotes, cakes, and cookies, and for flavoring hot punches such as mulled cider and Christmas wassail.

Allspice can be purchased as berries for home grinding or already ground. If a recipe calls for allspice, you can substitute a half teaspoon ground cinnamon and a half teaspoon ground cloves for a teaspoon of ground allspice, or you can use ground cinnamon, cloves, and nutmeg in equal amounts.

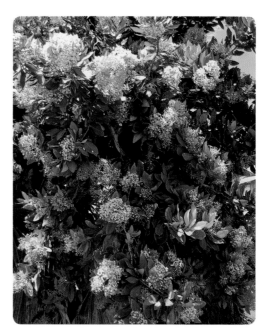

An allspice tree in full bloom. It may not flower outside its native range, but it makes a great small container tree, with attractive, aromatic foliage and whitish gray bark.

Medicinal Properties

The volatile oils found in the spice contain eugenol, which is a mild antimicrobial. Natural healers have prescribed it for treating stomach disorders and as a deodorant. Eugenol oil is also used as an anesthetic for toothaches.

History and Lore

» *P. dioica* was named by Dr. Diego Alvarez Chanca, a member of Columbus's crew, on his second expedition to the New World.
» The aroma of allspice, a rich mixture of cinnamon, cloves, and nutmeg, makes it perfect as a simmering potpourri.
» During the Napoleonic War of 1812, Russian soldiers put allspice in their boots to keep their feet warm—and banish odor. Since that time, allspice oil has been used in the scent and cosmetic industries for men's toiletries, especially anything with "spice" in its name.
» When walking sticks made of allspice shoots became the vogue in the late 1800s, Jamaica's allspice trees became threatened.
» The plant is propagated across the Caribbean and South America from seeds dropped by flying birds, but they are fertile only after they have passed through the avian gut.

Winter Wassail Punch

Flavored with allspice, this cheery hot libation is sure to please guests during the cold winter months. This recipe will yield 18 to 22 servings.

Ingredients
- 6 cups red wine
- 8 cups apple cider
- ½ cup packed brown sugar
- 2 teaspoons whole allspice
- 2 teaspoons whole cloves
- 6 orange slices, studded with cloves
- 3 cinnamon sticks, each about 3 inches long

Directions
In a large saucepan, bring wine, cider, sugar, and spices to a boil. Reduce heat, cover, and simmer for a minimum of 20 minutes. Strain into a glass punch bowl, and float orange slices on top. Garnish with sticks of cinnamon, if desired. ■

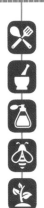

Aniseed

Pimpinella anisum

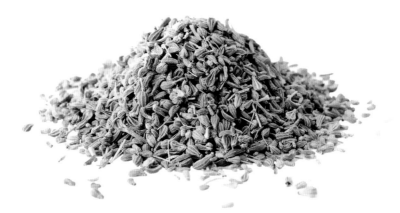

Anise, or aniseed, is best known for its licorice-like flavor, which can be mild or bold, sweet or savory. It has a long history, predating ancient Egypt, as a spice, fragrance, and natural cure.

This semi-hardy annual plant is a member of the parsley family, Apiaceae, related to caraway, dill, cumin, and fennel. It is native to the eastern Mediterranean region, Egypt, and the Near East, but now can be found worldwide.

The anise plant typically reaches two feet in height, with lobed leaves at the base and feathery, pinnate leaves along the stem. The tiny

> **DID YOU KNOW?**
>
> Anise, a member of the dill family, is prized for the flavor of its seeds, which are reminiscent of fennel, star anise, and licorice.

yellow-white flowers form dense umbels and produce small, oblong fruit that ripen to a gray-brown when ready for harvesting.

Culinary Uses

Aniseed, either whole or ground, possesses a licorice flavor that is sweet, aromatic, warm, and fruity. It has been enjoyed in baked goods, meat dishes, and confections from the days of ancient Egypt, Greece, and Rome up to modern times. Aniseed provides the flavoring for black jelly beans—it is often added to candy in place of licorice—as well as international cookies like Italian *pizzelle;* Australian humbugs; British aniseed balls; Mexican *bizcochitos;* Netherland *muisjes;* and German *Pfeffernüsse* and *Springerle.* It is also responsible for the heady taste and aroma of many liqueurs, including French absinthe, anisette, and pastis; Greek ouzo; Italian sambuca; Colombian *aguardiente;* Middle Eastern *arak;* Mexican *Xtabentún;* and German Jägermeister. Aniseed might also be one of the mysterious "secret" ingredients in French Chartreuse.

In Indian cuisine, the spice punches up the flavor of soups and fish dishes, while the whole seeds are eaten, like fennel, as a digestif. Italians and Germans add the seeds to bread and

Aniseed adds flavor to the traditional Italian waffle cookies called *pizzelle.* These crisp treats are popular during Easter and Christmas and are often served at Italian weddings.

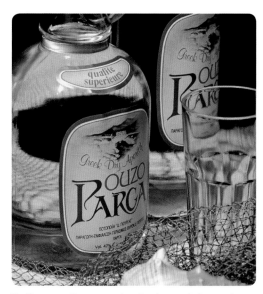

Mediterranean liqueurs, such as Greek ouzo, Italian sambuca, and French pastis, get their licorice-like taste from aniseed.

gingerbread dough. In Mediterranean cuisine, aniseed is often used in bakery items: cakes, cookies, and sweet rolls. It also adds a savory touch to sausage, tomato sauce, and pickles, and it enhances chicken, duck, and veal. The leaves can also be snipped off and used in salads or sprinkled over vegetable dishes.

The source of the spice's distinct flavor is a component of the essential oil called anethole, a phytoestrogen, which is found in both anise and an unrelated spice called star anise *(Illicum verum)*. Nutritionally, the seeds supply high levels of essential B-complex vitamins such as pyridoxine, niacin, riboflavin, and thiamin, as well as minerals like calcium, iron, copper, potassium, manganese, zinc, and magnesium.

CULTURAL CONNECTIONS

Roman Feasts to Wedding Cakes

Because anise was known to be a powerful digestive aid, the Romans served aniseed cakes, called *mustaceoe,* at the end of celebratory banquets. This practice of eating cake after a celebration eventually led to the preparation of a special cake for a wedding. The Romans, furthermore, broke bread over a new wife's head to bring bounty and good fortune to the couple; this also possibly influenced the tradition of serving wedding cakes— which are now a booming industry. ■

Healing Properties

Early Egyptian medical texts detail the use of anise as a diuretic and as a treatment for digestive issues and toothache. The Greeks took it to relieve pain and breathing problems and to ease thirst. In Rome, Pythagoras advised its use to ward off epileptic seizures, and Pliny recommended it for insomnia and halitosis. In the 1500s, herbalist John Gerard wrote: "the seed . . . consumeth winde . . . alaieth gripings of the belly . . . and stirrith up bodily lust."

Today, aniseed is employed as an expectorant and to decrease bloating and settle the digestive tract, especially in pediatric applications. Natural healers use it in higher doses as an antispasmodic and antiseptic to treat coughs, asthma, and bronchitis. The oil has also been effective against scabies, lice, and psoriasis.

History and Lore

» Romans paid taxes with anise and hung anise plants near their pillows to prevent bad dreams.
» In 13th-century England, a tax on anise paid for repairs to London Bridge.
» Anise serves as a food plant for the larvae of some Lepidoptera species, including the lime-speck pug and wormwood pug.
» Anise nectar is a favorite of bees, and when they won't feed on their sugar syrup, beekeepers add a few drops of anise oil to encourage them.

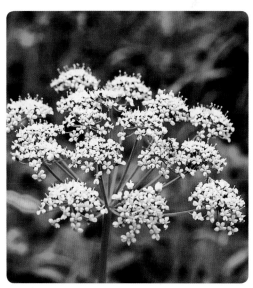

Anise, sometimes called sweet Alice, produces flowers typical of the Apiaceae: clusters of tiny blossoms on a hollow stem.

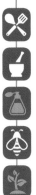

Cacao

Theobroma cacao

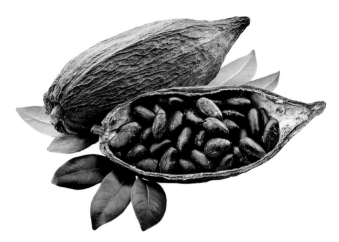

Few things are as universally popular as the rich, complex substance known as chocolate. Raw chocolate is processed from a seed, or bean, that grows on the cacao, or cocoa, tree. These delicate evergreen trees, members of the mallow family, Malvaceae, are native to the tropical forests of Central and South America. The trees reach between 15 and 25 feet in height, with alternate, unlobed leaves, and small whitish pink flowers that bloom up against the trunk in a manner known as cauliflory. The

DID YOU KNOW?

The cacao tree or cocoa tree is a small evergreen, which produces large seed-filled fruit. These seeds, known as cacao beans, are processed to create chocolate.

flowers are pollinated by tiny flies, *Forcipomyia* midges, and mature into ovoid, orange pods that contain from 20 to 60 seeds and can weigh a pound or more.

The tree's genus name, *Theobroma,* comes from the Greek *theos,* "god," and *broma,* "food," or "food of the gods." The species name, *cacao,* comes from the Meso-american word *kakaw,* or from the Aztec *xocoatl,* perhaps meaning "bitter water." Cultivation first took place some time around 1900 B.C., an estimate based on vessels found with the residue of cacao beverages in them.

Culinary Uses

Cacao beans, like coffee beans, display differences in taste depending on where they are grown. The three main varieties are *forastero,* hardy and prolific, with a strong flavor; *criollo,* complex but delicate and hard to grow; and *trinitario,* a hybrid of the two that occurred in Trinidad when *forastero* was introduced to the island's *criollo* crop. After the pods are harvested, the beans and pulp are removed and left to ferment for a week, so that yeast and gases can break down the sugars and proteins. The beans are then roasted and ground by a melangeur, huge granite rollers that produce

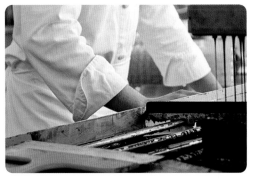

An artisan at work in a chocolate factory. Cacao beans must be processed and worked until they form a smooth mass. With the addition of cocoa butter or other fats and sugar, it will become the sweet chocolate that most of us love.

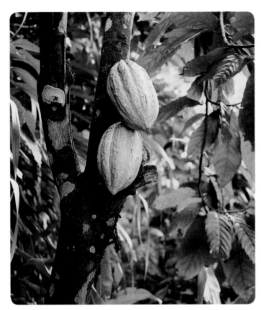

Unripened cacao fruits on the tree. The seeds are the main ingredient of chocolate. The fruit's pulp is often discarded, but in some countries it is used to prepare beverages.

a paste called mass. The mass is then pressed and split into solids and butter. Next comes conching, developed by Swiss chocolatier Rodolphe Lindt, the constant grinding and blending of chocolate until it is a smooth liquid. Finally comes tempering, heating the cocoa butter crystals to exactly the right size so they result in the smooth, hard finish chocolate lovers crave.

Modern cooks use cocoa powder to flavor cakes, cookies, puddings, ice cream, and candy. But this cornucopia of confections is not the way early Mesoamericans enjoyed chocolate—they consumed it as a hot frothy beverage seasoned with ground chili peppers. The Europeans were the first to add sugar and milk to the beverage, and much later chocolatiers like Henri Nestlé and Milton Hershey turned the sale of chocolate bars into candy empires.

Healing Properties

Cacao is considered a "superfood," containing more than 300 nutrients as well as phytonutrients and flavonoids. From the time it was first imported to Europe in the 16th century, it was prescribed for fever, heart ailments, kidney and liver disease, tuberculosis, anemia, and gout. More recently, research indicates that the antioxidant flavonoids in very dark chocolate can decrease the risk of heart disease, lower blood pressure, and reduce inflammation.

It is not a myth that chocolate makes people feel better, especially after suffering emotional distress—cocoa powder has mood-elevating qualities due to its theobromine, caffeine, and other compounds (including one similar to the chemical in marijuana) that create feelings of alertness and euphoria.

History and Lore

» In pre-Columbian Mesoamerica, cacao beans provided both a ceremonial beverage and a system of currency.

» Milton Hershey helped make chocolate a treat for the masses—at the turn of the 20th century, a Hershey's chocolate bar cost only a few cents.

» While most Americans consume up to 12 pounds of chocolate every year, the Swiss consume a hefty 22 pounds on average.

» Today, most of the world's cacao is exported from West Africa, especially the Côte d'Ivoire.

Chocolate is easily molded into shapes, such as the Easter bunnies that have become part of many festive springtime celebrations.

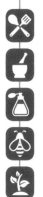

Cardamom

Elettaria cardamomum, Amomum spp.

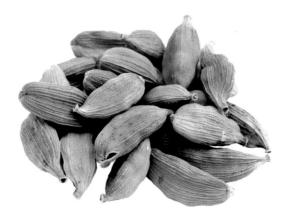

ardamom is certainly one of the world's oldest spices: ancient Egyptians chewed it to cleanse their teeth, the Greeks and Romans wore it as a perfume, and Viking traders who voyaged to Constantinople (Istanbul) introduced it to Northern Europe. The distinctive flavor of this spice still defines much of Scandinavian cuisine.

There are two main types of cardamom: green and black. When a recipe calls for cardamom. it usually refers to *Elettaria cardamomum*, the green version, which is, by weight, one of the most valuable of all spices. Fortunately, a little goes a long way, tastewise. The seeds of

black cardamom (*Amomum subulatum* and *A. costatum*) are large and strong, and they bestow a smoky, piney, camphor-like flavor.

Cardamom is native to the forests of the western ghats of southern India, where it can still be found. The plant, a member of the ginger family, reaches a height of ten feet or more and produces large leaves and white flowers tinged with pink, orange, and yellow. These blooms mature into pods that contain three rows of small, dark brown, sticky seeds. The plant also produces vast, fleshy rhizomes.

Culinary Uses

Green cardamom (shown above) has a cool, spicy-sweet taste, but it can also be included in savory dishes. While the Scandinavians use it to flavor sweet breads, like holiday *julekake* and Finnish *pulla*, in Arab countries, it is also added to strong coffee and to rice pilaf. Indian cuisine includes cardamom in curries and desserts, and in the beverage masala chai.

Green cardamom pairs well with fish, shellfish, chicken, duck, lentils, meat, peas, and squash. It adds complexity to baked goods—cakes, cookies, and stollens, and makes a delicious addition to mulled wine and other spiced drinks.

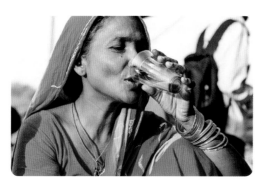

Indian masala chai. Cardamom is the dominant flavor note in this milky tea, now sold in coffee houses around the world.

Exotic Asian Potpourri

This warm, heady mixture with a hint of spicy sweetness is perfect for filling sachets, sleep pillows, or potpourri bowls throughout your home.

Ingredients
- ¼ cup cardamom seeds or flowers
- ¼ cup saffron seeds
- ½ cup small chunks dried sandalwood
- ½ cup cinnamon sticks in pieces
- ¼ cup anise flowers
- ¼ cup orange peel
- ½ cup lavender flowers, seeds, and leaves
- 20 drops jasmine essential oil

Directions
Make sure all plant ingredients are dry; if not, place on a tray in a sunny window for several days. Combine botanical ingredients in a large bowl, mixing lightly, then add the jasmine oil. Place all ingredients in a brown bag and close up tightly. Store the bag in a cool, dark spot for at least two weeks, gently shaking up the mixture occasionally. After two weeks, spoon the mixture into sachets, pillows, or bowls. ■

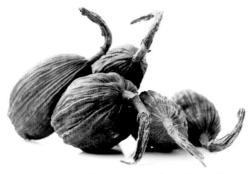

Black cardamom is dried over an open fire. Its intense flavor works well in recipes that call for slow-cooking.

In contrast to the green variety, black cardamon is considered a warm spice, and it is a bit brasher compared to its cousin. It is used to create bold savory dishes in Indian, Szechuan, and Vietnamese cooking. Mixed with coriander seeds, black pepper, cloves, and cinnamon, it forms the popular Indian blend garam masala, which literally means "warming mixture." It also makes an excellent grilling rub or marinade.

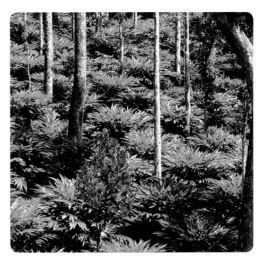

A field of green cardamom. This plant is widely cultivated in tropical regions, such as Indochina and Central America.

For maximum taste, purchase whole pods and grind the seeds at home. The seeds can also be lightly crushed and toasted before adding to recipes. Nutritionally, cardamom contains the minerals calcium, sulfur, and phosphorus.

Healing Properties

Cardamom oil has been used by Eastern cultures for centuries to treat digestive discomfort. Research confirms that the essential oil acts as an analgesic and an antispasmodic in rats and rabbits. Natural healers prescribe the oil for treating bad breath, tooth or gum pain, indigestion, and urinary problems. Two phytochemicals found in the seeds, IC3 and DIM, are also known to ward off hormone-responding cancers.

Aromatic Qualities

Green cardamom possesses a warm fragrance, like lemony eucalyptus with a little camphor. In aromatherapy, cardamom oils can be added to the bath to combat depression and reduce stress. Tea made from the ground seeds has similar benefits.

History and Lore
» According to folk herbalists, cardamom lends us wisdom when we are overburdened with responsibilities and encourages generosity in our dealings with others.
» Guatemala is the largest exporter of the spice, followed by India.

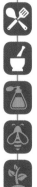

Carob

Ceratonia siliqua

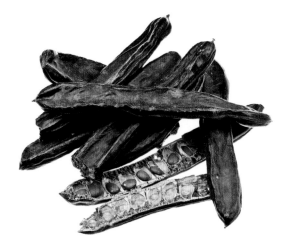

Best known nowadays as a low-fat, high-fiber, caffeine-free substitute for cocoa powder, carob has a long history in its own right as a food source and medicine. Also known as the carob tree, St. John's-bread, and locust bean, carob is a flowering evergreen in the pea, or legume, family, Fabaceae. It is native to the Mediterranean, North Africa, and the Middle East, where it has been farmed for more than four thousand years. The plant does well in harsh climates and poor soil and can now be found in many warm regions, including Florida and the American Southwest.

DID YOU KNOW?

A flowering evergreen, carob produces podlike legumes that, when dried, produce a sweet powder or syrup that is used in desserts, often as a chocolate substitute.

The word *carob* comes from Middle French *carobe,* taken from the Arabic *kharrūb,* or "locust bean pod." The ancient Greeks planted the trees both at home and in Italy. In the 1500s, Spaniards transported carob to Mexico and South America, while the British planted it in South Africa, India, and Australia.

Carobs are dioecious, having male or female trees, although some do produce hermaphroditic flowers. They can reach a height of 50 feet and feature glossy, leathery, dark green leaves and small orange or yellow flowers that form catkin-like racemes. After 8 to 15 years, carobs produce reddish brown foot-long fruit—or pods. These can take a full year to ripen and are the source of the pulp from which the carob powder is made. The seeds are considered inedible.

Culinary Uses

Carob's taste is sweet and mild, and it has a pleasing, earthy undertone. Besides hot beverages, it can be used to make cookies, cakes, brownies, candies, and puddings. It is delicious mixed into pancakes and muffin batter or sprinkled over ice cream, rice pudding, and espresso. Carob is also used to flavor herbal teas and intense artisanal brews such as stout.

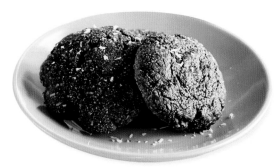

Carob coconut cookies. This plant product is a favorite with vegans because it lends itself to dairy-free baking and can also be used in raw recipes. Another bonus: it's caffeine free.

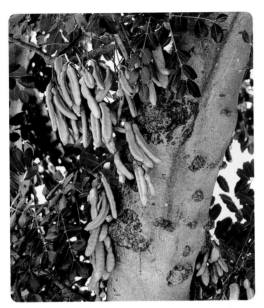

A carob tree produces masses of green legumes that when ripened and dried can be ground into a powdery spice.

When using carob in place of cocoa powder, the substitution ratio is 1:1. Remember to reduce the sugar—carob is naturally sweeter than cocoa. For a richer taste, use half cocoa, half carob.

During processing, carob pods are milled to separate the seeds from the pulp. The seeds are made into locust bean gum. This gum is used in the manufacture of confectionery items and can be employed as a stabilizer, emulsifier, and thickener, and to prevent sugar from crystallizing.

Healing Properties

Early healers used a decoction of carob leaves and bark for treating syphilis and other venereal diseases and epilepsy. Modern researchers have learned that the tannins in carob contain gallic acid, which works as an antiallergenic, analgesic, antibacterial, antioxidant, antiviral, and antiseptic substance. Carob can be used to soothe upset stomachs, help with nausea, and halt diarrhea. One tablespoon of carob powder in a cup of liquid is the recommended dosage.

Unlike cocoa, carob does not contain any caffeine or theobromine, another mild stimulant found in coffee. It contains no cholesterol, is high in protein, and is a great source of pectin, a soluble fiber. It supplies vitamin A and E, the B vitamins, and several important minerals, including three times the calcium of cocoa.

Worth Its Weight in Gold

Ceratonia siliqua, the scientific name for the carob tree, derives from the Greek word *kerátion,* from *keras* for "horn" and the Latin *siliqua* for "pod." Because traders in the Middle East weighed diamonds and other gems against the uniform seeds of the carob, merchants began to refer to the mass of a precious stone in carats. One carat was eventually fixed as 0.2 grams. In Roman times, a pure gold coin called the solidus weighed in at 24 carats (roughly 4.5 grams) and as a result, carats also became the standard measure for gold purity. Pure gold was 24 carat, while an alloy containing only 50 percent gold was 12 carat. ■

History and Lore

» Carob is an ancient species that survived the most recent ice age. It is actually a shrub that is trained into tree form by pruning.

» Carob gained the name St. John's-bread or locust bean because the pods were once believed to have been the "locusts" eaten by John the Baptist while in the wilderness. Bible scholars now believe he ate actual migratory locusts.

» Mohammed's army ate *kharoub*; Arabs planted the crop in northern Africa, while the Moors brought carob to Spain, along with citrus trees and olives.

» Carob was commercially introduced into the United States in 1854. Typically, plants with the finest fruit are bud grafted onto common stock.

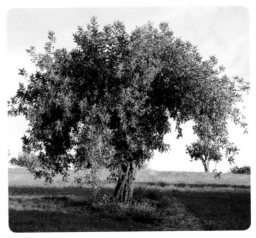

Though only of medium height, the carob is a lushly spreading tree. In some parts of the Mediterranean, it still grows wild.

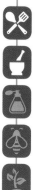

Cinnamon

Cinnamomum spp.

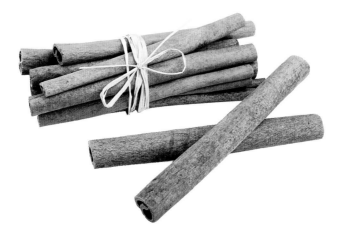

Cinnamon dates back to at least 2000 B.C. In Egypt, it was valued as a seasoning, as a medicine, and as a tool in the embalming art. Today, it is found in recipes around the world, in both sweet and savory dishes, and medical science has only begun to uncover its healing potential.

There are two main species of cinnamon: *Cinnamomum verum,* called Ceylon cinnamon, is considered the real or true cinnamon. *Cinnamomum aromaticum,* called cassia or Chinese cinnamon, originated in southern China and is less costly. The spice's botanical name comes from the Hebraic and Arabic term *amomon,* which means "fragrant spice plant."

Cinnamon was originally harvested from wild trees native to the Caribbean, South America, and Southeast Asia. This

DID YOU KNOW?
A favorite spice in cookery around the world, cinnamon is obtained from the inner bark of several trees from the genus *Cinnamomum.*

evergreen member of the laurel family, Lauraceae, produces thick oval leaves and bisexual yellow or green flowers on panicles, which are pollinated by tiny insects. Although mature trees can reach 60 feet in height, two-year-old trees are coppiced, which means that they are cut down to a few feet and covered in soil. This encourages them to spread out and become bushy. It is from these shoots that cinnamon is harvested—the inner bark is stripped and set out in the sun where it dries into curls, or quills.

Culinary Uses

Many cultures long valued cinnamon for its sweet, warm flavor and ability to preserve meat, due to its phenol content, which inhibits bacteria. The spice's strong aroma also obscured the smell of spoiled foods. Colonial Americans used cinnamon sticks as a digestive aid and to flavor or "mull" cider. In modern kitchens, ground cinnamon is used in baked goods, stewed fruits, vegetables, spiced teas, mincemeat, and coffees, and for preserves and pickling.

Ceylon cinnamon, the original spice, has a taste all its own—not as intense or sweet as cassia but warm and earthy,

Cinnamon is a favorite spice for breakfast treats and desserts, such as snickerdoodles. These rich cinnamon-sugar cookies are a holiday classic, with chewy middles and crisp edges.

214

The Spice of Control and Conflict

In the 1600s, while the Dutch were in control of Ceylon—a major source of cinnamon—they coerced a coastal Indian king to destroy his own cinnamon trees to preserve their monopoly on the spice. England then won the island in 1795 after ousting the Dutch, but by 1833, their cinnamon empire ended, after competing countries discovered that the trees would thrive in Java, Sumatra, Borneo, Mauritius, Réunion, and Guyana. Today, the spice is also grown in South America, the West Indies, and other tropical regions. ■

with notes of citrus and vanilla. Because it is more subtle, Ceylon cinnamon should be used in dishes where it is the featured flavor, such as cinnamon ice cream or crème brûlée.

Healing Properties

From ancient times, cinnamon was employed throughout Asia and the Mediterranean to treat coughs, arthritis, sore throats, and colds, and to aid circulation and digestion. Europeans of the Middle Ages considered it a cure-all, although its actual source remained something of a mystery to them. More recently, it has been used to treat muscle spasms, vomiting, diarrhea, loss of appetite, bacterial and fungal infections, cognition problems, and sexual dysfunction.

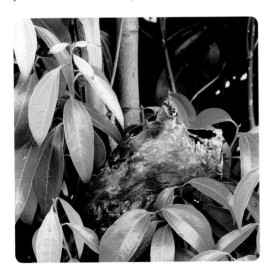

Cinnamon's thick oval leaves resemble those of other laurels. When harvesting the spice, workers allow stacked layers of the peeled bark to curl into "quills," or cinnamon sticks.

Modern research proves that the spice deserves its reputation—early studies indicates its ability to lower blood sugar in both type 1 and type 2 diabetes, while researchers at Tel Aviv University have found that an extract in the bark, CEppt, may inhibit the onset of Alzheimer's disease. Rush University Medical Center believes that cinnamon may halt the process of multiple sclerosis, and a study in India revealed that extracts of *C. aromaticum* have been effective against HIV. Cassia contains cinnamaldehyde—useful for fighting bacterial and fungal infections.

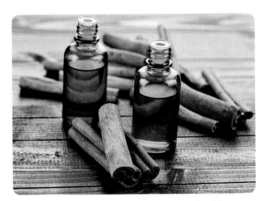

In aromatherapy, the essential oil of cinnamon is said to heighten spiritual vibrations and stimulate the senses, encouraging confidence and generosity.

Aromatic Qualities

Cinnamon, with its warm, spicy scent, has been used for millennia to process perfumes and sacred anointing oils. Powdered cinnamon was an ingredient of *kyphi,* a favorite Egyptian ceremonial incense, and it has long been a popular aphrodisiac in India and Europe.

History and Lore

» As a sign of remorse after murdering his wife, Poppaea Sabina, Roman emperor Nero ordered a year's supply of cinnamon to be burnt.

» This spice was so prized by Romans that it was used as currency. Pliny wrote of it being worth 15 times more than silver.

» Italians call cinnamon *canella,* or "little tube"— from the word for cannon—based on the shape of the quills.

» The phoenix bird of legend reputedly built its nest from cinnamon and cassia.

» In the Victorian language of flowers, cinnamon says: "My fortune is yours."

Cinnamon

215

RAISE YOUR GLASS!

Savor the many liqueurs flavored with spices and herbs.

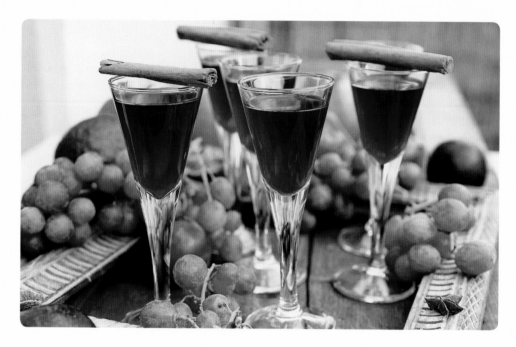

In many cultures around the world, people enjoy sipping a sweet alcoholic cordial after a large meal or simply while relaxing at a café or bar. These cordials—called liqueurs—are made from flavored distilled spirits and are bottled with the addition of sugar or high-fructose corn syrup.

What Is a Liqueur?

Liqueurs often contain less alcohol than liquor—most liqueurs range between 15 and 30 percent alcohol by volume, although some go as high as 55 percent. Flavors can be gained by infusing woods, fruits, herbs, spices, or flowers in water or alcohol, or by distilling aromatic agents. Although most liqueurs are not aged like other spirits, they are given time for the often complex flavors to blend. Typically sweet and syrupy, liqueurs are often served as or with the dessert course.

A Long History

Culinary historians believe that liqueurs evolved from early herbal medicines. They are documented as far back as the 13th century in Italy and frequently originated in societies of monks. In Germany, Kräuterlikör, a medicinal liquor made with spices or herbs and sugar, traces its lineage to the Middle Ages and is still produced today. As trade routes opened up over the centuries, a wider variety of spices—like ginger and chocolate—became available to distillers, resulting in a new array of flavors.

A World Tour of Flavorful Liqueurs

Liqueurs are popular just about everywhere in the world. Below is a sampling of the many herb- or spice-based liqueurs produced around the globe. Naturally, their distillers jealously guard the recipes for these commercial liqueurs, which contain complex blends of herbs, spices, and various other flavorings.

- **Anisette** (Mediterranean): Variations of this popular anise-flavored drink (which contains no licorice) is produced in Italy, Spain, Portugal, France, and Turkey

- **Bénédictine** (France): Promoted as the product of an old Benedictine abbey, this liqueur was created by Alexander Le Grand in the 19th century. Its secret recipe, known only to three people at a time, contains 27 plants and spices.

- **Campari** (Italy): This cherry-red mainstay of the Italian café scene is made of bitter and aromatic herbs, plants, and fruit.

- **Chartreuse** (France): This distinctive liqueur gave its name to a yellow-green color and has been made by Carthusian Monks since 1737. It contains an astonishing mix of more than 130 herbal extracts.

- **Drambuie** (Scotland): This whisky-based liqueur is made with Scotch, heather honey, herbs, and spices.

- **Galliano** (Italy): This sweet, woodsy liqueur is distilled from more than 30 botanicals, including vanilla, star anise, ginger, citrus, juniper, musk yarrow, and lavender.

- **Goldschläger** (Switzerland): This liqueur is flavored with cinnamon and contains flakes of real gold leaf. Danzig Goldwasser was the Polish forebear of this gold-flecked liqueur.

- **Irish Mist** (Ireland): The makers of the Emerald Isle's first liqueur began production in the 1940s using a thousand-year-old recipe for heather wine, which is a blend of aged Irish whiskey, heather and clover honey, aromatic herbs, and other spirits.

- **Jägermeister** (Germany): Popular with the bar shots crowd, this throat-warming liqueur is made from a blend of 56 herbs, including licorice, anise, poppy seeds, saffron, ginger, juniper berries, and ginseng.

- **Kümmel** (Russia): This Russian cordial, which hails from the 16th century, contains caraway seed, cumin, and fennel.

- **Mead** (Worldwide): Mead is created by fermenting honey with water and adding in various herbs, fruits, and spices.

- **Metaxa** (Greece): This brown spirit is a blend of wine distillates, Muscat wines, and an undisclosed combination of rose petals and Mediterranean herbs.

- **Pastis Ricard** (France): A south of France favorite, pastis is made by a process called maceration, combining aniseed and licorice.

- **Pernod** (France): After the banning of absinthe, French beverage distiller Pernod Ricard began producing the anise-based Pernod Anise.

- **Sambuca** (Italy): This popular after-dinner cordial is flavored with the essential oils of anise, star anise, and licorice, as well as elderflower (in Latin *sambucus);* it is sold in white, red, and black varieties.

- **Sorel** (Caribbean): A bright scarlet, hibiscus-infused liqueur, sorel is spiced with clove, cassia, ginger, and nutmeg.

- **Southern Comfort** (USA): This American favorite is a potent liqueur made from neutral grain spirits combined with whisky, peaches, oranges, and various spices.

- **Strega** (Italy): This potable yellow "witch" is formulated from more than 70 herbs and spices, including mint, saffron, and fennel and is drunk after dinner. ▪

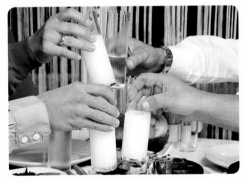

Drinkers who imbibe aniseed-based spirits such as pastis and sambuca often add water to dilute the thick syrupy liqueurs, which then causes the clear liquid to become opaque.

Cloves

Syzygium aromaticum

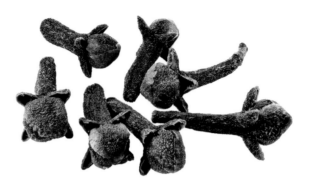

This diminutive spice has been prized as a flavoring and healing agent for more than two thousand years. Arab traders first introduced cloves to Europe around the fourth century, but they were not widely used until the Middle Ages, when their robust flavor made them valuable for covering up the taste of poorly preserved foods.

Cloves are actually the unopened flower buds of the clove tree, which are dried until they are brown and hard and resemble small tacks. The tree, an evergreen member of the Myrtaceae family, can reach 25 or 40 feet in height and produces large, glossy green leaves and creamy flowers in terminal clusters. Once established, the tree can bear buds for a century.

Clove trees were once exclusively found in the Maluku Islands, formerly the Spice Islands, of Indonesia. Today, they are also commercially cultivated

in Zanzibar, Sri Lanka, Madagascar, the West Indies, India, Pemba Island, and Brazil. More than a thousand tons of cloves are imported to the United States alone each year.

Culinary Uses

Cloves, with their sweet, earthy taste are key elements in classic spice blends used around the world—Chinese five spice, Indian garam masala, Moroccan *ras el hanout,* and French *quatre épices.* They flavor meats, curries, and marinades and complement fruit, puddings, cookies, and pies. In Mexican cooking, cloves are often combined with cumin and cinnamon.

Cloves make bland recipes come alive. An onion pierced with cloves adds tang to soups. Ground cloves and curry powder included in stir-fry recipes give them an instant Indian pop. Cloves add pleasing heat to applesauce, cider, and chai tea. They lend a savory boost to turkey stuffing when combined with walnuts and raisins. Cloves have an intense flavor, so they should be added sparingly. Whole cloves hold their flavor better than powdered ones and can be ground at home in a coffee grinder. Place them in water to check their quality—fresh cloves will float vertically, stale ones will float horizontally.

A branch of the clove tree with the ripening buds. Nutritionally, the buds contain more manganese than almost any other food. They are a good source of vitamin K, dietary fiber, iron, magnesium, and calcium.

Healing Properties

Cloves were used medicinally by early Roman, Indian, and Chinese civilizations. Modern natural healers often call cloves the "super spice"—in part because their antioxidants have a staggering ORAC (oxygen radical absorbance capacity) of more than 290,000, higher than any other therapeutic-grade oil. They also offer antiviral, anti-inflammatory, and antibacterial qualities and might be able to prevent adult-onset diabetes by stabilizing blood sugar. Eugenol, the spice's main constituent, combines with its other components to create a mild anesthetic, which made it especially beneficial in dentistry—during root canal therapy and for gum or toothache pain.

The essential oil of cloves is irritating to the skin and should be handled with caution.

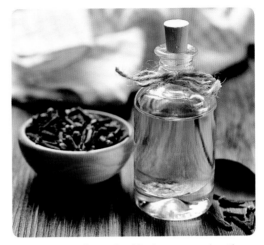

The essential oil of cloves is said to have memory-boosting properties. Oil of cloves is often used in dentistry to numb the gums, and aromatherapists use it as a mood enhancer.

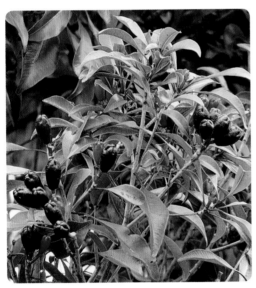

The fruits of the clove tree are elongated red berries. The tree's glossy, leathery green leaves are highly aromatic.

Aromatic Qualities

The scent of cloves is both spicy and sweet with additional hot and fruity notes. It was once believed that inhaling the fragrance would improve eyesight and fend off the plague. In modern aromatherapy, benefits include comforting the spirit, stimulating the mind, and lifting depression. The dried flower buds energize incense mixtures and increase their scent.

History and Lore

» Dating back to 200 B.C., Chinese courtiers would place cloves in their mouths before addressing the emperor in order to keep their breath fresh and not offend him.

» Cloves were said to be part of the "Marseilles vinegar" or "four thieves vinegar" used by grave-robbers to protect themselves during the plague in the 15th century.

» Cloves are used in a type of Indonesian cigarette called *kretek*.

MAKE IT YOURSELF

Orange-and-Clove Pomander

During the Middle Ages, it was common for city dwellers to carry a pomander, a round container with herbs inside, to combat the noisome odors of the refuse-cluttered urban streets. These pungent herbal scents were thought to ward off airborne diseases like the plague. Pomanders could also be hung in closets to discourage moths and other fiber-destroying insects.

An aromatic pomander ball to scent a room or drawer is easy to create with a container of cloves and a large, naval orange. Simply press the cloves into the orange in a pleasing pattern by using a thimble. As the orange dries out from within, the scent of cloves and orange peel will mingle for a year or longer. ∎

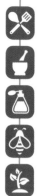

Ginger

Zingiber officinale

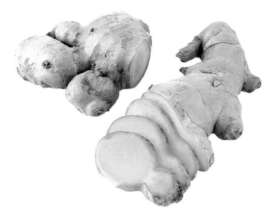

The power of ginger cannot be underestimated. The plant was of such value to early cultures—as a seasoning, medicine, and spiritual tonic—that it was referred to as a gift from the gods. The Koran describes ginger as a beverage of the "holiest heavenly spirits." In the kitchen, pungent ginger was a vital ingredient in many Asian dishes as well as in European bakery classics like gingerbread and ginger snaps. Medicinally, ginger has been employed as far back as 3000 B.C. to relieve gastric distress and as an aphrodisiac.

DID YOU KNOW?

Considered both a spice and a medicine, ginger is the rhizome of the plant *Zingiber officinale.* This versatile root is suitable for flavoring main dishes as well as desserts.

Ginger originated in Southeast Asia before naturalizing in China, India, and the Middle East. Wherever it was cultivated, it became a significant economic commodity, often resulting in great wealth for those who grew it. One of the first Asian spices introduced to Europe via India—possibly as early as the first century A.D.—by the Middle Ages, a pound of ginger was worth an entire sheep. Today's top producers include Jamaica, India, Fiji, Indonesia, and Australia.

This reedlike, perennial plant grows to three or four feet in height with leafy stems topped with clusters of pinkish buds that produce showy yellow flowers. The flesh of the rhizome, the source of the spice, can be white, yellow, or red. The plant's genus name come from the Sanskrit term *singabera,* or "horn shaped," referring to the rhizome.

Culinary Uses

Ginger comes from the same family as turmeric and cardamom, Zingiberaceae, but it has a distinctive taste—brisk and peppery. A versatile spice that once had a place on every European dinner table, like salt and pepper, it has become synonymous with Asian cuisine and is widely used in Arabic and Indian cooking as well.

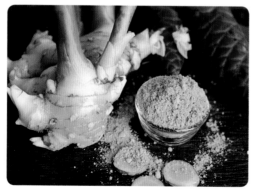

Ginger, in it many forms, has long been used by healers to calm the digestive tract. The juice from the roots also contains fragrant volatile oils that give ginger its distinctive tang.

Candied Ginger

Ginger makes a spicy confection—known as candied, crystallized, or glace ginger. Peel one pound of fresh ginger and slice it into one-eighth segments. Simmer in water over medium heat until tender. Keep a quarter of the cooking water. Weigh ginger and measure out an equal weight of granulated sugar. Place ginger and sugar in remaining water and heat until sugar syrup appears to recrystallize. Spread pieces out on cooling rack sprayed with nonstick spray. Once cool, transfer to airtight container. Keeps for two weeks. ■

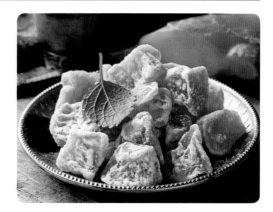

Ginger comes in several forms: fresh, dried, crushed, and powdered. Fresh ginger, the least potent, is peeled, and then sliced or grated. Dried ginger slices have a strong taste and keep well. They are used in soup stocks and curries. Crushed ginger provides the pungent taste of fresh ginger without the prep work and it is a mainstay of Asian cuisine. Tangy ginger powder is most often used in baking—for ginger snaps, gingerbread, pies, and muffins. It is typically added to Indian spice blends, Asian stir fry, pickling brine, mulled wine, and ginger ale.

Healing Properties

Chinese healers employed ginger to treat toothaches, colds and flu, and hangovers, while the Japanese found it relieved aching joints. In Europe, it was used as protection against the plague during the Black Death. Early 20th-century American physicians prescribed it for painful menstruation. But it is the rhizome's effectiveness as an antispasmodic for calming the digestive tract and expelling gas that it is best known.

Modern research confirms ginger's gut-soothing qualities and its antioxidant and anti-inflammatory effects. The latter is the result of a potent compound called gingerol, which is effective for treating arthritis and rheumatism. Ongoing studies indicate that gingerol might also combat colorectal cancer tumors. Whatever medicinal benefits ginger will reveal in the future, herbalists were in on the secret first—ginger remains a component of more than 50 percent of all traditional herbal remedies.

History and Lore

» A piece of the dried ginger root worn within an amulet is said to strengthen and protect the health of the wearer.

» How well ginger flourishes in a garden supposedly reveals the health of the gardener.

» Fifth-century Chinese sailors used ginger, with its high levels of vitamin C, to prevent scurvy on long voyages.

» In 19th-century England, barkeeps put out containers of ground ginger for customers to sprinkle on their ale—which is the origin of the beverage ginger ale.

» In aromatherapy, ginger's warm and earthy aroma, with a note of camphor, is used to improve digestion, ease headaches and joint pain, stimulate circulation, and break up congestion.

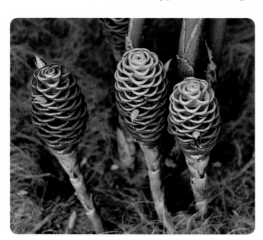

As they mature, the red-tinged buds of the ginger plant will burst into showy yellow flowers. Ginger adapts to many warm climates and, with the tropical foliage and exotic blossoms of some variations, is often used as a landscape or border plant.

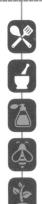

Mace/Nutmeg

Myristica fragans

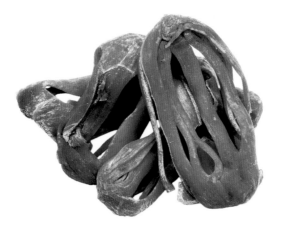

The nutmeg tree produces two distinct spices: nutmeg, the holiday seasoning, is the dried seed, while mace comes from the irregular, waxy, red sheath, or aril, that forms around the seed casing.

The tree is native to the Banda Islands, part of the Maluku Islands, in Indonesia, where spices have been harvested for centuries. This evergreen can reach 40 feet in height and produces large, dark green leaves, and waxy, pale yellow, bell-shaped flowers. Each tree has a specific gender, and even though both genders produce flowers, only the females mature into the fleshy fruit. Once the seed is exposed, the red aril (mace) is removed and left to dry, turning dark and brittle before it is ground. Meanwhile, the kernel, or nutmeg, takes two months to dry inside its shell.

During the Middle Ages, Arab traders sent these spices into the West via Venetian merchants, but carefully obscured their source. When the Portuguese conquered the Maluku Islands in 1511, they, and then the Dutch, tried to keep the trees restricted to two

DID YOU KNOW?

Myristica fragrans, an evergreen tree, is the source of two spices—nutmeg and mace—each with its own distinct flavor and aroma.

islands. By the late 1700s, however, nutmeg trees were growing in Africa and the Caribbean. Today, they are cultivated in many tropical regions.

Culinary Uses

Nutmeg—sweet, spicy, and nutty—is used in cakes, puddings, fruit pies, eggnog, French toast, and wine punch. It also makes a surprisingly tasty addition to savory dishes like stews, cream soups, sauces, pasta, meatballs, and sausage. It is an essential part of béchamel sauce and Greek moussaka, and it blends well with tomatoes, spinach, broccoli, beans, onions, and eggplant. It is used frequently in the cuisine of India, Indonesia, the Middle East, Italy, Holland, and Japan.

Mace is similar to nutmeg, but more delicate. The pale spice is used in custards, potato dishes, and cream sauces to add flavor without darkening them. Whole-blade mace is used in soups, sauces, pickling blends, and wine mulling mixes. Powdered mace is often found in sweet pound cake and doughnuts, as well as savory meatballs and barbecue sauces.

The spice nutmeg (left) is derived from the seed of the *Myristica fragrans* tree, and the lacy reddish orange covering of the seed is sold as the spice mace (above).

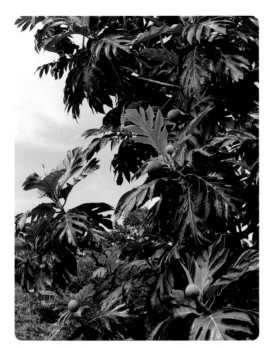

The green fruit of the evergreen nutmeg will turn yellow as it ripens, and then the outer husk will split open to reveal the lacy red covering around the seed inside.

Nutmeg loses flavor when heated, so it should be added at the end of preparation. Nutritionally, the spice is rich in B-complex vitamins, vitamin C, and vitamin A, and also supplies potassium, calcium, iron, and manganese.

Healing Properties

Nutmeg has been valued for centuries for its health benefits—in the Elizabethan era, it was even thought to ward off the plague. Natural healers use it as a sleep aid, as an antibacterial to protect teeth and gums (its eugenol content also alleviates toothache pain), to ease aching joints, to relieve stomach discomfort, and to boost kidney and liver function. A compound in the spice, called myristicin, shields the brain against degenerative conditions. When mixed into a paste with honey, nutmeg can brighten the complexion, heal acne, and reduce facial scars.

Aromatic Qualities

The steam-distilled essential oil of nutmeg is valued by the perfume and pharmaceutical industries as a natural flavoring in baked goods, syrups, beverages, and candies as well as toothpaste and cough syrups.

In aromatherapy, the warm, spicy oil makes an effective rub to relieve indigestion. Simply massage into the abdomen in a clockwise motion. A massage can also improve circulation in cases of arthritis, rheumatism, and gout, and relieve tension and mental fatigue. Potent nutmeg oil should always be used with a carrier oil.

History and Lore

» To keep nutmeg prices artificially high during the 1760s, the Dutch would intentionally burn warehouses full of the spice.
» Sam Slick, the pseudonym of a 19th-century judge and author, whose tales that crooked local peddlers sold carved wooden nutmegs in place of the real thing, may be the source of Connecticut's nickname, the Nutmeg State.
» The myristicin in nutmeg can reputedly make an individual hallucinate; due to this, nutmeg is banned in Saudi Arabia.

CURIOSITIES

Seasoning a Scots Favorite

The Scots are known for their eccentricities, one of which is their devotion to the gray, lumpen Scottish national dish, haggis. Haggis is a simmered meat pudding made of sheep's organs, onions, oatmeal, suet, and spices, including both mace and nutmeg, stuffed into a sausage casing. Food critics lament its unappealing appearance but praise the "nutty texture and delicious savory flavor." Although the dish is associated with Scotland, the first official recipe for "hagese" appeared around 1430 in Lancashire, England. ■

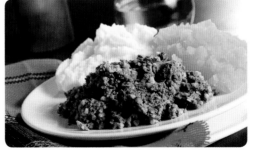

The Scots dish haggis, flavored with nutmeg and mace, is traditionally served removed from its casing with "neeps and tatties"—turnips and potatoes—and a dram of whisky.

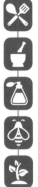

Poppy Seed

Papaver somniferum

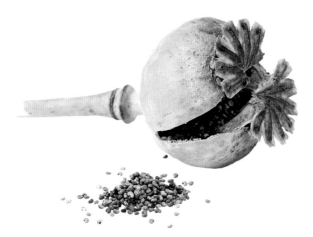

Poppy seeds are nutritious, nut-flavored oilseeds that are used in baking and in natural healing. The seeds are gathered from the dried pods of the opium poppy *(Papaver somniferum)*, a practice that possibly began as far back as six thousand years ago. The Greeks called the sap from the seed pod *opion*, which became the modern word *opium*.

Opium poppies are native to the Middle East, where they were cultivated for their seeds and for opium latex, which is the source of the analgesic and narcotic medicine morphine, as well as its derivative, the highly addictive street drug heroin. (In fact, the Latin name means "sleep-bringing poppy.") Opium has often been at the center of controversy, as in the wars fought between England and China in the mid 1800s,

DID YOU KNOW?

Often known as the opium poppy, *Papaver somniferum* is the source of culinary poppy seeds and poppy seed oil. It is also used medicinally to make opiate drugs such as morphine.

when the Chinese tried to stop Western traders from smuggling opium into their country.

Part of the family Papaveraceae, biennial opium poppies typically reach three feet in height. They produce lobed leaves at the base of long, sturdy stems, and flowers with four white, mauve, or red petals, although many varieties and cultivars appear in other hues. These blossoms develop into cup-shaped pods full of tiny seeds. The cultivation of poppies for seeds is the antithesis of cultivation for opium: seed harvesting requires the pods to dry out, while the pods need to be green and full of latex for extracting opium. The seeds are also pressed into valuable poppy seed oil, which has culinary, industrial, and medicinal applications. Due to its association with illicit drugs, many countries have banned the unregulated cultivation of this flower.

Culinary Uses

Poppy seeds, which have no narcotic effect, can be used whole or ground into a paste. In America, whole black poppy seeds are sprinkled on

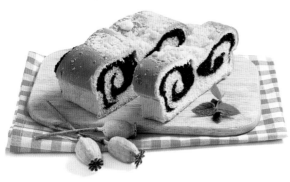

Poppy seed roll. The seed paste is a popular filling for stollens and strudels. The opium poppy is also called the breadseed poppy because of its common use in breads and cakes.

bagels and rolls or baked into muffins. In Eastern Europe, both black and white seeds are used on breads and soft buns. In Germany, they are used in desserts, and, in Poland, they are a featured part of the cuisine. Poppy seed paste—which can be flavored with vanilla, rum, lemon zest, cream, cinnamon, nuts, or raisins—is a popular filling for European strudel and stollen. During the observation of Purim, Jews eat *hamantaschen,* triangular pastries filled with poppy paste. In India, Iran, and Turkey, poppy seeds are known as *khashkhaash* or *haşhaş.*

These seeds are produced all over the world, including the Netherlands, Australia, Romania, and Turkey. Many cooks believe the tastiest seeds are the slate blue ones that come from Holland. Nutritionally, poppy seeds are high in calcium and magnesium and are a good source of iron and vitamin E.

Healing Properties

Poppy seeds were mentioned in Egyptian, Sumerian, and Minoan medical texts dating back thousands of years. Folk healers used them for treating asthma, insomnia, stomach ailments, and bad eyesight, and to promote fertility. Some even believed they bestowed the power of invisibility.

In modern times, medicinal opium—used to create poppy-based drugs called opiates—is produced in Australia (Tasmania), Turkey, and India.

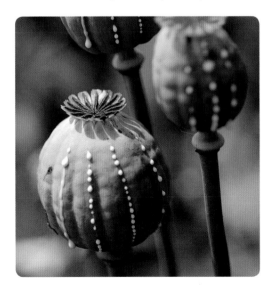

Opium poppy heads exuding latex. The hairless round fruits, called pods, will each yield abundant seeds, and they can also be dried to add interest to a cut-flower arrangement.

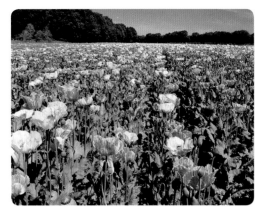

An impressive field of pink and white poppies in bloom. The flowers of opium poppies range from white to deep red, with many subspecies, varieties, and cultivars.

Because they are so addictive, these drugs are primarily reserved for treating extreme pain and for short-term sedation.

History and Lore

» Poppy seeds are miniscule; it takes 3,300 poppy seeds to make up a gram, and one pound contains between one and two million seeds.

» At one time, gold-covered poppy seeds were considered powerful talismans, and wearing them was thought to attract wealth.

» Quite fittingly, the opium poppy appears on the coat of arms of the United Kingdom's Royal College of Anaesthetists.

» In L. Frank Baum's *The Wonderful Wizard of Oz* and the 1939 film version of the novel, Dorothy and her companions must walk through a field of opium poppies, which send her and the Cowardly Lion into a deep sleep.

CURIOSITIES

A Scientific First

The drug morphine was isolated from opium latex in 1804 by German pharmacist Friedrich Sertürner. This is believed to be the first time in history that an alkaloid was isolated from a plant. Sertürner named his discovery morphium, after Morpheus, the Greek god of dreams. He continued to study the effects of the drug, and, around 1815, it finally began to be widely used. Merck started marketing it commercially in 1827. At the time, Merck, now a pharmaceutical giant, was a single chemist's shop in Darmstadt. ∎

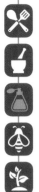

Sesame Seed

Sesamum indicum

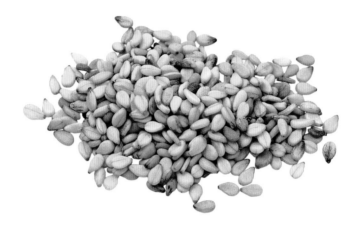

Sesame seed is one of the oldest seasonings known to humankind—it has been grown in the tropics since prehistoric times, and an early Egyptian tomb painting shows a baker adding sesame seeds to bread dough. Sesame was also one of the first crops cultivated for oil—around 3000 B.C., the Chinese burned the oil in lamps and used it to produce soot for ink-block printing. With their nutty flavor and light crunch, sesame seeds are a natural complement to many foods, but they are also known for their medicinal qualities.

DID YOU KNOW?

The flowering sesame plant is cultivated for its edible seeds. With their rich, nutty flavor, these seeds—and the oil made from them—are popular in the cuisine of many nations.

The sesame plant is a tall, annual herb in the Pedaliaceae family. It grows to roughly two to five feet in height and produces broad, opposite leaves and numerous white or pinkish foxglove-type blossoms. As the long, boxlike pods mature, a hundred or more seeds appear inside arranged in rows.

The plant was originally native to the East Indies, including Burma, China, and India. The name *sesame* derives from the Arabic *simsim,* the Coptic *semsem,* and the early Egyptian *semsent.*

Although sesame seeds were familiar to European cooks, they apparently traveled to North America with African slaves—who called them benné seeds—during the late 17th century. Documentation suggests that Thomas Jefferson grew benné seeds in test plots at Monticello. Today, the main commercial exporters of sesame seeds include India, China, Sudan, Ethiopia, and Mexico. Japan, where many recipes call for sesame oil, is the number one importer.

Culinary Uses

For millennia, sesame seeds have been used in baking, meat and vegetable dishes, sauces, dressings, and desserts. Modern cooks add them

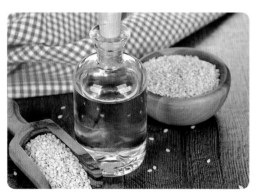

In the practice of aromatherapy, sesame seed oil is one of the most popular carrier oils for diluting herbal essential oils.

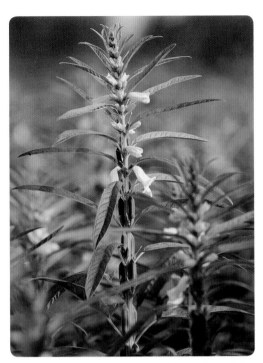
Sesame flowers are white or very pale pink, growing on hairy, single stems. The flowers will become fibrous capsules that each contain eight rows of tiny, flat pointed seeds.

to cakes and muffins, sprinkle them on roasted chicken with soy sauce or on broccoli, and blend them into vinaigrettes.

This staple of Middle Eastern cuisine is made into a paste called tahini sauce, which is used to prepare hummus, as well as the popular confection halvah. It is also found throughout Asian and Indian cooking in seed or paste form. Sesame oil is particularly valuable because it can be stored for long periods without becoming rancid.

Different cultivars of sesame produce seeds in different colors, including white, buff, yellow, black, and red. They can be purchased hulled or unhulled, either prepackaged or loose in bins. Hulled seeds need to be stored in the refrigerator or freezer. Sesame seeds are extremely nutritious, offering impressive levels of copper and manganese, calcium, magnesium, iron, selenium, phosphorus, zinc, vitamin B1, niacin, and fiber.

Healing Properties

Healers have always valued the seeds because they possess both curative and preventative qualities. They were a favorite medicine of Egyptian physicians, while women in ancient Babylon used a mixture of honey and sesame seeds to ensure their youth and beauty. Roman soldiers ate the same mixture—now a favorite sweet in health food stores—to furnish strength and energy.

The seeds contain two unique antioxidant compounds, sesamin and sesamolin, that belong to a group of beneficial fibers known as lignans. These have a cholesterol-lowering effect and can help prevent high blood pressure in humans and increase vitamin E levels in animals. Sesamin may also protect the liver from damage caused by free radicals.

History and Lore

» "Open Sesame!"—the magical command from the tale "Ali Baba and the Forty Thieves"—perhaps relates to the sesame seed pod, which bursts open when it reaches maturity.

» Rugged sesame, called a "survivor crop," will grow in drought conditions, in high heat, or even during monsoon rains. It is often the only thing that farmers can grow in the marginal soil at the edge of deserts.

IN THE KITCHEN

Honey Sesame Peanuts

This easy-to-make and crunchy snack combines two nutty flavors with the sweetness of honey.

Ingredients
- ¼ cup sesame seeds
- ½ cups honey
- 2 cups peanuts
- 2 tablespoons brown sugar

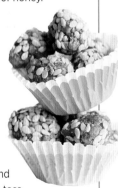

Directions
Preheat oven to 350° F. Line a baking sheet with parchment paper. Place peanuts on the baking sheet and roast for five minutes. Give them a toss, and then roast for another five minutes.

As the peanuts are roasting, melt honey and brown sugar in a small saucepan over medium heat until sugar is dissolved.

Pour honey mixture over nuts, tossing them thoroughly. Sprinkle on the sesame seeds until the peanuts are well coated. Bake for five to ten minutes, remove from oven, and cool completely before storing them in an airtight container. ∎

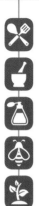

Star Anise

Illicium verum

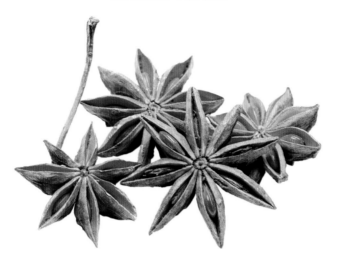

Star anise, with its eight-point snowflake shape and rich mahogany color, is surely one of the most ornamental spices. For more than three thousand years, it has been employed as both a culinary seasoning and a medicine.

Star anise is the fruit of a small evergreen tree in the magnolia family, Schisandraceae, which originated in China and Vietnam. The tree can reach 25 feet in height, and it takes five years to produce small, creamy flowers. It usually starts to bear fruit a year later and can continue to do so for a hundred years. The seed pods are harvested just before ripening and then sun-dried. Both pods and seeds are ground to make the spice.

DID YOU KNOW?

Long used as both a culinary and medicinal spice in Asia, star anise is now coming into its own in the West, adding anise-like flavor to both sweet and savory dishes.

The genus name *Illicium* comes from the from Latin *illicio*, meaning "enticement," referring to the attractive fragrance of these trees. Today, the trees are cultivated in Laos, the Philippines, Indonesia, and Jamaica.

Culinary Uses

Star anise was introduced to Europe in the 17th century and was quickly adopted for baking and to flavor fruit dishes and liquors. Its taste is more robust than Spanish anise, to which it is unrelated, although both spices contain anethole, which gives them their licorice-like flavor. The spice flavors the signature dishes of India, especially biryani, garam masala, and masala chai, and it enriches soup stocks and is part of the five-spice blend in China. In Southeast Asia, it plays a major role in Malay and Indonesian cookery and is a key ingredient in Vietnamese *pho bo* soup.

In the United States, where it is sometimes purchased as a lower-cost alternative to aniseed, star anise is used for baking; in barbecue sauces and meat rubs; to season pork, chicken, and duck; in rice pudding; and even for crafting. The stars are usually finely ground for most recipes; when whole stars are used, they should be discarded before serving.

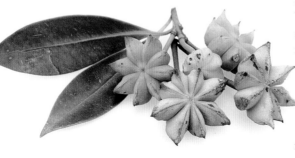

Illicium verum bears star-shaped fruits, which are harvested just before they ripen. They are dried to create star anise spice.

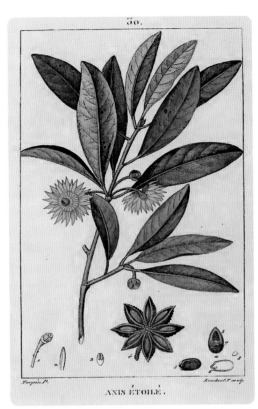

An illustration of star anise from *Köhler's Medicinal Plants,* published by Franz Eugen Köhler in 1887. Its glossy, leathery leaves grow in bunches of three to six.

Healing Properties

Traditional Chinese herbalists utilized star anise as a stimulant and an expectorant and to treat colic in babies and indigestion in adults. European folk healers recommended drinking it as a tea to soothe rheumatism and chewing the seeds as a digestive aid. It was also used to ease the birthing process, increase libido, and relieve menstrual cramping.

Modern medicine has only begun to tap the potential of this spice. Star anise is rich in shikimic acid, a compound that is one of the main ingredients—combined with quercetin—in the antiviral drug Tamiflu, used to fight influenza and bird flu. Extracts of star anise have also shown promise as antifungals, especially against *Candida albicans,* a form of yeast that can infect the mouth and throat and the intestinal and genitourinary tract. In Taiwan, four new antimicrobial compounds made

from star anise were recently found effective against 67 strains of drug-resistant bacteria. The spice, with its antioxidant qualities, has reduced the development of cancer tumors in lab animals. It is sometimes added to other medications to improve their flavor.

Aromatic Qualities

With a scent reminiscent of licorice, fennel, and anise, star anise is used to flavor liqueurs such as Galliano, sambuca, and pastis. In aromatherapy, its essential oil can be inhaled from a diffuser to ease symptoms of bronchitis, colds, and flu.

Studies have shown that the spice is also an effective insecticide against Japanese termites and adult German cockroaches.

History and Lore

» In Mandarin, the spice is known as *ba jiao hui xian,* which means "eight-horned fennel."

» In Chinese folklore, the spice was considered protection against the evil eye, while finding a star anise with more than eight points was considered good luck.

» A related species, Japanese star anise, *Illicium anisatum,* is a tree similar to *I. verum,* but its seeds are highly toxic. It is sometimes used in incense that is burned in temples.

CULTURAL CONNECTIONS

Chinese Five-Spice Blends

Like French cookery, with its numerous herbal combinations, Chinese cuisine also features a special mix that is known as five-spice powder, a piquant blend that offers a sweet counterpoint to meats. As Chinese culture spread to large cities throughout the world, the blend soon became incorporated into local cuisines.

In addition to star anise, the mixture traditionally contains cloves, Chinese cinnamon, black pepper, and fennel seeds. Variations might include anise seed, ginger, nutmeg, turmeric, cardamom pods, licorice, and Mandarin orange peel. Five spice is used as a rub on chicken, duck, pork, or seafood; as a marinade; in "red dish" cooking; and in stews, but more often in restaurants now than in Chinese homes. ■

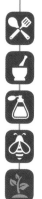

Vanilla

Vanilla spp.

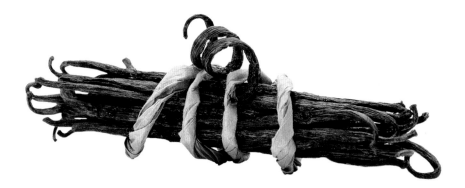

Vanilla is the second-most expensive spice in the world, behind precious saffron, but few tastes and scents are as recognizable—and intoxicating—as that of pure vanilla extract.

Vanilla "beans" are the fruit of a liana of the family Orchidaceae and are native to Central America. Although the white or yellow flowers are hermaphroditic, they need to be pollinated by hummingbirds or *Melipona* bees before maturing into long, green pods. After the ripened pods are harvested, they are "killed"—boiled, frozen, scratched, or sun-dried—to stop vegetative growth. The plant's entire growing environment—climate, soil, support trees or posts—is known as a terroir.

DID YOU KNOW?
Vanilla, a genera of fruit-bearing orchids, is the source of one of the world's classic flavorings.

As a spice of the Americas, vanilla was unknown to the rest of the world until conquistador Hernando Cortés carried it back from Mexico to Spain in the 16th century. Mexico then had a monopoly on its export until the mid-1800s, when growers in countries without *Melipona* bees realized that the plant could be successfully pollinated by hand. The word *vanilla* comes from the Spanish term for "little pod."

Culinary Uses

There are five main regions of cultivation and several different flavor profiles. Madagascar, a major exporter, grows the highest quality spice, *Vanilla planifolia*. Called Bourbon vanilla, it is creamy, sweet, and mellow, and can stand up to rich dishes. India and Indonesia, another export leader, also grow Bourbon vanilla. Mexican vanilla, *V. pompona*, is smooth, dark, and spicy; it goes well with chocolate and cinnamon. Tahitian beans, *V. tahitensis*, are flowery and fruity, with a touch of anise, and are a favorite of pastry chefs.

Today, vanilla is a dessert staple in many countries. It is also the main ingredient used to flavor chocolate. It can be purchased whole, powdered, as an extract—the macerated seeds are mixed with water and alcohol—and as a paste. Those

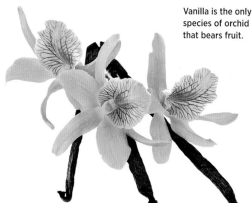

Vanilla is the only species of orchid that bears fruit.

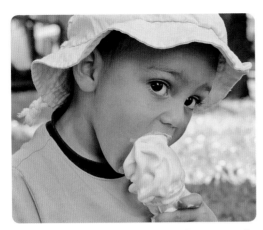

Vanilla routinely tops the list of best-selling ice creams, and the spice is also an ingredient in many other popular flavors.

black flecks in vanilla ice cream are remains of the flavorless seeds. Be aware that roughly 95 percent of vanilla products are artificially flavored with vanillin, which is derived from lignan.

Healing Properties

Vanilla has antioxidant, anticarcinogenic, antidepressant, fever-reducing, and sedative qualities. The Mesoamerican Totonacs, who first cultivated the spice, valued it as a treatment for poisoning, pulmonary diseases, and syphilis. The Aztecs of Mexico prescribed it for hysteria and depression. In 18th-century Europe, it was a nerve stimulant, and 19th-century physicians praised its ability to "exhilarate the brain and increase muscular energy."

The vanilloid it contains has healing properties similar to the capsaicin found in peppers and the eugenol found in cloves. The essential oil can help treat acne, ease symptoms of the flu, and combat morning sickness. Topically, it soothes burns and toothache.

Aromatic Qualities

This distinctive sweet, creamy fragrance is a popular "note" in most perfume mixtures and in many cosmetics. In aromatherapy, vanilla is both a relaxant and a stimulant. One study showed that inhaling the spice allowed seriously ill patients to cope better with stress. The scent also acts as a powerful aphrodisiac.

Vanilla is used as a base for other scents, blending well with the essential oils of orange, lemon, jojoba, chamomile, lavender, and sandalwood.

Treasure of the Totonacs

The Totonacs of Mexico, who lived in the Valley of Mazantla near modern-day Veracruz, first discovered the pleasures of vanilla. According to myth, the goddess Princess Xanat was forbidden to marry her mortal lover. The two fled to the forest, but were captured by her father, who ordered them both beheaded. Where their blood spilled onto the ground, the first vanilla vines grew. After the Aztecs conquered the Totonacs in the 15th century, they offered tribute in the form of vanilla beans instead of gold or corn. When Cortés conquered the Aztecs, he carried the spice to Spain. Soon it became the rage with European nobles, who combined it with cacao to make a delicious beverage. In 1602, Hugh Morgan, apothecary to Queen Elizabeth I, was inspired to use vanilla by itself as a flavoring. The aromatic spice then spread through European kitchens and beyond. ■

History and Lore

» Thomas Jefferson was introduced to vanilla beans while serving as ambassador to France; he is credited with bringing the spice to America.

» In the mid-1800s, Edmond Albius, a 12-year-old slave from Réunion Island, discovered how to speedily pollinate vanilla flowers by hand, opening the way to worldwide cultivation.

» The plant can only grow 10 to 20 degrees north and south of the equator.

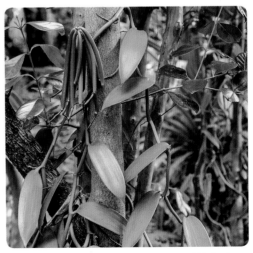

Green vanilla pods. *Vanilla planifolia* is a liana, which is a long-stemmed, woody vine that uses a tree as its vertical support.

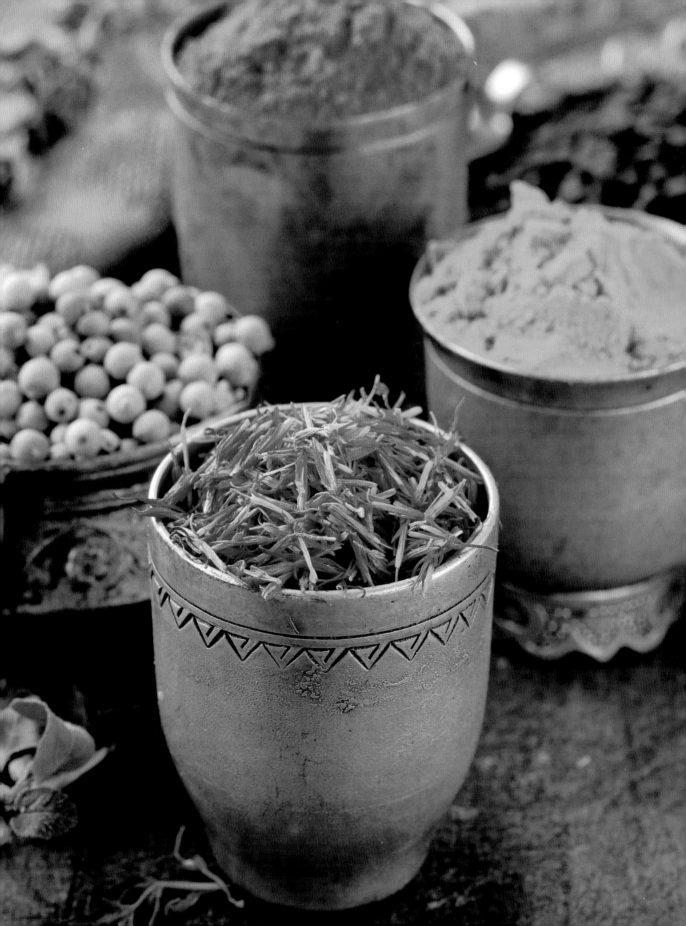

SAVORY SPICES

Opposite: Saffron (front), coriander (left), cayenne (back), and turmeric (right).

Walk on the Wild Side

SOME LIKE IT HOT AND PUNGENT

These are the zesty, fiery, or piquant spices that create what chefs call "complexity" in recipes—the nuanced layering of dissimilar flavors, a blending of two or more of the tastes we crave—sour, sweet, bitter, salty, and savory. These are the spices where a little goes a long way … but where brevity is the soul of a delicious dish.

Savory spices were eagerly sought after by many early cultures, including the Egyptians, Persians, Arabs, Greeks, Romans, Chinese, and Indians, who used them for cooking, healing, and preservation, and, in some cases, as perfumes and dyes. No matter their distant places of origin—the Far East, the Spice Islands, or Africa—these desirable seasonings were destined to journey to the bazaars of the Middle East and the metropolises of the Mediterranean.

ANCIENT FLAVORINGS

Spices that first found their way into the cooking pot were celery seed, revered by the ancient Egyptians and Greeks; coriander, used by Romans to flavor food and

The stigmas of the saffron crocus—the world's most expensive spice

wine; turmeric, the peppery golden spice carried from Asia to Europe by Alexander the Great; and black pepper, with a recorded history of more than four thousand years and bragging rights for consistent usage during every one of those years. Some spices, like saffron, go back to the very start of human culture—saffron pigment was found on fifty-thousand-year-old cave paintings discovered in Iran. Caraway was possibly the first spice used in Europe, based on archeological evidence collected at a Neolithic dwelling in Switzerland.

The early phase of the spice trade reached its peak in the first century A.D., when the demand for spices like black pepper grew exponentially. Spices actually accounted for 44 of the 80 classifications of goods imported to the Mediterranean from Asia and eastern Africa. It was the strategically located Arabs who profited most from the traffic with the Far East, at least until Rome

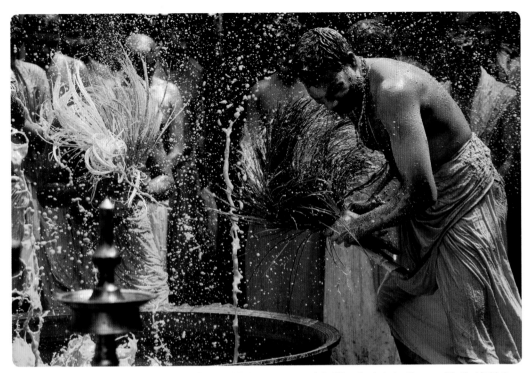

Devotees of the Hindu goddess Amman perform the Manjal Neerattu, a turmeric bathing ritual, during the annual festival held at the Amman temple in Chengannur, Kerala, India. Here, turmeric is not just a culinary spice, but it is also used as a purification agent.

began building ships capable of sailing from the Red Sea all the way to India. The spice markets of that country were soon so depleted that merchants had to import spices from Southeast Asia. Only decades later, the Chinese opened up what was called the Silk Road, carrying silks and spices to Rome, looking to trade for glassware, pottery, coral beads, gems, silver, and wine.

By the Middle Ages, exotic spices were entering gateway ports like Venice and Constantinople and traveling to the courtly halls of Europe. There, they were used to preserve meat, to offer novel flavors to the wealthy, and—in an age with no refrigeration—to disguise the aroma of spoiled food. Grains of paradise traveled up from West Africa, and cayenne pepper arrived from the New World, and both became kitchen favorites, the former as a less expensive substitute for black pepper.

> **"Spices are very hot, very hip. I love spices."**
>
> —*Todd English*

EARLY MEDICINALS

From our earliest history, humans have relied on certain savory spices to treat digestive and respiratory ailments, to heal wounds, and ease pain. Among the medicinals are caraway seeds, used to treat flatulence and indigestion; turmeric, known as an anti-inflammatory and antiseptic; sumac, used to lower fevers; paprika, beneficial to heart and circulatory health; and cayenne pepper, which contains capsaicin, a natural pain reliever for swollen joints and aching muscles.

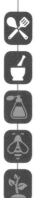

Black Pepper

Piper nigrum

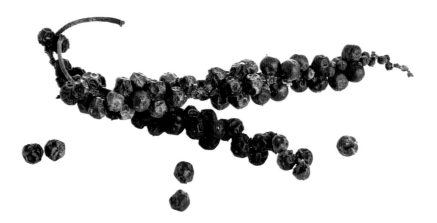

Often referred to as the "master spice" or the "king of spices," black pepper has a long and storied history. It was once used as a form of currency or for payment of ransoms—in the Middle Ages a pound of pepper was worth a pound of gold! It was even presented to the gods as a sacred offering. Native to Kerala, a southwestern state of India, pepper was in such demand throughout the Mediterranean and Europe that expeditions were formed to search for it in the distant Far East, and many merchant cities arose along the trade routes where it traveled.

DID YOU KNOW?

Long considered the "king of spices," black pepper has a host of both culinary and medicinal uses.

The pepper plant is a smooth, woody vine that can reach more than 30 feet in length. At three or four years, the vine produces clusters of small white flowers that mature into red berries called peppercorns. One plant can produce male, female, and bisexual flowers, and pollination is accomplished by rain. Currently, pepper is produced commercially in India and Indonesia.

Black, white, and green peppercorns all come from the same plant. The color variations are due to different times of harvesting and different methods of processing. Black peppercorns are picked half ripe and allowed to dry, green peppercorns are unripened, and the white ones are picked very ripe and soaked in brine to remove the dark shell. Black peppercorns, whether whole, cracked, or ground, have the most intense flavor.

Culinary Uses

Black pepper has seasoned dishes for more than four thousand years. Arabs and Phoenicians first traded for it with India, and it reached the Mediterranean around the fifth century B.C. Pepper was the first Far Eastern spice to reach Europe, and since that time it has become a key element in almost every national cuisine.

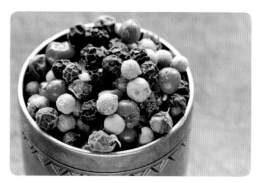

The *Piper nigrum* plant is the source of black, white, and green peppercorns. Pink peppercorns come from a different species—*Schinus molle*—that is related to ragweed.

Peppery Skin-Sloughing Scrub

Black pepper, with its anti-inflammatory and anti-bacterial qualities, makes a beneficial facial scrub. It will slough off dead skin, stimulate circulation, and help deliver nutrients and oxygen to the complexion. It can also prevent acne and other skin eruptions. Simply mix a half teaspoon of ground black pepper with a teaspoon of plain yogurt in a bowl and rub gently onto skin in a circular motion. For a more moisturizing scrub, replace yogurt with olive oil or almond oil. To avoid a burning sensation, apply only for a minute or two. ■

Modern cooks use pepper to add zest to meat and vegetable dishes, stews, soups, and casseroles, as well as fish and omelets. Cracked pepper makes a simple, tasty salad dressing combined with olive oil and lemon juice and can be added to many grilling rubs for both tang and texture.

Nutritionally, the spice is an outstanding source of manganese and vitamin K and also supplies copper, iron, chromium, calcium, vitamin C, vitamin A, flavonoids, carotenes, and dietary fiber. Ground pepper only remains fresh for three months, while whole peppercorns will keep almost indefinitely.

Healing Properties

The ancient Greeks valued black pepper more as a medicine than as a seasoning. For many centuries, European, Asian, and Ayurvedic healers have used black pepper to aid water loss, ease flatulence, cure earaches and vision problems,

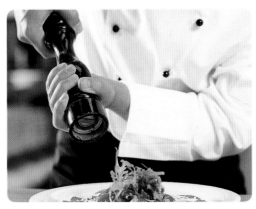

Because pepper loses flavor when heated, it should be added at the end of preparation or milled at the table.

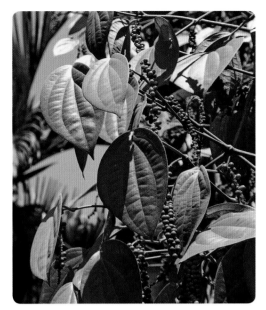

The fruits of the pepper plant first appear as cascades of tiny green spheres. For black pepper, they are harvested just as they begin to turn red, before they fully ripen, and then dried.

and induce sweating. Herbal healers prescribe it to treat respiratory infections, asthma, constipation, anemia, acne, impotence, muscle strains, dental diseases, diarrhea, and heart disease.

Medical research has confirmed black pepper's remarkable antioxidant, antibacterial, and anti-inflammatory qualities. The spice not only aids digestion, but the outer layer of the peppercorn also encourages the breakdown of fat cells, allowing for natural weight loss. Piperine, a key component of the spice, is being studied as a cancer preventative; it has also been shown to reduce memory loss and cognitive malfunction, making it of possible benefit to Alzheimer's patients.

Black pepper also promotes bioavailability, helping to transfer the benefits of other herbs and spices to different parts of the body. Adding black pepper to dishes not only improves their flavor, it also increases the healing potential of the foods we eat.

History and Lore

» In A.D. 408, when the invading king of the Visigoths held Rome for ransom, one of his demands was three thousand pounds of pepper.
» In 19th-century New England, scattering black pepper on furs and flannels before storing them for the summer supposedly kept moths away.

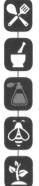

Caraway Seed

Carum carvi

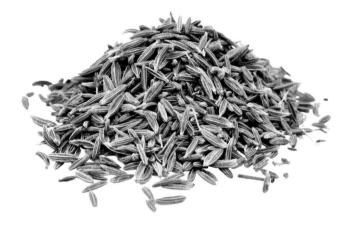

Perhaps best known as a pungent ingredient of rye bread, caraway seeds have a surprising number of other uses—including as a seasoning, healing agent, and aromatic agent.

The biennial caraway plant is a member of the Apiaceae family, which also includes parsley, dill, anise, fennel, and cumin, although caraway has its own distinct flavor. The plant grows to a height of two feet and produces feathery green leaves and umbels of small, creamy white flowers. These mature into crescent-shaped fruit, or seeds, that feature five pale ridges.

Originally native to Asia Minor—modern Turkey—the plant is now distributed throughout northern and central Europe and Asia. It is

cultivated commercially in England, Holland, Germany, Finland, Russia, Norway, and Morocco. Although it grows wild in North America, it is also an export crop in parts of Canada. The early Arabs were perhaps the first to utilize the seeds in cooking, calling them *karawya,* a name they still bear in the Middle East. It is also possible that caraway was the first spice used in Europe, based on evidence found in Switzerland at a five-thousand-year-old Neolithic lake dwelling.

Culinary Uses

Warm, pungent, sharp, and peppery tasting, caraway seeds have been used as a seasoning since the early Greeks, although it was later considered a "peasant spice." In German, Austrian, and Hungarian kitchens, the seeds flavor sausage, pork, brisket, sauerkraut, cheese, cabbage dishes, salad, and soup. Bakers use them in British seed cakes and Irish soda bread, and Eastern European cooks used them to garnish breads and rolls. The savory seeds are found in Middle Eastern curries and North African *harissa,* the hot chili paste used in soups, couscous, and stews. They also add flavor to liqueurs, like the Scandinavian spirit aquavit and the Russian and German Kümmel.

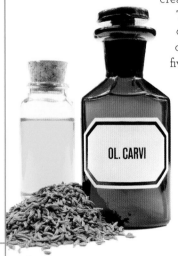

Caraway seed oil is used to scent soaps, lotions, and perfumes.

OL. CARVI

SAVORY SPICES

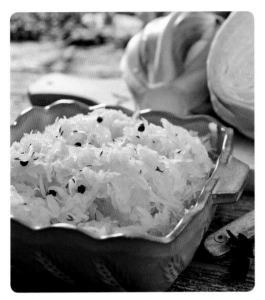

Sauerkraut seasoned with caraway. Strongly aromatic, caraway is a signature flavor in German, Austrian, and other Northern European cuisines. Usually used whole, the seeds have a pungent, anise-like flavor and aroma with a peppery twist.

Caraway leaves can be used like parsley in many recipes, and the root, which is similar to parsnip, can also be eaten. The seeds are used as a pickling spice and in recipes for making corned beef.

Nutritionally, caraway provides iron, copper, calcium, potassium, manganese, selenium, zinc, magnesium, and dietary fiber, as well as vitamins A, E, C, and many B-complex vitamins like thiamin, pyridoxine, riboflavin, and niacin. The seeds are sometimes used to flavor gargles and mouthwashes.

Healing Properties

Natural healers from the time of the Greeks have used caraway to treat flatulence, indigestion, and—especially—infant colic. The extract is sometimes added to traditional medications that ease sore muscles, clear up colds and bronchitis, and treat irritable bowel syndrome.

The seeds contain beneficial essential oils, including a number of volatile compounds that are known to have antioxidant, digestive, carminative, and antiflatulent effects. The seeds also provide flavonoids, antioxidants capable of eliminating free radicals—that can cause cancer, aging, infection, and degenerative neurological disorders—from the body.

A Dish of Caraways

Serving caraway seeds as an accompaniment to baked apples has a long tradition. In Shakespeare's *Henry IV,* for instance, Squire Shallow urges Falstaff to partake of "a pippin and a dish of caraways." In Trinity College, at England's Cambridge University, roasted apples are still served with a small dish of caraway seeds. ■

History and Lore

» The plant is also know as meridian fennel and Persian cumin.

» Roman physician Dioscorides prescribed that caraway oil be taken by "pale-faced girls."

» Folklore claims that caraway seeds, placed inside a valuable object, prevented it from being stolen . . . by making the thief unable to leave the house.

» In Scotland, when buttered bread is dipped into caraway seeds, it is called salt water jelly.

» Caraway was also thought to keep lovers from straying, and the seeds were use to stir up love potions. They supposedly also had the same effect on pigeons, so owners of tame birds would feed caraway to their flocks.

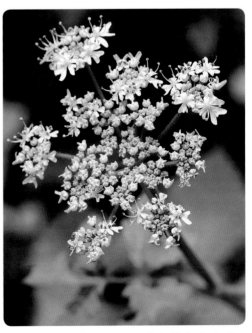

A member of the Apiaceae, caraway plants display the family characteristic of delicate white flowers blooming in umbels.

Caraway Seed

239

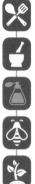

Cayenne

Capsicum annuum

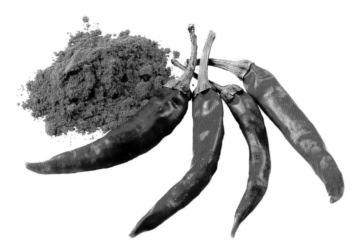

Cayenne pepper, or chili pepper, is the fruit of the chili pepper plant, a cultivar of *Capsicum annum*. It is native to Central America, where it provided heat and flavor to Mesoamerican and Mexican food for millennia—archeological remains indicate that *Capsicum* was a Mexican dietary staple nine thousand years ago. Spanish and Portuguese explorers carried the plant to Europe in the 1600s, where it was adopted into Mediterranean cuisine and embraced by most of Asia, especially India. It is still grown there commercially today, as well as in Pakistan, China, Argentina, and the United States.

> **DID YOU KNOW?**
>
> A spicy staple of cookery around the world, cayenne peppers are often ground as a spice, and the fresh or dried fruit is used whole.

Cayenne is a member of the nightshade family, Solanaceae, which also includes tomatoes, eggplant, and potatoes. This perennial shrub grows to a height of three feet or more, with dark green foliage and small cream-colored flowers. These evolve into long seed pods that start out green and mature to a bright red.

Culinary Uses

Red peppers can be purchased as fresh vegetables or dried—whole, flaked, or powdered. Fresh cayenne is used in Asian and Indian cuisine to make curries, stir-fry dishes, soups, sauces, chutney, spicy water, and pickling brine. The powdered form, which is preferred by Mexican, Mediterranean, and American cooks, is a key ingredient in salsa, taco powder, chili powder, Cajun spice mix, buffalo wings, tomato sauce, and many grilling rub and marinade recipes.

Cayenne's fiery heat comes from three active alkaloid compounds: capsaicin, capsanthin, and capsorubin. The intensity of hot or spicy foods is measured on a scale called Scoville heat units; cayenne registers a hefty 30,000 to 50,000 SHU, while bell peppers register 0 SHU. When slicing or dicing fresh chilies, it is best to wear protective gloves and avoid touching the eyes.

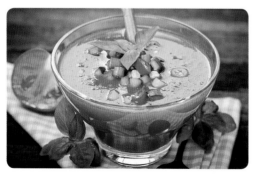

Gazpacho, the classic cold soup from Spain, gets heats from cayenne and other peppers, such as poblano and tabasco.

Pollinating Peppers

Although cayenne peppers are self-pollinating, to be assured of a healthy crop of vegetables, it helps to pollinate them by hand. This process can also be used to crossbreed peppers, which can end up offering your garden—and dinner plate—some interesting results.

1. Hold the base of the cayenne pepper plant and gently shake it to dislodge the pollen, which will correct any lack of fruiting due to a failed pollen tube. Shake the plant at midday when the weather is warm, still, and dry.
2. Insert a clean cotton swab into the flowers. Probe the yellow, pollen-coated stamens to collect the pollen by twirling the swab.
3. Carefully remove the swab and insert it into a neighboring flower and twirl it against the pistil, the central structure inside the flower.

After pollination, mist the flowers to increase humidity and keep the pollen in place. ■

These nutritionally rich vegetables contain substantial amounts of vitamin A, vitamin C, and B-complex vitamins, including niacin, pyridoxine (vitamin B6), riboflavin, and thiamin (vitamin B1), They also contain high levels of iron, copper, zinc, potassium, manganese, magnesium, selenium, and antioxidant flavonoids.

Healing Properties

Natural healers value cayenne for its many benefits, including its anti-irritant, antifungal, antiallergen, and antibacterial uses. It has been used as a decongestant flu and cold remedy and to treat upset stomachs, ulcers, sore throats, coughs, diarrhea, delirium, gout, paralysis, tremors, fever, dyspepsia, flatulence, hemorrhoids, nausea, tonsillitis, scarlet fever, and diphtheria.

This spice stimulates muscle movement throughout the digestive tract, which increases secretions and aids in the absorption of nutrients. It also increases circulation, especially to the extremities. For these reasons, cayenne is often added to other medicines—it helps to carry them throughout the body. It is also a catalyst that enhances other treatments. Because cayenne boosts metabolism, the spice can be a useful aid for weight loss. A radical detoxifying juice fast, called the Master Cleanse, involves drinking nothing but cayenne and maple syrup in water, tea, or lemonade.

Studies in Loma Linda University in California found that cayenne may help prevent lung cancer in smokers—possibly due to the high levels of capsaicin it contains it does not allow tumors to form. Capsaicin also makes this spice an effective pain reliever when used as a rub or liniment on aching joints. Because cayenne helps to keep blood pressure normalized and LDL cholesterol and triglycerides low, the spice also promotes a more healthy heart

History and Lore

» Cayenne is also known as Guinea spice, cowhorn pepper, aleva, and bird pepper.
» In Central Africa, the spice is used to make a calming, stress-relieving tonic.
» A mascot named Cayenne is the "spirit leader" for the Ragin' Cajun athletic teams of the University of Louisiana at Lafayette.

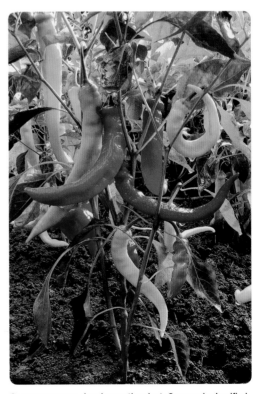

Cayenne peppers ripening on the plant. Cayenne is classified in the fiery Longum group of *Capsicum annuum,* which also includes jalapeño, serrano, and poblano peppers.

HOT AND HEALTHY

Hot peppers furnish natural relief to aching joints and muscles.

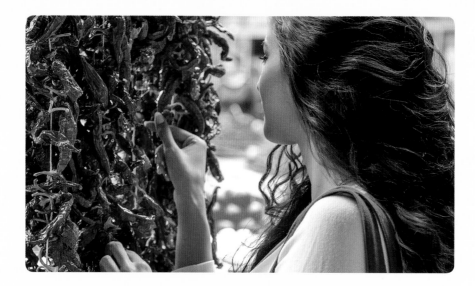

Central American cultures began using chili peppers for treating pain more than six thousand years ago . . . and the Old World eventually caught on. It may seem odd that something that causes pain—intense explosions of heat inside the mouth or on the skin—could also be a potent pain reliever, but pepper's beneficial effects have been well documented.

This pain-killing ability is due to capsaicin, a fiery phenolic resin found in peppers that triggers the nerve endings to release a neurotransmitter called substance P. Substance P sends feelings of pain to the brain, causing the burning sensation. Yet, once substance P is depleted, the area remains pain free. This makes capsaicin a natural analgesic for treating chronic conditions like osteoarthritis, rheumatoid arthritis, bursitis, and diabetic neuropathy, or short-term muscle, joint, or nerve pain. It has also been used to ease painful psoriasis, herpes zoster, and neuralgia.

Studies are currently underway to determine if capsaicin prevents the growth of cancer tumors, though it's not just the capsaicin that contributes to this goal, say researchers. Hot peppers also contain carotenoids and flavonoids that scavenge cancer-causing free radicals in the system. Research may be ongoing, but one thing medical science does agree on is that capsaicin is the "purest and most certain stimulant in the herbal materia medica."

There are five main species of *Capsicum*: *C. annuum* includes cayenne, jalapeño, and bell pepper; *C. frutescens* includes tabasco, malagueta, and Thai; *C. baccatum* includes *ají* and *criolla sella*; *C. pubescens* includes *rocoto*; and *C. chinense* includes habanero, naga, and Scotch bonnet.

A Natural Defense

Capsaicin possibly developed in peppers to ward off predators like hungry animals or destructive fungi. In 1816, German pharmacist Christian Friedrich Bucholz first extracted the compound and named it after the pepper's genus *Capsicum*, from the Greek *kapto*, "to bite." Capsaicin is concentrated in the white inner pith, rather than in the flesh of the fruit. The seeds do not contain capsaicin, allowing birds to eat them and pass them, so they can spread and germinate.

Capsaicin is also used in police pepper sprays and to repel animals and insects. Pure capsaicin extract is rated higher than 15 million Scoville heat units (the measurement of the pungency of chili peppers)— never apply it directly to the skin or mouth.

Going Nuclear

Recently, tasting hot, torrid pepper sauces—and their corresponding peppers—has developed into a social trend, and hosts throw "Go hot or go home!" parties for guests to experience escalating levels of bottled heat. The allure, say those who indulge, is that there are 20 minutes of agony followed by 40 minutes of blissful endorphin rush. Dedicated fresh pepper tasters, or chiliheads, favor "superhots" and "nuclears"—cultivars that register more than one million units on the Scoville heat scale (SHU).

These include the 'Carolina Reaper', the hottest pepper according to the 2014 Guinness Book of Records; the 'Trinidad Moruga Scorpion', the 2012 record holder; the '7 Pot Brain Strain', the '7 Pot Primo'; the 'Naga Viper'; and the venerable 'Ghost Pepper', the first to test over one million SHU. Yet, even the most infernal of hot peppers still manages to provide pain-relieving and antioxidant benefits.

Below is a sampling of some common peppers and where they measure on the heat scale. ■

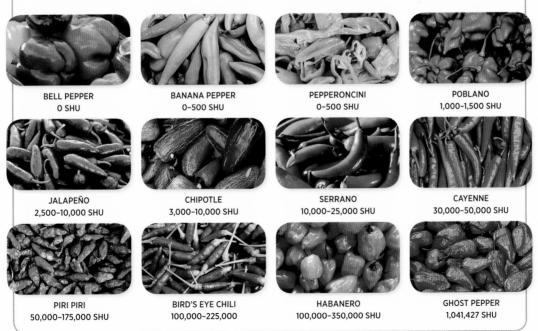

BELL PEPPER 0 SHU	**BANANA PEPPER** 0–500 SHU	**PEPPERONCINI** 0–500 SHU	**POBLANO** 1,000–1,500 SHU
JALAPEÑO 2,500–10,000 SHU	**CHIPOTLE** 3,000–10,000 SHU	**SERRANO** 10,000–25,000 SHU	**CAYENNE** 30,000–50,000 SHU
PIRI PIRI 50,000–175,000 SHU	**BIRD'S EYE CHILI** 100,000–225,000	**HABANERO** 100,000–350,000 SHU	**GHOST PEPPER** 1,041,427 SHU

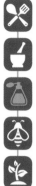

Celery Seed

Apium graveolens

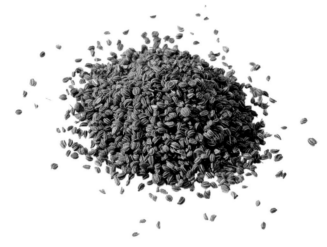

Warmly fragrant celery seed is not as popular in American kitchens as some savory spices, but it is slowly gaining advocates. On the medicinal side, this ancient seasoning continues to show great potential against several serious diseases.

Succulent celery is a member of the Apiaceae family of umbellifers. It is native to Southern Europe, although wild celery "cousins" are found in Africa and North and South America. The plant dates back at least to ancient Egypt, where woven garlands of wild celery have been found in tombs. In the 17th

DID YOU KNOW?
Another member of the Apiaceae family, celery is grown not only for its edible leaf stalk, but also for its tiny fruits, which are used as a flavoring or spice, either as whole seeds or ground and mixed with salt.

century, the Italians experimented with the cultivation of the plant as a vegetable, gaining stable, solid stems and losing any bitter taste. Today there are two varieties of stalk celery—self-blanching or yellow celery, and green or Pascal celery.

Celery grows to an average height of three feet, with segmented leaves and white flowers that form graceful umbels before producing ovoid seeds. The name derives from the French *céleri,* in turn from the Italian *seleri,* which comes from Late Latin *selinon,* the latinization of the Greek *selinon,* or "parsley."

Culinary Uses

The seed, which tastes like a concentrated version of celery stalks, is found in the cuisines of Germany, Italy, Russia, and Asia, and in modern Jewish cookery. It is used to make pickles, mustard, and chutney, to season thick soups and chowders, and to enhance rich seafood, such as salmon. It can be rubbed on fresh beef or pork at a measure of a half teaspoon per pound of meat. The seeds add a piquant flavor to salads, sandwich meats, and bread or rolls.

Nutritionally, celery seeds are a good source of vitamins A, C, and folate, as well as dietary fiber,

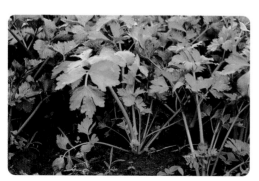

Celery can be tricky to grow, but it is a great kitchen garden plant, yielding a tasty vegetable and seeds to use as a spice.

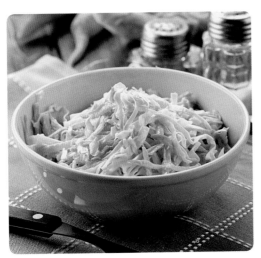

Celery seed is often one of the ingredients of coleslaw salad, a classic side dish in diners and delicatessens across America.

iron, manganese, calcium, phosphorus, copper, and zinc. Be aware that the celery seeds in commercial gardening packets have been treated with chemicals and should not be consumed.

Healing Properties

Celery seed was known to many early cultures, including the Greeks and Romans, as a versatile healing agent. It was prescribed by Hippocrates and Aulus Cornelius Celsus, and valued by herbal healers in China and Japan. In Ayurvedic medicine, the seeds were used to treat liver ailments, colds and flu, indigestion, water retention, and arthritis. During medieval times, they were a popular treatment for toothache, lumbago, and rheumatism. Later, in America, the cure for joint pain was to wear a bag containing celery seeds—and a wedding ring—around one's neck.

Celery seeds are thought to possess carminative, antibacterial, antirheumatic, antiseptic, aphrodisiac, hypotensive, sedative, stimulant, and diuretic qualities. Recent research also confirms that they are a rich source of antioxidant phytonutrients, and coumarins—a beneficial chemical compound responsible for their taste and scent. They are being studied as a possible treatment for high blood pressure, nervous conditions, and even cancer. Celery seeds contain a flavonoid called luteolin that researchers believe may possess anti-cancer properties, specifically by suppressing cancer cell "survival pathways."

Aromatic Qualities

Herbalists recommend the essential oil of celery seeds as a liver tonic and to treat gout, arthritis, indigestion, and pain. Commercially, the oil is used as a fragrance component in soaps, cosmetics, and perfumes.

History and Lore

» Celery was considered a sacred plant in classical Greece; it was worn by the winners of the Nemean Games, similar to the bay leaves presented at the Olympic Games.

» *Apium,* the genus name for the celery plant; Apiaceae, its family name; and apiary, a collection of beehives, all come from the same Latin word, *apis,* meaning "of bees," referring to flowers that attract bees.

FOR YOUR HEALTH

Blood-Pressure Breakthrough

Drugs that normalize high blood pressure are among the most prescribed in the United States, yet celery seed extract seems to have a similar effect on hypertension—and without side effects. Recent studies of celery seed at the University of Chicago Medical Center identified one of its compounds—3-n-butylphthalide, or 3nB—as the factor responsible for this health benefit. Conventional drugs, like beta blockers, decrease the amount of blood flow to the brain, reducing the chance of stroke. The downside is that patients often feel tired, forgetful, depressed, and dizzy. Based on the study's results, celery seed may be the best option for lowering blood pressure of any natural product available at this time. ∎

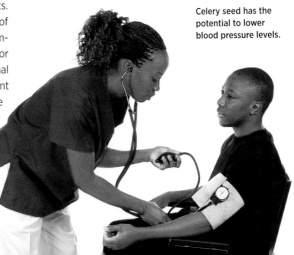

Celery seed has the potential to lower blood pressure levels.

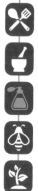

Coriander
Coriandrum sativum

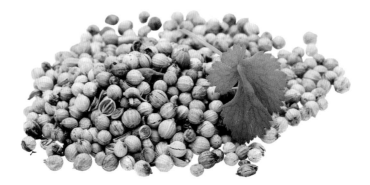

A lthough it comes from the same plant as the herb cilantro (the green leaves), the spice coriander (the fruit or seed) has its own distinct flavor, a combination of citrus and sage. Beyond its value in the kitchen, it has been used as a healing agent and an aphrodisiac for centuries.

The cilantro plant, a member of the Apiaceae family, grows to a height of one or two feet and bears clusters of small white, pink, or pale lavender flowers. These mature into green, and then brown, aromatic fruits. A native of

the Mediterranean and Asia Minor, the plant dates back at least five thousand years—it was mentioned in Sanskrit writings and placed in Egyptian tombs. Its popularity in European cookery decreased during the Middle Ages after the arrival of exotic Eastern spices. Meanwhile, in early 17th-century Massachusetts, coriander became one of the first herbs cultivated by the colonists. Around the same time, the French distilled coriander to make liquor. Today, the plant is cultivated in tropical and subtropical regions around the world, with the majority being produced in Morocco, Romania, and Egypt, followed by China and India.

Culinary Uses

Not only did the early cultures of the Mediterranean basin add coriander to both food and wine, Bronze Age invaders carried it to Britain, where it was used it to flavor gruel and mixed with cumin and vinegar to preserve meat. After Spanish conquistadors introduced the spice to Central and South America, it was quickly absorbed into local native cuisines—where it is still in evidence.

Unlike cilantro, with its slightly soapy taste, coriander offers a pleasant citrus flavor that is valued by Asian, Indian, Mexican, Tex-Mex,

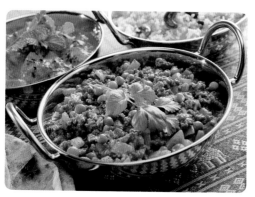

Coriander spices many Indian dishes, including the classic chicken tikka masala (left) and keema matar, a minced lamb and pea dish. This northern favorite is garnished with cilantro.

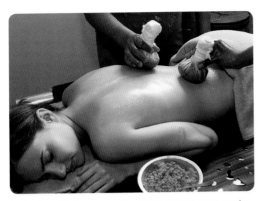

Coriander, with its warm, nutty, slightly orange scent, can be used in aromatherapy massage to release emotional fears and to combat addictions and cravings.

Chinese, African, South American, and Scandinavian cooks. It is also mixed into several spice blends, including curry powder, chili powder, garam masala, and *berbere*. It goes especially well with lentils, beans, onions, potatoes, sausages, pork, seafood, lamb stews, and pastries. The seeds are used in brewing Belgian wheat beers and in preparing Middle Eastern falafels.

Many American chefs have not yet discovered the delights of coriander, but as more home cooks become exposed to new seasonings via TV cooking shows, it's only a matter of time before coriander becomes as popular as its "plant-mate"

cilantro. Nutritionally, coriander contains vitamins A, C, and K, dietary fiber, and substantial amounts of calcium and potassium.

Healing Properties

Early healers believed that anything that smelled as distasteful as the "old sock" odor of cilantro had to have powerful medicinal qualities. Roman physician Dioscorides noted that coriander seemed to increase a man's sexual potency, while Chinese healers prescribed it to treat hernias, dysentery, measles, and nausea. In India, it is still widely used to prepare health tonics and cough medicines. The spice also has a long tradition as a cure for flatulence and a treatment for arthritis and rheumatism.

Coriander contains beneficial phytonutrients and antioxidants. It is believed to help cleanse the body of harmful heavy metals and toxic substances. Diabetes research at Cairo University indicates that the essential oil can normalize glucose and insulin levels and support the pancreas. In general, however, medical science is just beginning to investigate the healing potential of this venerable spice.

History and Lore

» The Chinese believed that eating coriander seeds conferred immortality.

» According to writings from 1550 B.C., fragrant coriander was used to scent the wondrous Hanging Gardens of Babylon.

» If consumed in excess, coriander seeds can have a narcotic effect; this led to the spice being nicknamed dizzycorn.

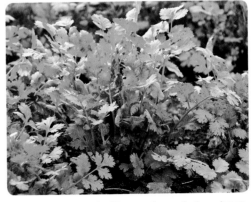

In contrast to the airy, fernlike upper leaves, the lower leaves of coriander are lobed and look a little like curly-leaf parsley.

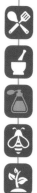

Cumin

Cuminum cyminum

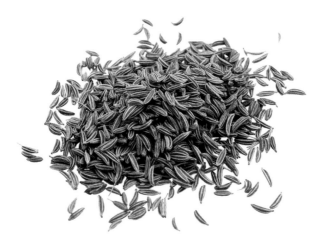

Cumin is the second-most popular spice in the world, after black pepper, but it has only recently entered the kitchens of American home cooks. This annual plant was originally native to the Mediterranean, and its cultivation dates back more than five thousand years to ancient Egypt, where it was both a seasoning and an embalming spice. The Greeks kept a container on the dinner table, as Americans do with salt and pepper, a tradition still seen in Morocco. Cumin's value as a medicine was so great, according to the Bible, that it was used as currency.

DID YOU KNOW?

A staple of both Mexican and Indian cuisine, cumin adds nutty, peppery flavor to dishes, while also delivering powerful health benefits.

Readily available during the Middle Ages, unlike imported spices, *Cuminum cyminum* could often be found growing in monastery gardens. The Celts used it to season fish dishes. It was first introduced to the Americas by Spanish and Portuguese settlers and was quickly adopted in both hemispheres. The spice can now be purchased either whole or ground in most groceries.

A member of the Apiaceae family, cumin grows to a height of 20 inches and produces threadlike leaves and dark green stems that all attain the same height, creating an even canopy of white or pink flowers. The ovoid fruits, or seeds, from which the spice is made, are yellowish brown with pale ridges.

Culinary Uses

Cumin's intense flavor—nutty, peppery, sharp, and slightly bitter—has made it popular across the globe. It has been a key ingredient of Indian cuisine—curry powder, kormas, masalas, and soups—for many centuries, and is also found in the ethnic dishes of Nepal, western China, North Africa, the Middle East, Brazil, and Mexico. Cumin is used in grilling rubs and to season stews, egg dishes, vegetables, cheeses, and breads.

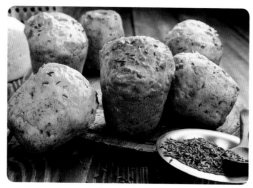

Cumin adds a savory note to lightly sweet cornbread muffins, making them the perfect accompaniment to a bowl of chili.

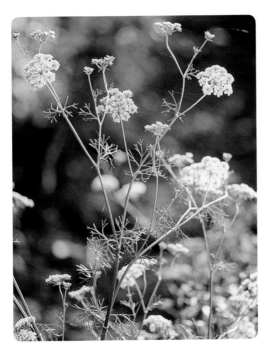

Cumin is a small, slender member of the parsley family, with airy threadlike leaves alternating on hollow stems. The blooms are borne in umbels of tiny white or pale pink flowers.

Nutritionally, cumin is rich vitamin C and E and in iron, which increases hemoglobin production and blood flow, making it helpful for treating anemia and problems with concentration or cognition.

Healing Properties

Herbal healers use cumin to treat indigestion, cure skin eruptions, improve immunity, and treat hemorrhoids. Its high dietary fiber content and antifungal and antimicrobial properties make it a natural laxative. The presence of caffeine makes it an ideal decongestant for respiratory problems.

Cumin is a valuable antioxidant and all-purpose health booster, and it may also prove effective in treating cancer—research shows that the spice possesses chemo-preventive properties and speeds up the secretion of detoxifying and anticarcinogenic enzymes from the glands. It might also be useful in combating diabetes—early studies report that cumin, among other spices, can reduce the chances of developing hypoglycemia.

Aromatic Qualities

The scent of the essential oil aroma is strong—musky, warm, and masculine, with spicy-sweet notes of anise. In aromatherapy, it is used as a general tonic and antiseptic and to lower blood pressure, ease cramps, and treat fatigue. On an emotional level, it is both a relaxant and a stimulant.

History and Lore

» In Europe, cumin was once a symbol of fidelity and was supposed to keep both chickens and lovers from wandering off. Couples who carried cumin seeds at their wedding ceremony were guaranteed happiness.

» The Arabs created what they considered to be a powerful aphrodisiac by mixing cumin with honey and black pepper.

IN THE KITCHEN

Traditional Garam Masala

The term *garam masala* comes from the Hindi words for "hot" and "mixture of spices." Recipes vary, but always use freshly ground ingredients to get the sharpest flavors, although high-quality packaged spices will come close to the real thing.

Ingredients
- 1 tablespoon ground cumin
- 1½ teaspoons ground coriander
- 1½ teaspoons ground cardamom
- 1½ teaspoons ground black pepper
- 1 teaspoon ground cinnamon
- ½ teaspoon ground cloves
- ½ teaspoon ground nutmeg

Directions
Thoroughly mix all the spices together, transfer to an airtight container. Keep in a cool, dry spot. ■

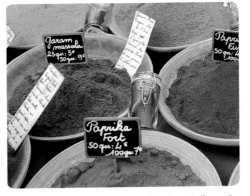

Garam masala is an important part of Northern Indian and South Asian cuisine and is used to flavor curries, biryanis, chicken, lamb, fish, rice pilaf, and baked goods.

GRILLING RUBS AND MARINADES

Make your barbecue memorable with spicy blends.

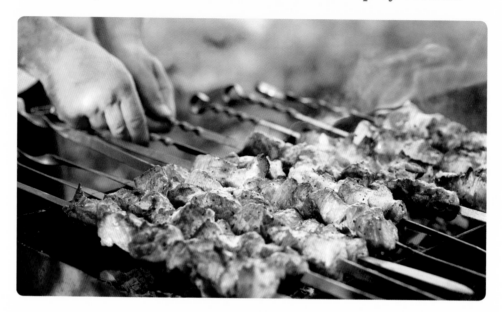

Whether the main course at your cookout is being fire-grilled or slow-cooked in the smoker, most meats benefit from some type of spicy rub or marinade. Marinades are meant to enhance flavor and tenderize tougher cuts of meat, while rubs are meant to impart a distinctive taste profile.

Perhaps the best part of preparing your own rubs and marinades is how easy it is to customize them to your specific taste preferences with the addition of herbs and spices. Marinades and rubs can lend a true regional feel to your grilled meats (and even vegetables), from American Cajun, Tex-Mex, Kansas City, and Memphis barbecue to world profiles like Mexican, Asian, and Moroccan. Some rubs are geared to specific cuts of meat, brisket, say, or baby back ribs. And don't forget that when it comes to grilling, sweet and savory make the perfect complementary pairing.

Year-Round Barbecuing

With the advent of propane grills that can be fired up and ready to go in minutes, many home cooks are making use of their barbecues all year long, even during the colder months. Grilling fans are also exploring another popular feature: the smoker, which is a closed unit that slow-cooks meat and poultry until it is tender to the bone.

Get Your Grill On with the Taste of Summer

You can add summertime flavor to your grilled meats any time of year. Below is just a sampling of simple, flavor-packed rub and marinade recipes.

Grilling Rubs

For best results, pat the mixture on by hand or place meat and rub in a plastic bin and shake.

- **Memphis Rib Rub:** Combine ¼ cup paprika, 1 tablespoon each of salt, onion powder, black pepper, and cayenne with 1 teaspoon each of dry mustard, garlic powder, and celery salt. Perfect for pork ribs.

- **Universal Rub:** Mix 4 tablespoons each of sugar and salt, 2 tablespoons mustard powder, 1 tablespoon paprika, ½ teaspoon ground black pepper, a pinch of dried oregano, and a pinch of dried thyme. Works well on chicken or beef.

- **Brown Sugar Brisket Rub:** Combine ⅓ cup each of brown sugar, coarse salt, paprika, chili powder, and ground black pepper with 1½ teaspoons dry mustard. Grill brisket on lower heat to avoid burning sugar. Also great on pulled pork.

- **Cajun Blackened Rub:** Mix 1½ tablespoons paprika and 1 tablespoon each of garlic powder, onion powder, ground dried thyme with 1 teaspoon each of ground black pepper, cayenne, dried basil, and dried oregano. This salt-free rub works on meats, poultry, and seafood.

- **Pungent Asian Pork Rub:** Mix 6 tablespoons ground cumin, 4 tablespoons hot chili powder, 2 tablespoons each of kosher salt and ground coriander, 1 tablespoon paprika, and 1½ teaspoons each of ground allspice and ground black pepper. Use 1 tablespoon of the rub per serving.

- **Kansas City Ribs Sweet Rub:** Mix ½ cup brown sugar and ¼ cup paprika with 1 tablespoon each of chili powder, garlic powder, onion powder, black pepper, salt, and cayenne. Grill ribs on lower heat to avoid burning sugar. A classic with pork ribs, but can also be used on brisket. Serve with a tomato-and-molasses barbecue sauce.

Marinades

In addition to herbs, spices, and oils, these flavor-infusing recipes feature at least one acidic component to break down the tissues of the meat.

- **4-Star Steak Marinade:** (Yields approximately 2 cups) Mix 1 cup vegetable oil, ½ cup soy sauce, ⅓ cup red wine vinegar, ¼ cup fresh lemon juice, 3 tablespoons Worcestershire sauce, 2 tablespoons Dijon-style mustard, 1 tablespoon freshly ground black pepper, 1 onion (sliced), and 2 cloves garlic (minced). Cover steak with mixture, and marinate for 8 hours in refrigerator.

- **Tasty Teriyaki Marinade:** (Yields 1 cup) Mix ⅓ cup each of water, brown sugar, and soy sauce with 1 teaspoon crushed garlic and ½ teaspoon ground cinnamon. Can be used on all meats and poultry, especially good for kebabs. Marinate 2 hours in refrigerator.

- **Korean BBQ Poultry Marinade:** (Yields 3 cups) In a saucepan, mix 1 cup each of sugar, soy sauce, and water with 1 teaspoon each of onion powder and ground ginger. Whisk together over high heat, and bring to a boil. Cool, and add 1 tablespoon lemon juice and 3 teaspoons hot chili paste (optional). Cover chicken with mixture, and marinate for 4 hours in refrigerator. Can also be used as grilling sauce. ◼

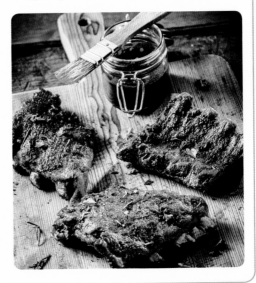

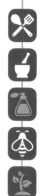

Grains of Paradise
Aframomum melegueta

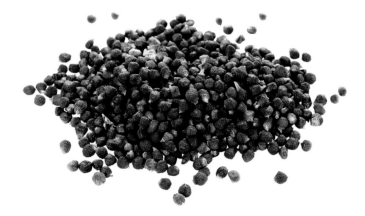

This African spice, with its exotic-sounding name, has remained unfamiliar to most American cooks until very recently. Now, more and more home chefs are beginning to discover its rich mélange of flavors. In other parts of the world, grains of paradise, also known as Melegueta pepper, guinea grains, and alligator pepper, is used to enhance meats and vegetables and is included in many spice blends. It is also a frequent flavoring in beers and liquors. In addition, the spice has a long history of use by natural healers.

A native of the "Grain Coast" of West Africa, it was exported to Europe starting in the ninth century as a more easily obtained substitute for black pepper. The spice was given its fanciful name in the 14th century, perhaps as a marketing ploy by traders to increase demand. Once pepper became more available, however, grains of paradise fell out of favor in most European kitchens.

A member of the ginger family, Zingiberaceae, the grains of paradise plant is short-stemmed and prefers marshy terrain. It produces narrow, palmlike leaves and fragrant, pinkish orange trumpet flowers. The fruit, or pods, contain the numerous brown seeds that are dried to make the spice.

Culinary Uses

The taste of the spice has been described as a woodsy blend of ginger, cardamom, and black pepper with a floral hint or nutty citrus with a kick of jasmine. It is used in West African cuisine, in the curried dishes of North Africa and the Middle East; in the Moroccan *ras el hanout*—meaning "top of the shop"—spice blend; in European paellas and cassoulets; and to flavor beers and liquors, including ale, aquavit, and gin. It is

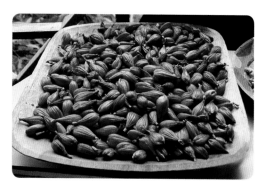

Aframomum melegueta pods, the source of grains of paradise, at a market on São Tomé Island in the Gulf of Guinea. There, the fruits, called *ossame* by the locals, are eaten raw.

The Grain Coast

For centuries, Europeans merchants viewed the African continent as if it were a vast treasure chest of rare and exotic seasonings that was theirs for the taking. Yet, of all the spices that traveled north and east from Africa to markets in Europe, the Middle East, and Asia, it was grains of paradise that gave its name to an entire region. The western coast of the Gulf of Guinea, from Cape Mesurado to Cape Palmas (in present-day Liberia), hosted a thriving trade in grains of paradise overseen by African and Portuguese merchants and it was thus known as the Grain Coast. ■

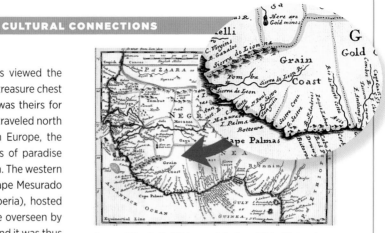

A map of the Gulf of Guinea, originally published in London in 1727, shows the so-called Grain Coast of West Africa.

great in vinaigrettes, added to fish and vegetable marinades or potato salad, or as a seasoning for sausage, lamb, steak, and shish kebab. For those who like a bit of spice with their sugar, grains of paradise can be added to desserts like cobblers, bread pudding, spice cookies, or apple pie.

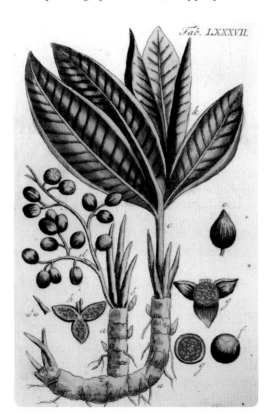

The parts of a grains of paradise plant shown in a Dutch book of botanical illustrations published in 1813. Its natural habitat is swampy land along the West African coast.

Grains of paradise can be substituted for black pepper in many recipes. The grains are typically ground just before use, although whole grains are sometimes added to soups to provide a milder flavor. The spice can be purchased at many Asian groceries, brewing supply stores, or online.

Healing Properties

The spice has been used by West African herbal healers as a stimulant, diuretic, and aphrodisiac—in recent studies on lab rats, grains of paradise did increase their libido—and as a remedy for leprosy and measles. In the 1500s, English herbalist John Gerard recommended the spice for stomach problems. It has also been used to treat parasitic infestations, to purify the blood, and ease constipation.

During a Rutgers University study, biochemists found a powerful anti-inflammatory compound in grains of paradise seeds, possibly the most powerful anti-inflammatory compound yet discovered. The spice is also being considered as an inexpensive, phytomedical alternative to costly, hard-to-access allopathic medicines in certain tropical regions.

History and Lore

» Grains of paradise was one of the favorite spices of Queen Elizabeth I, and it remained popular during the Renaissance.
» Lowland gorillas eat grains of paradise in the wild, and the seeds are believed to improve their heart health. Gorillas in zoos, who do not get the seeds, often have poor cardiovascular health.

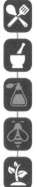

Juniper Berry
Juniperus communis

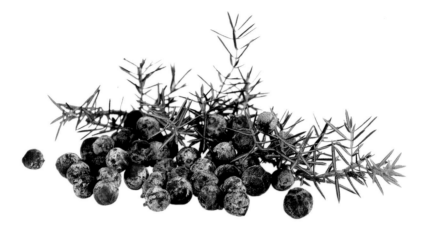

Juniper berries may be best known for flavoring gin, but the berries and branches of the *Juniperus communis* tree have been a part of natural and spiritual healing for thousands of years. Ancient Greeks, Romans, and Arabs used juniper more as a medicine than as a seasoning, and the berries were considered a cure for snakebite, plague, and pestilence during the Renaissance.

The juniper can be either a bushy shrub or an erect tree. It is a member of the cypress family, or Cupressaceae, and it is native to Asia,

Canada, Northern Europe, Scandinavia, and Siberia. It is believed that prehistoric peoples who lived near juniper forests used these evergreens as a source of food, fuel, and wood for shelters. The juniper tree, which can live for more than two thousand years, grows to a height of 30 feet and features hard, blue-green needles and small yellow flowers. The so-called "berry" is actually a female seed cone, which starts out with leathery scales. After three seasons, it matures into a blue-black berry with a white bloom.

Culinary Uses

Juniper berries make an excellent addition to stews, sauces, hearty soups, and savory meats—they counteract the strong taste of venison and game birds and cut the fatty taste of pork and duck. They are favored in Scandinavian, German, Austrian, Czech, and Northern Italian cuisines—especially in alpine regions where the trees grow in abundance. The berries add complexity to sauerkraut, stuffing, vegetable pâtés, and tea, and they make a delicious meat marinade with wine or a pungent smoky rub when combined with coriander. They even go well with fruit tarts and compotes.

A juniper tree lures wildlife, such as the red squirrel *(Sciurus vulgaris),* to your backyard. The prickly foliage makes a safe shelter for many small mammals and birds, which will also feast on the berries that ripen from green to blue or black.

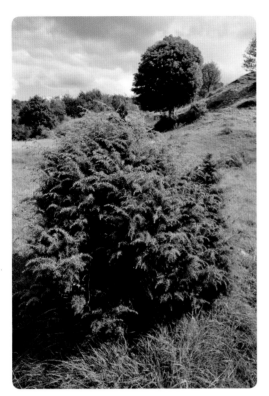

Juniper is a slow-growing evergreen shrub or small tree that thrives on open wooded hillsides, maritime escarpments, and on exposed slopes and plateaus in dry and rocky soil.

Nutritionally, juniper berries contain vitamin C, as well as copper, chromium, calcium, iron, limonene, phosphorous, magnesium, and potassium.

Healing Properties

Juniper's role as a medicine goes back at least to ancient Egypt—a remedy to treat tapeworms was discovered on a papyrus that dated to 1550 B.C. Since then, healers have used juniper—with its antiseptic, astringent, and antispasmodic qualities—for urinary infections, enlarged prostate, kidney stones, digestive and liver problems, respiratory infections, arthritic and rheumatic conditions, and to calm anxiety, nervous tension, or mental exhaustion without any sedative side effects.

In Europe and Asia, juniper was employed to combat contagious diseases such as cholera, typhoid fever, and the plague. Indians in the Pacific Northwest made tonics from the branches to treat colds, flu, arthritis, and kidney problems. The oil is effective against skin conditions like acne, weeping eczema, psoriasis, and dandruff.

Aromatic Qualities

The distinctive aroma of the essential oil is piney, fresh, and crisp. Juniper was used by Native Americans to make incense, as well as to welcome guests and cleanse horses. It can purify a space for prayer or meditation, and, when sprayed in a mister, can help kill airborne germs. In aromatherapy, the oil is used to treat addictions, hangovers, and indigestion; to stimulate the nervous system; and to boost the spirit. As a blended massage oil or diluted in the bath, it can treat adult colic, arthritis, cellulite, cystitis, swollen joints, liver problems, and muscle fatigue. Juniper is grown commercially in Austria, Canada, the Czech Republic, Slovenia, France, Hungary, India, and Italy. The oil can be extracted from the berries, the needles, and the wood.

History and Lore

» Juniper branches and berries were burned as offerings in ancient Sumeria and Babylonia. They were considered sacred to the Sumerian goddess Inanna and her successor, the Semitic goddess Ishtar.

» In the Middle Ages, juniper was used to create antitheft spells, rituals of protection, and love sachets. It supposedly attracts healthy energies and positive spirits.

CULTURAL CONNECTIONS

Getting Gin from Jenever

For centuries, juniper berries have been used to flavor gin, a popular modern liquor that originated as an herbal medicine in Europe in the Middle Ages. Gin is based on an earlier beverage made by crudely distilling malt wine. The result was not very palatable, so medicinal herbs, especially juniper berries, were added to improve the flavor. This led to the drink being called jenever, from the Dutch word for "juniper." Today, there are several versions of the liquor: Traditional gin contains natural flavorings that are added to a neutral spirit of agricultural origin. Distilled gin re-distills the spirit with juniper and other flavorings. London gin, or dry gin, is the most popular variety—it contains limited added sugars, but has a higher alcohol content and is often flavored with citrus peel. ■

255

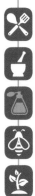

Paprika

Capsicum annuum

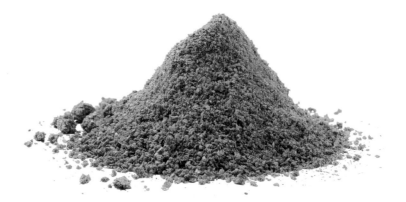

Ground paprika derives from same species of pepper as the fiery cayennes and jalapeños, but it typically contains a larger proportion of sweet and mild red bell peppers. In cookery, this spice is versatile and nuanced, and it is available in a variety of intensities. Medicinally, it has been used to reduce joint pain, ease digestion, and maintain circulatory and heart health.

Native to the New World, this member of the nightshade family, Solanaceae, likely originated in South America and was first cultivated in Mexico. Columbus brought the plant back with

DID YOU KNOW?

Forever linked with Hungarian cuisine, paprika is a bright red-orange spice made from ground, air-dried red peppers.

him to Spain, and Spanish and Portuguese traders introduced paprika to all of Europe—and subsequently Asia and Africa. By the 1560s, it had made its way to the Balkans, where it was called *paparka*. Central European paprika was hot and spicy until the 1920s, when a grower in Hungary discovered a plant that yielded sweet peppers, which became the source of a milder paprika. Today, the major producers of paprika peppers are Spain, the Netherlands, Central Europe, and the United States.

Culinary Uses

This spice is most often made from dried, ground red bell peppers, yet any pepper can be made into paprika. It adds a rich, ruddy hue to dishes, and the taste can be intensified by lightly sautéing the powder in oil. Paprika is identified with Hungarian cuisine, but it is also used in Spain, Turkey, and the Balkans, as well as in South Africa and Morocco. There are several varieties of paprika, each with a different taste and aroma profile. In general, sweet paprika has more than half the pepper seeds removed; hotter paprikas contain more seeds, plus calyces and stalks. Smoked paprika is created by slowly smoking red peppers over a wood fire for two weeks.

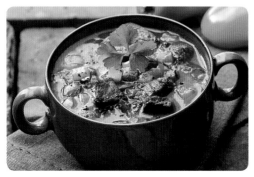

Hungarian goulash, which began as a hearty peasant soup, is now known throughout the world. Although there are many recipes for this dish, paprika is always on the ingredient list.

Keeping Flamingos in the Pink

Many zoos add paprika to the diet of flamingos to help them maintain their peachy pink plumage, which can fade in captivity. In the wild, the striking color of these wading birds would normally come from the tiny carotenoid-rich mollusks and crustaceans they consume in tidal shallows. Even though these small shellfish and crustaceans are often blue or green, when they are digested, their carotenoid pigments dissolve in fat and are deposited in the new feathers. This same phenomenon is seen when greenish shrimp are boiled and turn a bright pink. ■

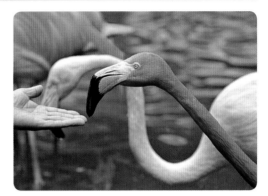

Without their natural carotenoid-rich diet, flamingos will fade to near white. Adding paprika can restore their rich coloration.

Sweet Hungarian paprika has a zesty flavor and is best used for seasoning goulash, chicken paprikash, stuffed peppers, deviled eggs, potato salads, fish, marinades, and salad dressings. Smoked sweet paprika, cool to the taste, is found in Mediterranean gratins, fish or bean dishes, on leafy greens or on crisp potatoes. Smoked bittersweet paprika gains its taste from a type of pimiento; it is a cornerstone of Spanish and Hungarian cuisine—sausages, paella, grilled meat, and stews. Smoked hot paprika offers only a moderate heat factor; it is used with beans and soups, and on pork and chicken or shrimp. It also adds punch to garlic mayonnaise or deviled eggs. Spanish paprika—or *pimentón*—is available in three strengths—mild, medium spicy, and very spicy. In Hungary, there are eight grades of paprika, ranging from mild deep red to spicy light brown.

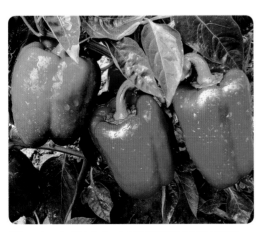

Although many *Capsicum annuum* peppers can be used to make paprika, sweet bell peppers are a traditional choice.

Paprika also lends color and flavor to a host of popular spice blends, including grilling rubs, marinades, and seasoned salts. It is loaded with healing nutrients, including carotenoids that contain vitamin A and give the spice its color; potent antioxidant vitamin C; vitamin E, vitamins B1, B2, and B6, and iron.

Healing Properties

Due to its lower levels of capsaicin—the disease-fighting substance found in peppers—paprika is not as medicinally powerful as, say, cayenne or jalapeño peppers. Still, it offers antibiotic, anti-inflammatory, antioxidant, and anti-aging benefits. Paprika can help normalize blood pressure, improve circulation, and increase production of saliva and stomach acids to assist digestion. Natural healers in Spain mix it with alcohol and cucumber juice to treat upset stomachs and cramps, while Hungarians add it to fruit brandy as a cure for colds and fevers.

History and Lore

» Paprika is famous for being the substance from which vitamin C—called L-ascorbic acid, for its antiscorbutic properties—was first identified by Hungarian physiologist Albert Szent-Györgyi. Szent-Györgyi won the 1937 Nobel Prize in Physiology for his discovery.

» Paprika powder can be used along with henna to add a reddish tint to the hair.

» If a red, orange, or reddish brown food is labeled "Natural Colors," chances are the hue comes from paprika.

Paprika

GLOBAL FLAVORS

Discover a new world of exotic herbs and spices.

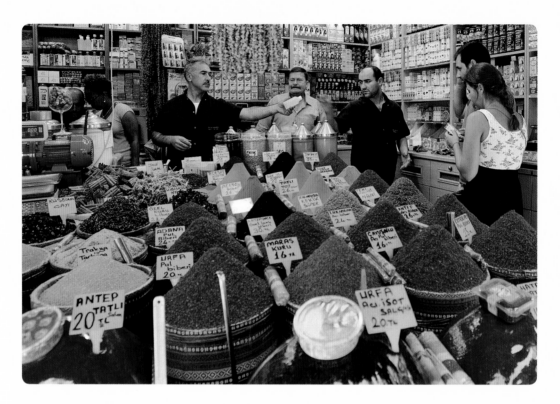

It started with Julia Child. Once the American host of *The French Chef* had introduced television viewers to the intricacies of *coq au vin* and *boeuf bourguignon,* many home cooks across the country were no longer satisfied making chicken casserole and meat loaf. Their cooking became more adventurous—they began bandying about terms like *braising* and *filleting* and started investigating the vast array of seasonings beyond black pepper and cinnamon.

In response to this home-cooking revolution, gourmet shops and specialty food stores selling a wide range of spices eventually sprang up in larger cities, while Latino, Asian, and Indian groceries began to appear in ethnic urban neighborhoods. Today, the revolution continues, with the Internet opening up a world of spices.

A New Spice Palette

Having mastered the basic seasonings of ethnic cuisine, like cumin and ginger, home cooks continue to discover even more ways to "internationalize" their menus. They now require a new palette of exotic spices and blends to complement their increasingly global dishes.

Stretch Your Culinary Boundaries

If you are interested in stretching your culinary boundaries, here are some promising additions to your spice rack. Any that cannot be found at local specialty shops can usually be ordered online.

- **Ajwain seeds:** This cousin of coriander and cumin starts out hot, but tastes like thyme or caraway after cooking. Small quantities—to avoid bitterness—are added to Asian, Arabic, Ethiopian, Indian, and Pakistani dishes. It is also used to relieve gas.
- **Amchur powder:** Made from sliced, unripe mangos that have been sun-dried and ground, amchur is used as a souring agent in Northern Indian cuisine.
- **Anardana:** The dried, sticky seed of wild pomegranates, *Punica granatum,* is used in Persian and Indian cooking as a souring agent, and it is typically included in chutneys. Its tart, fruity flavor makes it a good addition to seasoning mixes for fish and poultry, or try it as a tangy marinade for game.
- **Asafoetida:** The dried gum resin of the ferula root *(Ferula assa-foetida),* this herb combines the aroma of onions and garlic. Found in Indian, Afghani, and Pakistani cuisine, it is also used as an aid to digestion. In Western medicine, it is a respected antiviral and antimicrobial that has been used to treat influenza outbreaks.
- **Epazote:** This licorice-like herb, *Dysphania ambrosioides,* has been used in Central American cooking for thousands of years to flavor bean dishes, eggs, rice, salad, soup, and meat, and to make tea. It helps curb the gas-causing effect of beans.
- **Filé powder:** Sassafras leaves are the source of this flavoring and thickening powder that is the heart of Creole cuisine. It is used in chowders, gumbos, and other Creole dishes.
- **Gochugaru:** This Korean red pepper is known for its hot, sweet, and slightly smoky flavor.
- **Kaffir lime leaves:** The leaves of the kaffir lime *(Citrus hystrix),* used either fresh or dried, have a unique citrus taste that is hard to replicate. Native to Southeast Asia, they create a signature flavor note in Thai dishes and are also found in Balinese and Javanese cuisine.

- **Kala jeera:** Also known as black cumin or nigella, these small crescent-shaped seeds, members of the parsley family, have a nutty, grassy flavor. They are used in rice and meat curries and tandoori dishes in Northern India, and to flavor Pakistani naan bread.
- **Kiyuzu:** This tart, aromatic Japanese seasoning comes from the rind of a Chinese citrus fruit. It is used to flavor soy sauce, vinegar, and miso, and it is added to Japanese stew, sushi, sashimi, and cooked fish dishes. It also flavors a wide assortment of sweets.
- **Laska leaves:** These crushed leaves are sprinkled on Vietnamese laksa soup. They have a peppery taste reminiscent of mint and cilantro and can be substituted for either.
- **Loomi:** This sour spice, also called black lime, is ground from dried limes and used in many Middle Eastern dishes.
- **Mahleb:** Derived from the pit of the St. Lucie cherry, *Cerasus mahaleb,* this spice offers the flavor of almond with a hint of rose and cherry. Mahleb is used for baking—especially breads—and general cookery in Greece, the Middle East, and the Mediterranean. ∎

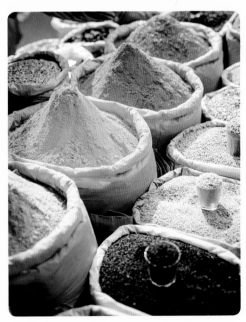

A traditional spice market in India sells spices by weight.

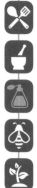

Saffron

Crocus sativus

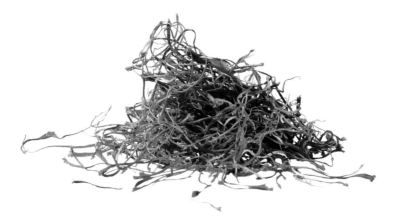

Harvesting saffron requires so much delicacy and care, that it is, by weight, the most expensive spice. Saffron comes from the three red stigmas, or threads, of the fall-flowering saffron crocus. They are traditionally picked by hand, and it takes roughly 75,000 flowers and 20 hours of work to make one pound of saffron. Fortunately, just a few threads of the spice can season an entire dish. In addition to offering a sublime taste of bitter honey, the strands create a golden hue in many dishes, including paella, Indian pilaus, and Cornish saffron buns.

DID YOU KNOW?
A delicate purple crocus is the source of saffron, the most costly of spices. Each tiny red thread is really the hand-picked stigma of the flower.

This native of West Asia was first cultivated more than four thousand years ago, possibly as a healing resource—it is mentioned in a Chinese medical book dating from 2600 B.C. The Egyptians used it as medicine, in perfumes, as a dye, and for cooking. The Persians believed saffron tea cured depression. The fragrant spice was strewn in Greek courts and baths and scattered in the streets of Rome when Nero made an entry into the city. In the eighth century, the conquering Muslims introduced the spice—*az-zafaran*—to Spain, beginning a rich culinary association that continues to the present. During the Renaissance, the spice was actually worth its weight in gold.

This bulbous perennial is a member of the iris family, Iridaceae; it grows to about eight inches in height, and produces upright pale purple flowers with the three distinctive red stigmas. Today, saffron is cultivated in Spain (three-quarters of world production), as well as in Italy, France, Greece, Turkey, Iran, and India.

Culinary Uses

Perhaps best known for giving Spanish paella its distinctive taste and color, saffron is also used to flavor French bouillabaisse; Indian rice,

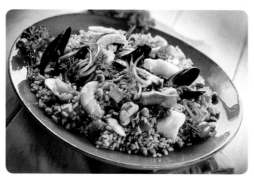

Paella, a complex rice dish from the Valencian region of Spain, can include a mix of many meats, vegetables, and seafood, but authentic paella always gets its golden hue from saffron.

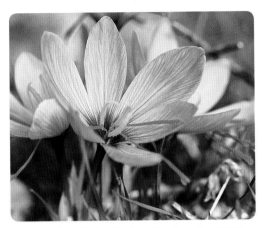

Only grown in cultivation, the late-blooming saffron crocus has been bred over time to produce very long stigmas.

sweets, and ice-cream; Milanese risotto; the Swedish bread served on St. Lucia's day; and Saudi Arabian coffee. Other cultures use saffron to enhance soups, stews, meat, seafood, breads, egg dishes, and vegetables. When adding saffron to recipes, remember that the flavor will be stronger on the second day.

Spanish Coupe Grade Saffron (*coupe* means "cut"), considered the finest saffron, consists exclusively of deep-red threads. Nutritionally, saffron supplies vitamin A, folic acid, riboflavin, niacin, and vitamin C, as well as the minerals copper, potassium, calcium, manganese, iron, selenium, zinc, and magnesium.

Healing Properties

Both Eastern and Western folk healers used saffron as a sedative, expectorant, and aphrodisiac, prescribing it for sore gums, indigestion, heart and lung disease, smallpox, colds, kidney stones, alcoholism, cramps, insomnia, diabetes, asthma, and depression. Its anti-aging properties led to its addition to many beauty potions—including, supposedly, those of Cleopatra.

Modern medicine acknowledges saffron as a potent antioxidant that can relieve both pain and inflammation. The spice contains more than 150 volatile and aroma-yielding compounds, ensuring years of study before all its healing secrets have been unlocked. Early research has indicated its ability to lower blood pressure, strengthen the heart, relieve menstrual distress and depression, and possibly even slow the progress of Alzheimer's disease and cancer.

Aromatic Qualities

Saffron has a woodsy, haylike bouquet with hints of honey. In aromatherapy, the essential oil is used to massage aching joints, lower blood pressure, treat migraines, and boost the appetite. Studies have shown that just a whiff of saffron can alter hormone levels in young women—increasing estrogen and decreasing cortisol—and help reduce anxiety.

History and Lore

» The crocus was considered a sacred symbol of the sun on Crete and was used to dye foods yellow as part of sun worship rituals.

» Henry VIII of England threatened death to anyone who attempted to adulterate saffron with less expensive spices.

» Buddhist monks traditionally wear saffron-colored robes to signify holiness—although today the robes are dyed with turmeric.

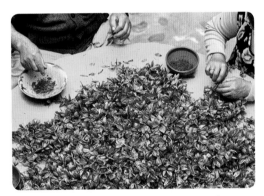

Gathering saffron is a painstaking process, with workers plucking each crocus flower's threadlike stigmas by hand.

CULTURAL CONNECTIONS

A Spice as Old as Time

The use of saffron goes back to the dawn of human history. In northwest Iran, archeologists found caves with 50,000-year-old images that contain traces of saffron pigments. On the Greek island of Thera, in the Aegean Sea, 3,500-year-old frescoes depict a Minoan goddess overseeing the manufacture and application of a medicine made from the crocus flower. An Egyptian text from 1500 B.C. describes crocuses growing in the palace gardens at Luxor. Even the name *saffron* is likely derived from Sumerian, a 5,000-year-old language of Mesopotamia. ■

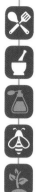

Sumac

Rhus coriaria

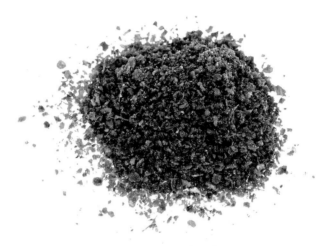

Tangy, lemony sumac is possibly one of the most under-rated spices in American kitchens, even though it is a staple of Middle Eastern cuisine. This deep-red spice is ground from the dried purplish fruit, also called berries or drupes, of the sumac bush—also known as Sicilian sumac, elm-leaved sumac, and tanner's sumach.

Although the plant is a cousin to the noxious poison ivy of North America, *Rhus coriaria* is safe to eat or touch. The spice was included in recipes by the ancient Romans, who also used it

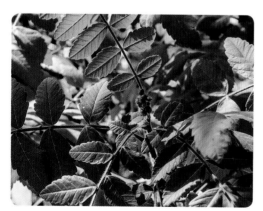

Sumac's pointed oval leave resemble those of the elm tree, giving it one of its common names, elm-leaved sumac.

DID YOU KNOW?
A deciduous shrub, sumac has a long history of medicinal use, and the dried and crushed fruit is a popular spice in the Middle East.

medicinally to lower fevers. Sumac supplied a tart element to many Arabic dishes in the days before the Romans introduced lemon trees to the region, and Europeans used it as a spice and medicine as well as a dye during the Middle Ages.

A member of the Anacardiaceae, or cashew family, *R. coriaria* originated in the Mediterranean. The bush grows to a height of 20 feet and produces pinnate leaves and tiny green, white, or red flowers that form dense spikes reaching nearly a foot in length. Sumac grows in many subtropical or temperate regions, including Africa, Southern Europe, Afghanistan, and Iran.

The common name comes from the Old French word *sumac,* meaning "red."

Culinary Uses

Sumac has a complex fruity flavor that is milder than lemon juice or vinegar. It enhances the taste of many recipes without overwhelming them, and it is not at all acidic. Tart, lively sumac works best with fish and chicken dishes, cheese and yogurt, salad dressings, and rice pilaf. The spice is widely used in Turkey, the Middle East, Syria, and Lebanon to season kebabs, hummus, and tabbouleh. It is mixed with thyme and sesame

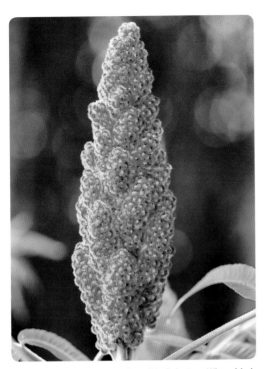

The tart fruit of sumac grows in pointed clusters. When dried and crushed, the fruit is mixed with ground dried oregano, thyme, or marjoram and toasted sesame seeds to make the popular Middle Eastern spice mixture *za'atar*.

seeds to create *za'atar,* the Middle Eastern table-top condiment that is sprinkled on *fattoush* salad. Try using sumac in grilling rubs, hot vegetable dishes, and cold bean or beet salads—anywhere that fresh lemon juice might be used.

Nutritionally, the spice contains high levels of vitamin C, as well as protein, dietary fiber, potassium, calcium, magnesium, and phosphorus. Sumac is available ground—and sometimes whole—in most Middle Eastern markets, specialty food stores, or online.

Healing Properties

While it is not bursting with health benefits, like the "superfoods," sumac is known to have antimicrobial, antifungal, and antioxidant properties, and it is a digestive aid. Natural healers have employed it as a diuretic, for bowel complaints, to reduce skin inflammation, and to ease respiratory conditions. Meanwhile, medical research is still uncovering possible health benefits. One study showed that sumac mixed in water was able to rid fresh fruit and vegetables of the harmful *Salmonella* bacteria.

History and Lore

» Sumac drupes were found in an 11th-century shipwreck discovered off the coast of Rhodes, indicating they were being used as either a food source or a medicine.

» Certain types of sumac yield tannin, a substance used in the tanning of leather that is intended to make it flexible and light.

» In North America, two related species *(Rhus glabra)* and staghorn sumac *(R. typhina),* are used to prepare a tangy cooling drink known as sumac-ade, Indian lemonade, or rhus juice.

IN THE KITCHEN

Middle Eastern Sumac Salad

Considered an essential for cooking in much of the Middle East, ground sumac is still new to the American culinary scene. This salad combines fresh cucumber, tomatoes, and red onions with the lemony counterpoint of ground sumac and cilantro to make a refreshing summer meal or a year-round side dish.

Ingredients
- 2 large cucumbers
- 1 large ripe tomato
- ½ red onion
- 1 tablespoon sumac
- 4 tablespoons minced cilantro
- 1 tablespoon virgin olive oil
- salt, to taste

Directions
Peel and slice the cucumbers into chunks, and then chop the tomatoes into bite-sized pieces. Slice the onions into small pieces. Place all vegetables in a bowl, along with minced cilantro, and drizzle with olive oil. Sprinkle on sumac and season with salt. ■

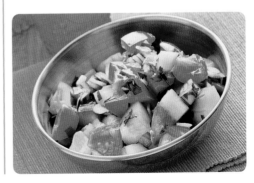

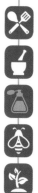

Turmeric

Curcuma longa

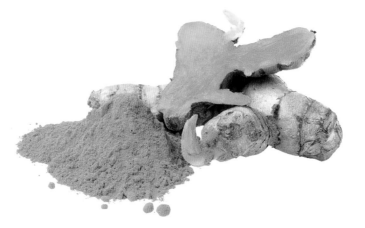

Turmeric has recently gained wide media recognition for its many restorative and preventative qualities. This is not surprising, considering that natural healers have been prescribing it for four thousand years to treat a variety of ailments. A symbol of auspiciousness in Hindu philosophy, turmeric surely deserves its nickname, "the golden spice," for its versatility as a foodstuff, medicine, textile dye, and cosmetic.

This tropical perennial, a member of the ginger family, Zingiberaceae, likely originated in Southern Asia. It spread to the Middle East and Mediterranean around 330 B.C., after Alexander the Great conquered Central Asia. Turmeric is estimated to have reached China around the year A.D. 700, East Africa by 800, and West Africa by 1200. It was first seen in Jamaica in the 1700s.

The plant grows to a height of three feet and produces long, oblong leaves and clustered yellow flowers topped by a pink or white bract. The thick, tuberous rhizome of the plant is the source of the spice after being dried and ground into a yellow-orange powder. The common name derives from the Latin words *terra merita,* or "meritorious earth," which refers to the yellow-orange color of ground turmeric.

> **DID YOU KNOW?**
>
> Known for its antioxidant powers, turmeric is the crushed and ground rhizome of *Curcuma longa.* A versatile spice, this staple of Indian food is also used for dyeing.

Culinary Uses

While warm, peppery turmeric is sometimes used as a less expensive alternative to saffron, the spice brings a lot to the table in its own right. It is a key ingredient in curry powder, and it is used in the Middle East and North Africa to flavor and color sauces, syrups, rice dishes, meats, and vegetables. Turmeric is essential to the Arab *ras el hanout* spice blend and to Indian masala spice mixtures. Worldwide, it is used as a coloring in commercial foods like canned beverages,

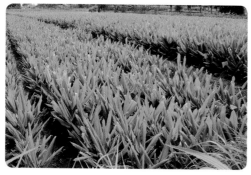

Rows of turmeric plants stretch into the horizon at a farm in India. India grows up to 85 percent of the world's turmeric and also consumes about 80 percent of the spice.

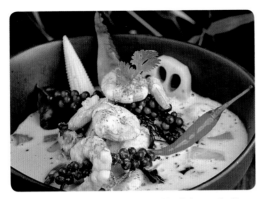

Thai Green Curry with Shrimp. Thai cuisine is known for its wide variety of curries. Fresh turmeric rhizomes are used to prepare the classic yellow and green curries.

dairy products, ballpark mustard, cereals, chips, cheese, butter, baked goods, ice cream, yellow cakes, orange juice, popcorn, cake icings, cereals, sauces, and gelatins. The turmeric root can also be eaten raw or cooked and has a sweet, nutty, slightly bitter flavor.

Nutritionally, it contains significant quantities of vitamins C, E, and K, folate, niacin, pyridoxine, and potassium electrolytes, as well as calcium, copper, iron, magnesium, manganese, phosphorus, and zinc.

Healing Properties

Turmeric possesses potent antioxidant, anti-inflammatory, antibiotic, antiseptic, and analgesic qualities. Indian and Chinese healers have used it for centuries, especially to treat rheumatoid arthritis, eye ailments, conjunctivitis, skin cancer, small pox, chicken pox, digestive disorders, loss of appetite, wounds, urinary tract infections, and liver ailments. Many South Asian countries still use it as an antiseptic for cuts, burns, and bruises. Although the ancient Greeks were aware of turmeric, it never intrigued Western culture as a seasoning or medicine the way ginger did. As a result, very little was written about the spice, and it did not attract the attention of Western herbal healers until the 20th century.

Modern science, on the other hand, has marveled at the spice's potential for combating chronic diseases. Its active ingredient, curcumin, may prove helpful in treating cancer, diabetes, allergies, arthritis, bowel disorders, and Alzheimer's disease. (India, which consumes the most turmeric, has some of the lowest prevalence rates for the disease.) Turmeric is also believed to lower cholesterol, heal ulcers, relieve depression, aid in the metabolism of fat, and reduce the side effects of chemotherapy.

Aromatic Qualities

Turmeric has a mild, but delicious, fragrance, slightly reminiscent of orange and ginger. The essential oil, like the spice itself, acts as an anti-inflammatory and antioxidant.

History and Lore

» The South Indian state of Tamil Nadu, the largest producer of the spice and its major trading center, is also known as "Yellow City," "Turmeric City," or "Textile City."

» In Hawaii, turmeric is called olena and is employed in the magical arts.

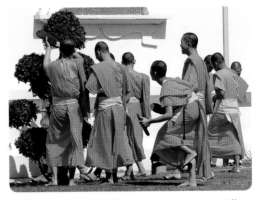

Buddhist monks traditionally wear what are known as saffron robes. In keeping with their vows of poverty, they do not use the highly expensive saffron to dye the cloth the deep yellow-orange color, but instead use the far cheaper turmeric.

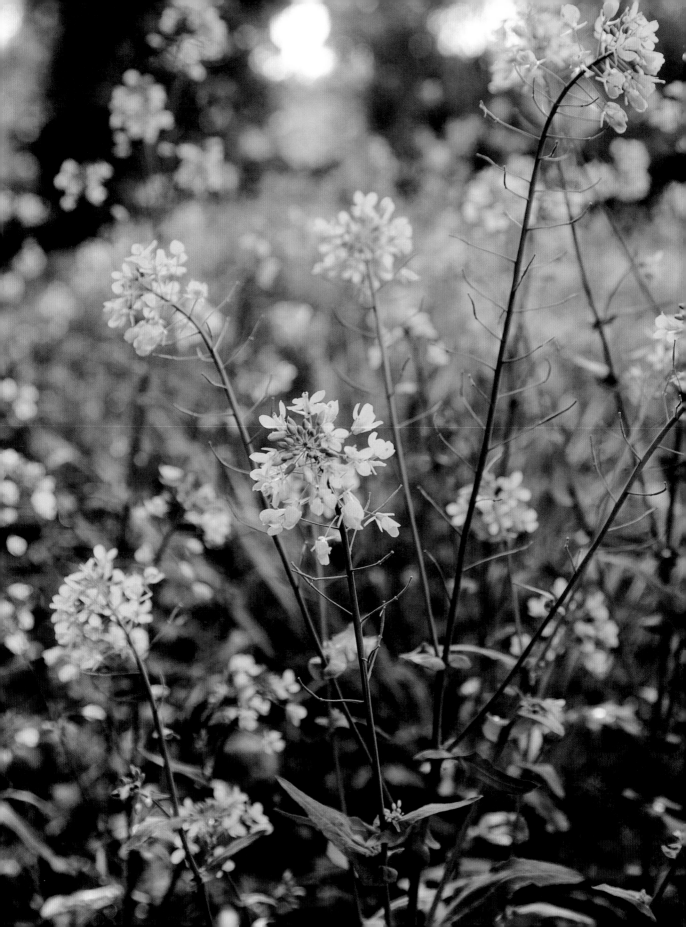

SEASONINGS

Opposite: **Mustard**

Finishing Touches

TOPPING OFF YOUR RECIPES IN STYLE

After a meal is cooked, the ritual of preparation is not always over. A dish may require a soupçon of something more—a bit of vinegary tartness or the aromatic aura of garlic, the bite of mustard, the crisp contrast of onion, or the satisfying sweetness of sugar.

Then again, some of these flavorings can be used during the preparation of a recipe or sprinkled on at the table, like salt. Regardless of when they are applied or how they are used, these are our seasonings, our condiments—not leafy herbs or exotic spices, but rather the tasty, welcome additions to mealtimes around the world.

Auguste Escoffier, legendary French chef and the man who popularized traditional French cooking methods, classified both seasonings and condiments in his 1903 book, *Le guide culinaire*. He broke seasonings down into four groups: saline, including salts and spiced salts; acids, including lemon juice and vinegar; hot seasonings, such as black pepper or paprika (presented as spices in this book); and saccharine seasonings, including sugar and honey. Condiments include the pungents—alliums and horseradish; hot condiments— mustard, capers, gherkins, Tabasco, and wines for braising; and fats—including lard, butter, edible oils, and margarine.

GOING WAY BACK . . .

Many condiments go back to the dawn of civilization—archeologists recently found the residue of garlic-mustard seeds on six-thousand-year-old pottery shards in Denmark and Germany; garlic and onions, too, date back at least that far, especially in China. Salt has a long and colorful history and was first extracted from water around 4000 B.C. in Romania and China. Sugar cane was "the sacred reed" of India for millennia, but its spread to the West was relatively slow, and it was not widely available in Europe until around A.D. 1200. Perhaps the no-cal sweetener stevia sounds new to a lot

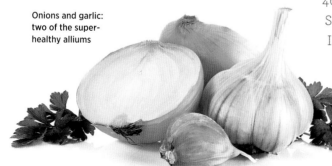

Onions and garlic: two of the super-healthy alliums

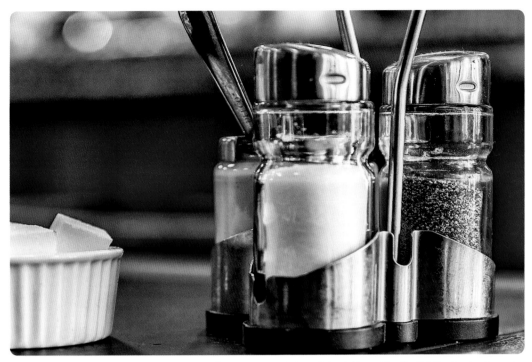

Condiments, like salt and pepper, sugar, and mustard, are ever present at our dining tables, adding the finishing touches to meals.

of us, but the indigenous people of Paraguay have used this naturally sweet plant as food and medicine for centuries.

Seasonings go in and out of style for reasons of culinary fashion or health awareness, and authentic-tasting substitutions for sugar and salt—without their purported negative side effects—are always being sought. In the days of ancient Rome, garlic was considered too potent for the well-bred diner, and so it became a staple of the working class for centuries. When Americans began to embrace ethnic cuisines, like Italian or Korean, garlic again became fashionable. These days, consuming garlic as part of a heart-healthy, Mediterranean diet is an established practice.

> **"It's hard to imagine a civilization without onions."**
>
> *—Julia Child*

MEDICAL MARVELS

Many seasonings are effective disease fighters, with health benefits that at times even eclipse herbs and spices. The allium family alone boasts at least two antioxidant-packed "superfoods"—the aforementioned garlic, which can lower triglycerides and cholesterol, and prevent the formation of blood clots, and onions, which can lower the risk of certain cancers. Another allium, ramps, when grown with increased levels of selenium, might help to combat asthma and cystic fibrosis. Both mustard and horseradish contain cancer-fighting agents called glucosinolates, with the latter supplying ten times more of that phytonutrient than broccoli.

Finishing Touches

269

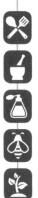

Garlic

Allium sativum

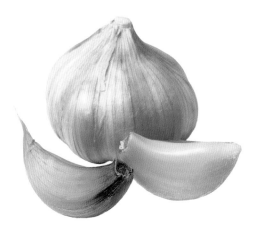

Known to Asian cultures at least six thousand years ago, garlic is an ancient herb, but its exact origins are lost in the sands of time. What is known is that the Egyptians worshipped the plant, and while the Greeks and Romans fed it to athletes and soldiers for strength and courage, the patricians called it the "stinking rose," and declared it fit only for laborers. It was again looked down upon in the early 20th century but had revived by century's end. Americans now consume more than 250 million pounds of garlic every year.

DID YOU KNOW?
Garlic is renowned as both a pervasive seasoning and a potent medicinal resource that is only beginning to be tapped.

The plant's common name comes from the Old English word *garleac,* which means "spear leek." It is a member of the lily family, or Amaryllidaceae, and it is a cousin to onions, leeks, and scallions. Garlic plants can grow to a height of about two feet and feature globular pinkish white flowers. The bulbs that grow and mature underground can be harvested in late summer, bundled together, and hung up to dry.

Culinary Uses

Garlic does more than complement a recipe—it lends its essence to the present moment and lingers afterward. Garlic is vital to the pungent cuisine of many regions, from Mediterranean and Indian to Chinese and Southeast Asian. While it can "lift" a dish in small amounts, it can obliterate other flavors if applied with a heavy hand. Some recipes, however—like French and Spanish aioli and Greek *skordalia*—specify a liberal quantity. Garlic makes a perfect accompaniment to beef, pork, venison, poultry, and seafood, and can enhance soups, salad dressings, grilling rubs, marinades, sausage, and pasta sauce.

Nutritionally, garlic is rich in vitamin B6 and magnesium. It is also a good source of selenium and vitamin C.

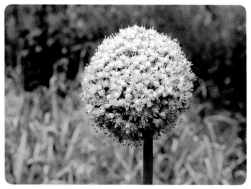

Garlic will produce a pretty globe of white to pinkish white flowers, but to harvest the largest edible bulbs, cut off any flower shoots when they emerge in spring.

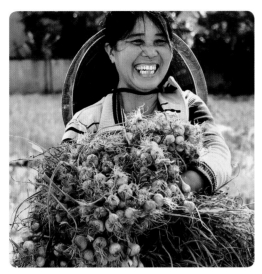

A farm worker in Vietnam harvesting bunches of garlic. These bulbs are a very popular seasoning in many Asian cuisines.

Cancer researchers have determined that a high intake of garlic can lower the risk of all cancers, except prostate and breast cancer. The operative word here is *high,* as in eating some garlic every day.

Garlic is also justifiably renowned for its antibacterial and antiviral properties. It has the ability to control both bacterial and viral infections, as well as those caused by fungi, yeasts, and worms. Researchers are exploring the possibility that garlic can combat overgrowth of the bacterium *Helicobacter pylori,* a key cause of stomach ulcers.

One way to help garlic do its job as a disease fighter is to let it sit a while after cutting it, allowing its beneficial enzymes to work. Immediate cooking has been shown to decrease their protective qualities.

Healing Properties

Since antiquity, garlic has been touted as a cure for various ailments, including heart conditions, infections, indigestion, and lack of libido. In the Middle Ages, it was even thought to combat the Black Plague and leprosy.

Faith in the plant was not misplaced: garlic's high levels of powerful sulfur-containing compounds—responsible for its intense odor—are the source of its health-promoting qualities and help to regulate blood pressure and maintain levels of sulfur. Like other hearty-healthy alliums, garlic can lower triglycerides and cholesterol; limit the oxidative stress that damages blood vessels and causes inflammation; and prevent the formation of blood clots.

Aromatic Qualities

In aromatherapy, garlic is used as a syrup to relieve coughing, as an ointment to ease swollen joints, as a vinegar to treat skin outbreaks, and as a lotion for stimulating the hair and scalp.

History and Lore

» According to Arab legend, garlic grew from the footprint the Devil left behind after he fled Eden.
» Garlic was believed to protect children or farm animals from sorcery, to keep seafarers safe, and to ward off the jealous nymphs who terrorized pregnant women and engaged maidens.
» During World War I, the Russians used garlic to treat battle wounds and infection.

The Bane of Vampires

In addition to its mellow, nutty flavor, garlic's other claim to fame in many cultures is its ability to repel evil. British author Bram Stoker incorporated this traditional theme into *Dracula,* his story of a charismatic vampire—one of the "undead" who lives on human blood and takes the form of a bat. In Stoker's story, garlic, along with holy water and the Christian cross, were said to keep the bloodthirsty creature at bay. As recently as the 1970s in Slavic countries, a corpse's nose, mouth and ears were stuffed with garlic cloves to keep out evil. ■

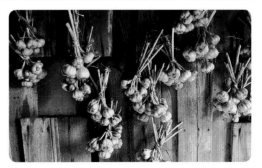

Along with the ability to ward off devils, werewolves, and vampires, according to European folk belief, garlic hung over a doorway would keep envious people from entering.

271

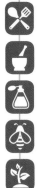

Horseradish

Armoracia rusticana

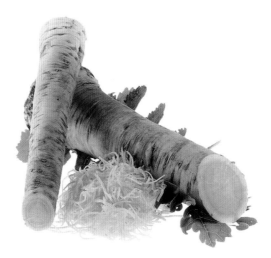

Fiery horseradish, which adds punch to so many dishes, is one of the newly christened "superfoods." Considering this root's long history as a popular seasoning and a powerful healer, it's not surprising horseradish is experiencing a renaissance.

The plant is possibly native to Hungary or to a larger area that ranged from Finland all the way to the Caspian Sea. In many parts of Europe, it grows wild as a garden escapee. It traveled to America with the European settlers, and both George Washington and Thomas Jefferson mentioned it in accounts of their gardens.

A member of the mustard family, or Brassicaceae, the horseradish plant reaches three to four feet in height and produces large, rough, green basal leaves and clustering white flowers. The large, white, tapered root has little

In summer, clusters of white, four-petaled flowers appear atop the leggy stalks of horseradish.

scent until it is processed—and then releases the intense, eye-watering aroma of hot mustard.

The word *horse* in the plant's common name indicates "strong" or "coarse," and was originally used to distinguish *Armoracia rusticana* from the edible radish, *Raphanus sativus.* Ironically, the plant is poisonous to horses.

Culinary Uses

In 16th-century Europe, horseradish was strictly a medicinal plant except in Germany and Denmark, where it was used as a condiment. By the mid-1600s, England too was serving it at the table. Once the French began to eat it, they referred to it as *moutarde des Allemands,* or German mustard.

Horseradish is popular in Poland and in Great Britain, especially served with roast beef. Tewkesbury mustard, mustard combined with horseradish, has been enjoyed in England since medieval times. In American kitchens, traditional horseradish accompanies stews, horseradish sauce prepared with mayonnaise is spread on sandwich meats, and horseradish cream (horseradish blended with sour cream) is served with prime rib. Prepared horseradish is also added to Bloody Marys and to cocktail sauce.

Stimulating Scalp Massage

In aromatherapy, the essential oil of horseradish is considered very effective for keeping the scalp healthy. It can even slow down the process of hair loss by stimulating the hair follicles. To make a beneficial scalp massage, combine two table-spoons of soya oil, a half fluid ounce of grapeseed oil, 2 drops of wheat germ oil, and 30 drops of horseradish oil. Apply to the scalp, and massage in with the fingertips. Leave on scalp for an hour or more, and then rinse out with a mild shampoo. ◼

When the grated root is mixed with vinegar, the result is a creamy white sauce. In many Slavic languages, this sauce is called *kren.* Sometimes beets are added, giving *kren* a bright magenta hue—Poles call this version *ćwikła.* European Jews serve it with gefilte fish, and it accompanies Easter lamb in Transylvania.

Nutritionally, horseradish is rich in vitamin C, folate, vitamin B6, riboflavin, niacin, dietary fiber, and the minerals sodium, potassium, manganese, iron, copper, zinc, and magnesium. Homemade horseradish keeps for months in the refrigerator.

Healing Properties

Healers utilize almost every part of this anti-biotic and antifungal plant. The root makes an expectorant tea, a sinus-relieving extract, and a poultice for joint pain. The flowers can be brewed into a cold-busting tea, and the raw leaves can stop headache discomfort when pressed against the forehead.

Recent scientific revelations continue to elevate the plant's stature as a healing agent. Many cruciferous vegetables, like broccoli and cabbage, contain cancer-fighting agents called glucosinolates, but horseradish contains ten times more of this compound than broccoli. (Glucosinolates are also responsible for the heat in horseradish, mustard, and wasabi.) They also increase the liver's ability to detoxify carcinogens, and may also suppress the growth of existing tumors.

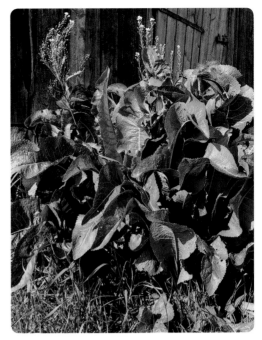

Planted in a sunny, out-of-the-way spot, rugged horseradish plants will thrive with very little care. Just one year after planting, horseradish will be ready for its first harvest.

History and Lore

» Horseradish is also known as mountain radish, great raifort, and red cole. In northern Italy, it is called *barbaforte,* or "strong beard."

» The plant's alternate species name is *Cochlearia armoracia.* This genus name comes from cochleare, which is a type of old-fashioned spoon that horseradish leaves were said to resemble.

» Folklore advised couples to put a slice of horse-radish under their pillows to determine the gender of an unborn child. If the husband's slice turned black before the wife's, the child would be a boy, and vice versa.

» Horseradish is the plant most often used as the bitter herb, or *maror,* that is eaten during the Jewish Passover seder as a reminder of the Israelites' enslavement to Egypt.

A passover seder plate with the traditional six symbolic food items arranged in their places, including a dab of horseradish (top center) as the bitter herb.

Horseradish

273

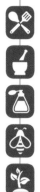

Mustard

Brassica spp., *Sinapis* spp.

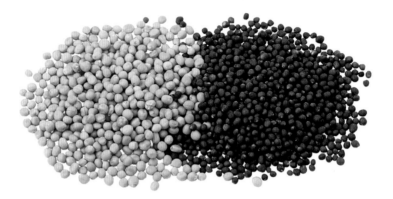

Mustard, which dates back to the tombs of the pharaohs, is now the second-most popular seasoning in the United States—after black pepper. Three plant species produce seeds that are used as a condiment: *Sinapsis alba,* or white mustard, is native to Europe and has been cultivated since antiquity. It grows wild in North Africa, the Middle East, and the Mediterranean. *Brassica nigra,* or black mustard, originated in the Middle East and is now grown in Argentina, Chile, the United States, and Europe. *B. juncea,* brown or Indian mustard, originated in the Himalayan foothills and is now cultivated in India, Canada, the United Kingdom, Denmark, and the United States.

Mustard plants are members of the Brassicaceae family, which also includes cabbage, broccoli, and horseradish. Black mustard is the tallest of

Often considered a weed, black mustard (Brassica nigra) is a winter annual in warm climates.

them, growing from two to eight feet in height, while white mustard reaches only a foot or so. They all bear four-petaled, yellow flowers that cluster on erect stems. These blossoms mature into narrow seed pods, with seeds that range in color from beige to dark brown.

The common name of the plant came from the Roman habit of steeping mustard seeds in must, or new wine, with the resulting mixture called *mustrum.*

Culinary Uses

In addition to home kitchens, mustard seeds are used commercially in the preparation of meats, sausages, vegetables, and relishes. Whole or processed, they will yield ground mustard, powdered dry mustard, prepared mustard, and mustard paste. All three color versions can be blended to achieve a balance of flavors.

White mustard seeds have fewer volatile oils than the black and are milder—this is the seasoning that flavors bland yellow mustard. Black has a stronger taste, though little aroma. In India, the seeds are used in curry and as the source of cooking oil; when sautéed, they pop open and develop a nutty taste. In Ethiopia, the seeds, shoots, and leaves are all

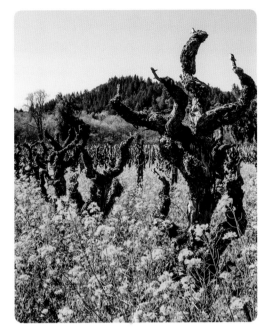

Golden mustard blossoms spill in riots of color between resting grapevines in California's Napa Valley. During this flowering plant's blooming season in February and March, local vineyards hold the annual Napa Valley Mustard Festival.

consumed. Brown mustard seeds, with their acrid, pungent taste, are the source of tangy Dijon mustard. The leaves are used in Japanese, Chinese, and African cookery, while the leaves, seeds, and stems are a staple of Indian and Nepalese cuisine. In American soul food, mustard greens are slow cooked and flavored with smoked pork.

Nutritionally, mustard is a good source of vitamins A, B1, and K, omega-3 fatty acids, selenium, magnesium, phosphorus, and copper.

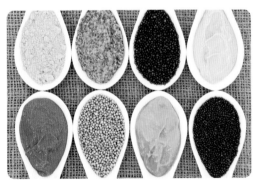

A few of the many varieties of mustard: Top row, from left: powdered, whole grain mustard, black mustard seeds, Dijon mustard; bottom row: English mustard, white mustard seeds, American yellow mustard, and brown mustard seeds.

Healing Properties

Both the Greeks and Romans used mustard to treat inflammation. In Eastern Europe, the ground seeds are mixed with honey and prescribed as a cough suppressant. Placing a poultice of ground mustard, flour, flax seed, and water on the chest is still a popular folk cure for treating respiratory infections.

Modern research indicates that mustard seeds contain beneficial phytonutrients called glucosinolates that are broken down into cancer-fighting isothiocyanates; these inhibit the growth of existing cancer cells and help to prevent the formation of new ones. The seeds can also help to ease the symptoms of asthma and rheumatoid arthritis, lower blood pressure, and reduce the frequency of migraines.

Aromatic Qualities

The essential oil of mustard is very strong, but it can be used externally to treat rheumatism, sciatica, and lumbago. In theory, mustard oil draws blood to the surface of the skin by irritating it, thus relieving the swelling of deep tissues.

History and Lore

» According to Greek myth, humankind received mustard from Aesculepius, the god of medicine, and Ceres, the goddess of agriculture.

» Both England and France are noted for the production of specialty mustards.

» It is possible that mustard seeds with high oil content can be used in the production of biodiesel, a renewable fuel similar to diesel fuel.

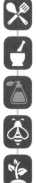

Onion

Allium cepa

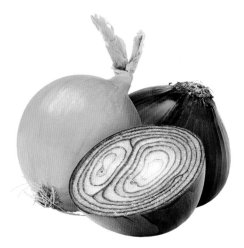

Onions are one of humankind's oldest foods—consumed by Bronze Age tribes and grown in Chinese gardens more than five thousand years ago. Early healers also employed them for treating bronchial ailments and joint inflammation.

The plant's origins are cloudy—*Allium cepa* has been cultivated for so long in Europe and Asia, it is difficult to determine where it first grew wild. Ancient civilizations revered these alliums, and, during the Middle Ages, onions were so valued, they were sometimes given as wedding gifts. The Spanish introduced them to the West Indies and European settlers brought them to North America, where the Indians were already using wild onions as food, medicine, and dyes.

Like other alliums, onions produce attractive globular flowers that appear singly on rather weak stalks.

The onion is a member of the lily family, or Amaryllidaceae. The plant reaches a height of about eight inches and features a fan of blue-green leaves that grows directly out of the developing bulb. This bulb can be harvested in the fall after the foliage dies back. If not harvested, the following spring a long, hollow stem will sprout and produce a globular umbel of tiny white flowers. The common name of this allium comes from the Latin *unio*, meaning "single large pearl," after the flower's shape and color.

Culinary Uses

Onions were one of the three main vegetables available in medieval Europe along with beans and cabbage—and they can now be found in most cuisines throughout the world. Savory or hearty dishes benefit from the addition of onions—their strong, pungent flavor mellows as they cook, and once fully caramelized their taste can only be described as sublime. When heated, they improve stews, soups, casseroles, gravies, and pasta sauces; served raw, they add bite to salads, hero sandwiches, hamburgers, and marinades.

There are more than a thousand kinds of onion, but a few have become kitchen favorites. White

No More Tears

Many cooks find slicing onions a trial, mainly because of the tears they generate. Unfortunately, cutting into an onion releases *syn*-propanethial-*S*-oxide, a chemical that triggers a powerful blinking and tearing reflex. Yet, there are methods for accomplishing this task without the waterworks. The first is to cut onions underwater in a small basin. Another trick is wearing swim or ski goggles to protect your eyes. Or try super cooling the onion for a few minutes in the freezer. Perhaps the most novel suggestion is to hold a piece of bread in your mouth—it can absorb the fumes before they reach your eyes. ■

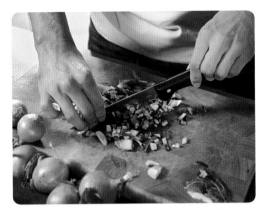

The eye-stinging and tear-inducing aroma of onions keeps cooks on the search for a tear-free chopping technique.

onions are mild and sweet, an intrinsic part of Mexican cooking. All-purpose yellow globe onions are robust, but sweet, and the choice for French onion soup and for standing up to liver. Red onions are mild, usually served raw. Versatile Spanish onions are large, yellow, and mild. Vidalia, or sweet, onions are pale and flat, ideal for those sensitive to onions.

Nutritionally, onions are an excellent source of vitamins C and B6, folic acid, and fiber, and also supply calcium, magnesium, phosphorus, potassium, and manganese.

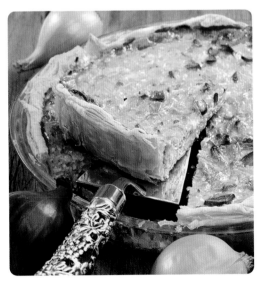

Along with its use as a seasoning for other foods, onions can take center stage, as in the traditional onion tart from the Alsace region of France that features caramelized onions in a base of savory custard and creamy Gruyère cheese.

Healing Properties

Natural healers have employed onions for millennia. Early cultures believed eating them improved strength. In medieval Europe, they were used to treat headache, snakebite, and hair loss. In China, they were prescribed for angina, coughs, and bacterial infections.

Modern research has discovered that onions are rich in phytonutrients called polyphenols, which are powerful antioxidants. Most of this beneficial goodness lies in the bulb's outer layers, however, so only peel away the papery skin. Onions contain a flavonoid called quercetin that is effective for slowing oxidative damage to cells. In studies, four or five servings of onion per week reduced the risk for certain cancers, including colorectal, laryngeal, and ovarian. Ideally, one allium vegetable a day should be included in the diet.

History and Lore

» To early Egyptians, the concentric rings of the onion symbolized eternal life; they often placed a stack of them in burial tombs—wrapped up in bandages like little mummies.

» Ancient Greeks believed onions balanced the blood; athletes competing in the Olympic games ate onions by the pound, drank onion juice, and even rubbed it on their bodies.

» Onions have inspired many folk cures, including binding a cooked onion over the ear to relieve earache, placing it under the pillow to cure insomnia, and chewing a raw onion to keep colds at bay.

Onion

277

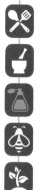

Ramps

Allium tricoccum

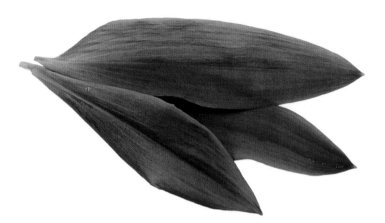

Ramps, also called wild leeks, spring onions, ramsons, wood leeks, and wild garlic, are another relative of the onion and still grow wild in many places. They are found in cool, shady glades with damp, rich soil, often along with early-spring bloomers like trillium, black cohosh, blood root, trout lilies, hepatica, and mayapple.

Perennial ramps are native to the Appalachian Mountains of the eastern United States, and they currently range all the way from South Carolina to Canada. The plant's small bulb

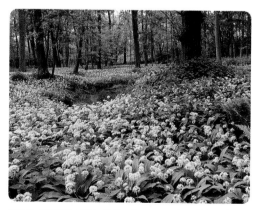

During springtime in North Carolina, a covering of blooming ramps forms a green-and-white carpet on the forest floor.

DID YOU KNOW?

Found growing in rich, moist, deciduous forests, this petite member of the amaryllis family is a wild onion that is harvested in spring for its garlic-onion flavor

is similar to that of a scallion, but its flat, broad green leaves—with reddish bases—distinguish the ramp from its cousin. The leaves emerge from the perennial bulb in early spring—usually late March or early April—and die back by late May. The flowers appear in June as a dome-shaped cluster of small white blossoms on a leafless stem.

The plant's common name, which is almost always used in its plural form, comes from the word *rams* (or *ramson*), which was Elizabethan dialect for wild garlic. English colonists were most likely familiar with the European ramp or bear leek (*Allium ursinum*), a plant related to the American species, which was found in abundance in Great Britain and was often used there as a vegetable.

Culinary Uses

Ramps have a sweetly pungent flavor and make a tasty addition to egg dishes, like quiche or frittatas, pizza, and pesto. They can be blended with potatoes or other vegetables in soup, added to green salad, chicken or tuna salad, or mixed into hamburger meat, cornbread batter, rice, or chili. They are delicious caramelized in butter or bacon fat and served as a side dish with trout.

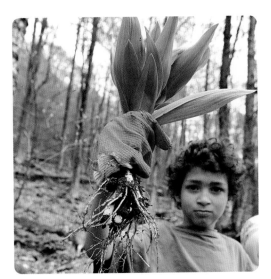

In spring, foragers—people who seek out edible food in fields and woodlands—scour East Coast forests in search of ramps.

To prepare ramps for cooking or salads, simply cut off the roots, rinse thoroughly, and pat dry. Fresh ramps have a short season, but extra bunches can be purchased, blanched, and frozen for later use. Nutritionally, ramps are a rich source of vitamins A and C and choline, as well as the trace mineral selenium and the essential mineral chromium.

Healing Properties

During colonial times, March ramps were the first "official" greens of the season and were considered a health tonic—their vitamins and minerals were especially valuable after a winter without fresh vegetables. Cherokee Indians used the bulbs to treat coughs, colds, and the flu, and they possibly shared this knowledge with the settlers. Natural healers also use the antibiotic qualities of ramp bulbs to combat colds and flu and to lower blood pressure.

Like other alliums, ramps are packed with antioxidants that are effective for balancing blood sugar levels and reducing the risk of cancer. Some clinical studies indicate the selenium in ramps may reduce the risk of prostate cancer. With this in mind, hydroponic cultivation can create enriched ramps with increased concentrations of the mineral. Selenium's antioxidant effects might also be effective in relieving the symptoms of asthma, cystic fibrosis, high blood pressure, and a number of other conditions.

CULTURAL CONNECTIONS

Ramps—Trending and Dwindling

Many East Coast states look forward to the early spring arrival of ramps, and some, like North Carolina, West Virginia, and Tennessee, are home to annual festivals honoring this little allium. These events grew in size once they began attracting tourists, and they became a key source of funding for local fire departments, rescue squads, and other civic organizations. When celebrity chefs began promoting ramps on television, they became trendy. Unfortunately, due to the large quantity of wild ramps consumed at the festivals, and the added demand from restaurants, native populations are now dwindling. Scientists are also collecting ramps for cancer research, compounding the problem of disappearing plants—especially considering that after one seasonal harvest it can take years for a given population to recover. Perhaps the United States needs to take a cue from Canada—due to excess harvesting, it has designated ramps a vulnerable species, and they are no longer available commercially. ■

History and Lore

» In the 1600s, a town near Lake Michigan took the Indian word for ramps, which grew beside the lake, as its name: *shikaakwa*—better known as Chicago.
» Food writer Jane Snow insists that ramps smell like "fried green onions with a dash of funky feet."

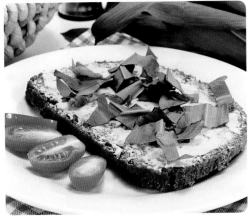

Chopped ramps can be used as a sandwich green to add a healthy kick of flavor, but they give off a pervasive garlic-onion odor that lasts for days, so use them sparingly in your dishes.

VERSATILE VINEGAR

Explore its many uses—from salad dressing to disinfectant.

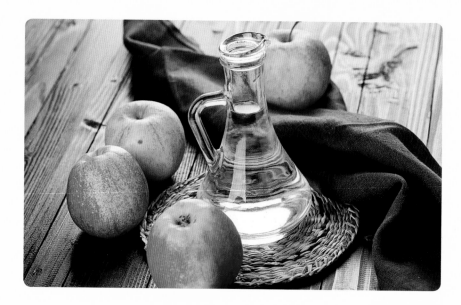

This humble kitchen condiment has been benefiting humans for more than ten thousand years. The discovery of vinegar—concurrent with the production of wine—goes back to the Neolithic period, 8500 B.C. to 4000 B.C., when the residents of present-day Egypt and the Middle East began farming crops for food.

The Safe Sanitizer

Vinegar is composed of acetic acid—CH_3COOH—and requires the fermentation of a sugar (fruit, honey, grain, sugar cane, or even cellulose) into alcohol using yeast, and then the further fermentation of alcohol by acetic acid bacteria (acetobacters). This process would have happened naturally if wine in a damaged clay jar was exposed to oxygen. Over time, the sweet wine would turn to sour vinegar, or *vin aigre*, French for "sour wine."

This metamorphosis was doubtless discovered accidentally by early civilizations like the Babylonians, who put the "mistake" to good use as a health tonic, disinfectant, food preservative, and seasoning. The mass production of vinegar became one of the earliest commercial industries in world history; by Roman times, the refreshing combination of water and vinegar called *posca* was a part of every meal. Today, vinegar is an ingredient in prepared mustard, mayonnaise, and ketchup.

Herbalists have always sworn by its curative and wound-healing abilities, but, so far, modern science only allows that vinegar aids in the absorption of minerals, including calcium, and that it shows promise in normalizing blood sugar levels in type 2 diabetes sufferers. Further research is ongoing, however.

The Safe Sanitizer

Due to its antiseptic and disinfectant properties, vinegar—especially a white or distilled variety—makes an effective and inexpensive cleansing agent. It is guaranteed to leave surfaces sanitized and gleaming, with the acid in vinegar cutting through any grease or germs. For most uses, simply add equal parts of vinegar and water, and sponge down sinks, faucets, countertops, vanities, windows, mirrors, appliances, pet mats, tubs, toilets, and shower stalls. After the initial acrid smell, vinegar leaves behind no lingering scent, just a streak-free shine. Best of all, it is safe to use around pets and children, unlike most commercial cleansers.

The Many Varieties of Vinegar

Vinegar gets its intense flavor from a wide variety of ingredients, usually with a base of either apples or grapes, although it can be made from any fruit or substance containing sugar. Other vinegar variations use beer, cane, coconut, palm, tea, and sherry wine. Vinegar quickly takes on herbal, floral, or spicy overtones, so any number of botanicals can be infused into it—including basil, rosemary, raspberry, and garlic. There are, however, several prepared varieties no kitchen should be without.

- **Apple cider vinegar**: Processed from apple must—pressed fruit juice—this vinegar is reddish brown in color, and the unfiltered and unpasteurized versions have an intense aroma. It goes great over salads, but diluted with fruit juice or sweetened with honey, it can also be consumed as a healthy drink.
- **Wine vinegar:** Less acidic than most vinegars, wine vinegar is made from red or white grapes and is a favorite of Central European and Mediterranean chefs for salad dressings, marinades, and sauces. The better brands are aged for two years in wood casks.
- **Balsamic vinegar:** This trendy aged and aromatic vinegar comes from the Italian provinces of Modena and Reggio Emilia. The best varieties are made from the must of white Trebbiano grapes and gain their rich, dark color and sweet, complex flavor from aging in

a succession of casks made of oak, mulberry, chestnut, cherry, juniper, ash, and acacia wood.
- **White or distilled vinegar:** White vinegar is not itself distilled—it is made from distilled alcohol. It is a favorite for pickling, cooking, baking, meat preservation, and cleaning. In the United States, corn is often used as the starting material.
- **Rice vinegar:** This light vinegar adds subtle Asian notes to any seafood, rice, or vegetable dish. In Japan, it is available in white and red varieties; in China, black vinegar is preferred.
- **Malt vinegar:** This is a light-brown variety made by allowing ale to sour. It is popular in Great Britain and Canada for sprinkling over fish and chips. ■

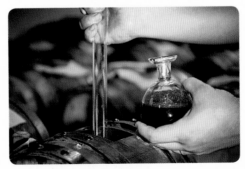

Balsamic vinegar being sampled from the cask. It gains its color and characteristics from the different kinds of wood the casks are made of, with some balsamics taking about 15 to 30 years to age properly.

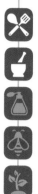

Salt

Sodium chloride

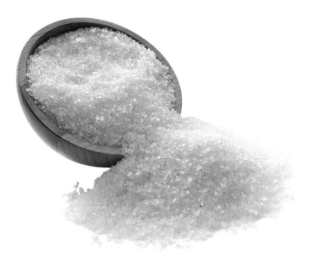

The condiment we call common table salt was once a precious seasoning sought after by the rich and powerful of Israel, Egypt, Greece, Rome, and Byzantium. Caravans and merchant ships transported it great distances, and fortunes were made by traders who brought it safely into the hands of the wealthy. Even the Incas of Peru established saltworks high in the Andes. Salt not only made food taste better, it was also a preservative, preventing meat from spoiling during a time when refrigeration consisted of a stone larder or a springhouse.

DID YOU KNOW?

One of the oldest seasonings in the world, salt brings out the flavor of food and is also used as a preservative.

Salt is a mineral composed of sodium and chlorine that in its crystalline form is known as halite or rock salt. It is also the main mineral constituent of ocean water. Salt is not only necessary to animal life, it is one of the five taste sensations humans crave—along with sweet, sour, bitter, and umami, or savory/meaty. Historians believe salt was first processed around 4000 B.C., when both the Romans and the Chinese began extracting it from water.

Today, salt is mined from sedimentary deposits or processed from seawater or spring water through evaporation. Only 6 percent of the world's salt is consumed in food. The bulk is used in industry, in the manufacture of plastics and other products—and in water conditioning, highway de-icing, and agriculture.

Culinary Uses

It is hard to imagine a savory dish without a dash of salt, but many modern staples, including bread, cereal, processed meats, and cheese, already contain added sodium. While salt is used in the cuisine of most nations, it is not quite so prevalent in East Asian cooking, where sodium-rich condiments like soy sauce, fish sauce, and oyster sauce furnish a similar flavor.

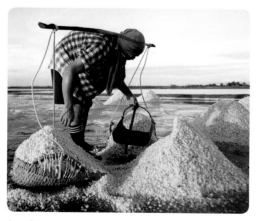

A worker collects salt at a saltworks in the Canary Islands.

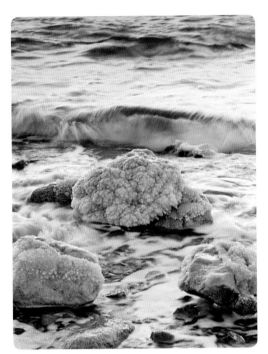

Salt forms naturally, such as in these deposits in the Dead Sea. Along the coast of this hypersaline body of water, the world's first health resorts sprang up to take advantage of salt's healing properties. People also use the salt and the minerals from the Dead Sea to create cosmetics and herbal sachets.

Iodized salt, first sold in American in 1924, was intended to supply the valuable micronutrient iodine—the lack of which can cause enlarged thyroid, or goiter. Kosher salt, which is not iodized and has larger crystals, is a popular alternative.

Designer Salts

American cooks, always seeking new tastes and textures, have recently discovered a variety of gourmet salts from around the globe. Some outstanding examples include *sel gris,* or gray salt, which is coarse and moist, perfect for meats or roasted root vegetables. *Fleur de sel* is made from brine and carries regional flavors. Hawaiian sea salt, red, gray or black, is full of trace minerals and goes well with pork and seafood. Korean "bamboo" salt is roasted inside bamboo cases. Murray River salt is a mild, flaky pale apricot variety from Australia. Himalayan salt ranges from white to pink to red. It is mined from ancient sea salt deposits in Pakistan and is considered one of the purest of salts, making it a kitchen and spa favorite. ■

Healing Properties

For centuries, humans have equated salt with improved health. People suffering from a variety of ailments took advantage of the benefits of sea air, while natural healers valued salt's antibiotic effect, especially on resistant respiratory problems. They also relied on its antiseptic qualities and prescribed it as a gargle for sore throats and as a topical treatment for skin conditions.

Yet, in recent decades, the overconsumption of salt has become linked to the risk of stroke and cardiovascular disease. The high sodium content in packaged foods, from which Americans take in 77 percent of their sodium, has exacerbated this problem. Still, sodium is necessary for human health—it allows nerves and muscles to function properly and helps regulate the fluid balance in the body. The World Health Organization recommends less than 2,000 mg of sodium—or 5 g of salt—per day for adults.

But which salt? Refined table salt is stabilized and chemically cleaned, making it inorganic and impossible to digest. Unrefined salt, similar to the sodium that occurs naturally in our bodies, is the healthier choice.

History and Lore

» After defeating Carthage during the Third Punic War, Roman general Scipio Africanus razed the city and sowed it with salt.

» The word *salary* comes from the Latin *salarium*—the money paid to Roman soldiers to purchase salt. The Latin word *salad* means "salted," based on the Roman habit of salting vegetable greens.

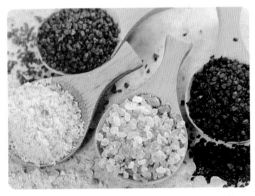

The variety of salts now available continues to expand. Above (counterclockwise from top left) are Red Hawaiian, Murray River, Pink Himalayan, and Black Hawaiian salts.

Scallion

Allium fistulosum

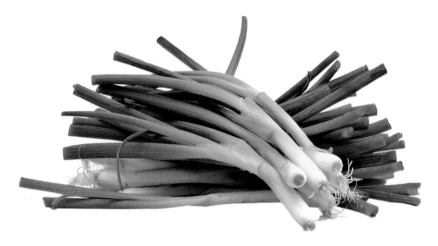

Also known as Welsh onions, scallions consist of the bulb, stem, and greens harvested from an immature onion plant. Crops are even planted close together to stunt the growth of the bulb, keeping it petite and sweet.

This perennial member of the lily family originated in Central Asia, but it is now cultivated throughout Asia, Europe, and the Americas. It has a long history as a food source and a medicinal plant—and recent research indicates it may possess many of the same healthful properties as garlic and onions.

A scallion plant features a long, slender, erect stalk and hollow tubular leaves that rise from a small, elongated bulb. In cross section, these leaves are round, as opposed to other alliums that have semi-circular tubules. In the second year, the flowers appear as white, pink, or lilac umbels. In some varieties, the bulbs will not regenerate. For those, it is best to let a few flowers grow the following season to produce seeds for future propagation.

The plant's common name evolved from a town in Israel, Ashkelon, where centuries ago a shrewd farmer supposedly began growing these exotic Far Eastern alliums.

DID YOU KNOW?

With a sweet and light onion flavor, scallions are harvested before the bulb begins to fully form.

Culinary Uses

With their sweet, mild flavor, scallions are often enjoyed raw, which is the optimal way to receive their health benefits. Whole scallions are served as a vegetable, but they can also be sliced or minced and used as a seasoning in omelets, soups, salsa, casseroles, and many Asian recipes.

Nutritionally, this leafy green plant is low in calories, but provides more dietary fiber than onions and shallots. It contains healthy amounts

Scallions form globes of tiny white blossoms in midsummer, which attract pollinating insects. The flowers are edible, and can be added raw to salads. Stalks of scallion flowers make attractive additions to cut bouquets, too, but keep in mind that they will give off a mild odor of onions.

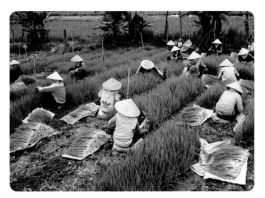
Vietnamese farmers harvesting a crop of scallions. Scallions are an important ingredient in *dua hành,* a dish of fermented onions served for Tet, the Vietnamese New Year.

of vitamin A and B-complex vitamins and the minerals copper, iron, manganese, and calcium. The greens contain pyridoxine, folic acid, niacin, riboflavin, thiamin, and vitamin C, and are an excellent source of vitamin K, which limits neuronal damage in the brain.

Asian Scallion Pancakes

These savory pancakes can be made as a breakfast, lunch, or light supper treat. Serves four.

Ingredients
- 2 cups all-purpose flour
- 1 cup boiling water
- ½ cup sliced scallions
- 1 tablespoon sesame oil
- ½ cup canola oil
- salt and black pepper to taste

Directions
Sift flour into bowl, and then slowly add water while mixing with wooden spoon until ball is formed. Let ball relax for 30 minutes under damp cloth. On a floured surface, roll out dough into a thin rectangle. Brush on sesame oil, cover with scallions, and season with salt and pepper. Roll dough into a spiral, like a jellyroll, and cut into four pieces. Twist each piece several times, then make a ball, roll again, and flatten into a five- or six-inch pancake. Coat a hot nonstick pan with canola oil, and sear both sides of pancakes until golden brown. Serve with a ginger-soy sauce and garnish with sliced scallions. ■

Healing Properties

Over the centuries, scallions have been used to treat respiratory problems: they can be brewed into a tea to relieve colds or combined with cayenne and garlic in a sinus-clearing broth. As a poultice, they help heal skin wounds and abscesses.

Scallions, like other alliums, contain antioxidant flavonoids. In particular, the plant's carotenoids are thought to help the body protect itself from lung and oral-cavity cancers. When scallions are sliced, the plant's enzymes create the powerful organosulfur compound allicin, which has antiviral, antibacterial, antifungal, and antiprotozoan properties. Allicin also decreases blood vessel stiffness—lowering blood pressure and blocking the formation of blood clots—reducing the risk of stroke.

History and Lore

» Scallions are known by many names: green onions, spring onions (in Britain), salad onions, table onions, green shallots, onion sticks, long onions, baby onions, precious onions, yard onions, gibbon, syboes, or scally onions.
» In Mexico, *cebollitas* are grilled scallions sprinkled with salt and lime juice, a popular side dish with barbecued meats.
» During the Passover seder dinner, when the word *dayenu* is read, Persian Jews lightly whip each other with scallions, symbolizing the Egyptians whipping their Israelite slaves.

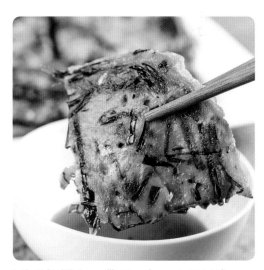
In the United States, scallion pancakes are a common item on Korean and Chinese restaurant menus. In both these countries, street vendors often sell these easy-to-make treats.

HEALTHY TRADES

Herbs and spices boost diet menus and vegetarian dishes.

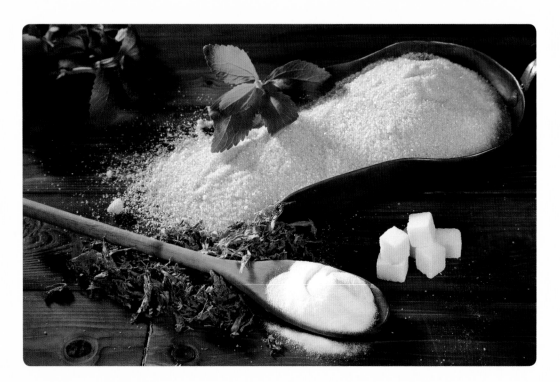

Whether health-conscious individuals are cutting down on sugar as part of a diet, limiting salt intake for medical reasons, or have made the decision to give up meat and follow a vegetarian lifestyle, they should gain enough supplemental flavor from herbs and spices to keep them on track.

A Sweet, Low-Cal Solution

Ever since saccharin, the first commercial artificial sweetener, was proven to have carcinogenic effects, chemists have been seeking a safe substitute for cane sugar as if it were a culinary Holy Grail. With all of sugar's

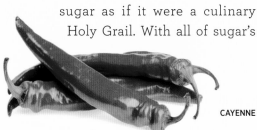

CAYENNE

drawbacks—that it has no essential nutrients, leads to tooth decay, overloads the liver, causes the conversion of fructose to fat, is highly addictive, creates insulin resistance, and can even lead to cancer—it has become the bane of dieters and non-dieters alike. And while subsequent generations of sweeteners, like Nutrasweet (aspartame) or Splenda (sucralose), scored well in the taste department, they fell short in the "safe" department.

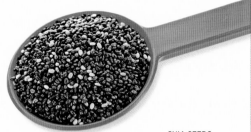
Enter stevia. This natural sweetener, extracted from the leaves of the stevia plant, has zero calories and few, if any, side effects. It is available in a powdered form of concentrated sweetness and a liquid form that is more palatable. Its only drawback is that it does not do well in baking. Other relatively safe options include sugar alcohol sweeteners, like xylitol, sorbitol, and erythritol, made through the fermentation of corn or sugar cane. Organic raw honey and mineral-rich blackstrap molasses are also good substitutions.

Limiting Salt

Many packaged or canned foods use staggering amounts of salt or sodium, the main element in salt, as a preservative—so much so that people on low-sodium diets are shocked by reading the nutrition charts on canned soup, say, or chili. Yet, a big part of a heart-healthy lifestyle involves reducing sodium, and here is where herbs and spices come to the rescue, either substituting for salt or replacing its taste with something almost as satisfying.

While nothing tastes quite as good as salt, some flavorful swaps include black pepper, cinnamon—which also regulates blood sugar—a combination of cardamom and cumin or coriander, pungent basil, sunflower seeds, and garlic powder, especially on meat or fish.

Excite the Taste Buds

Hot or hearty seasonings like cayenne pepper, fresh garlic, ginger, onion powder, and bay leaves can transform a bland dish into a rewarding dining experience. Low-sodium soy sauce can also be used; even though it does contain some salt, it has high nutritional value.

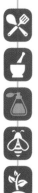

Stevia

Stevia rebaudiana

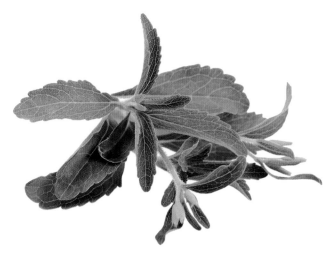

Stevia is a small perennial plant native to tropical regions from Mexico to South America. Although utilized by the local tribes for centuries, it has recently made food headlines as an alternative to artificial sweeteners with no known side effects.

Stevia was first identified in 1887 by Swiss-Italian botanist Mosè Bertoni. His research brought the plant to the attention of herbalists in Paraguay. During World War II, the British investigated the plant as a possible sugar substitute, but research stopped when the war

DID YOU KNOW?

A small wild shrub in the daisy family, *Stevia rebaudiana* is now widely cultivated for the intense sweetness of its leaves.

ended. The Japanese started cultivating stevia in hothouses in the 1950s and began using it in place of sugar in the 1970s. They are now the biggest consumers of the extract.

This member of the daisy family, Asteraceae, is also known as sweetleaf, sugarleaf, or honey leaf plant.

It can reach four feet in height and produces slender, branched stems and fibrous, serrated green leaves. In the fall, delicate white flowers appear. All parts of the plant taste sweet, but the leaves contain the highest concentrations of the sweetening agent glycoside stevioside. Yet, they give off no distinctive scent.

The plant still grows wild in Paraguay and Brazil, and it is currently cultivated commercially in Japan, Thailand, Paraguay, Brazil, and China—the leading exporter.

Culinary Uses

Stevia's flavor has been likened to honeysuckle nectar, although there are some who think the plant has a slight licorice or even a bitter aftertaste. Stevia's leaves are 300 times sweeter than cane sugar, and, in Japan, they are used to sweeten gum, soy sauce, soft drinks, and tea. Stevia is also frequently used in Indian, Eastern Asian, and South American cuisine.

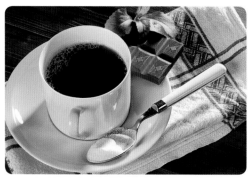

Stevia is available in powdered, liquid, and tablet forms for sweetening coffee or any foods that you would normally sweeten with sugar. It is also being used in manufactured foods, including Belgian chocolate.

A Taste of Honey

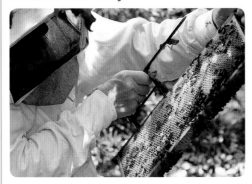

A beekeeper collecting combs of honey

Stevia is being touted as a safe, natural sugar substitute, but for millennia bees have furnished humans with the original natural sweetener—honey. The metamorphosis begins when bees use their long tongues to take nectar from blossoms. The nectar in their stomachs then mixes with enzymes that make it stable for long-term storage—important, since honey is kept in honeycombs as emergency food for the hive. Bees then fan the honey with their wings to evaporate any moisture until it turns thick and golden. The combs are then sealed with a secretion from the bee's abdomen that hardens into beeswax. Honey's flavor and color is determined by the nectar source—mainly flowers, trees, and herbs. Dark, rich buckwheat honey tastes far different than light, sweet clover honey. ■

The plant contains many nutrients—including vitamins A and C, rutin, and dietary fiber, as well as the minerals calcium, phosphorous, sodium, magnesium, and zinc—that are absent from sugar. It also has no calories, a long shelf life, high heat tolerance, and is nonfermenting.

Healing Properties

In South America, where it is known as *caa-he-éé* or *kaa jheéé*, stevia has been used for centuries by the Guarani of Paraguay to aid weight loss, treat wounds, relieve inflammations, and reduce swelling in the legs, and as a tonic to treat depression. Natural healers prescribe it to treat skin outbreaks, dandruff, and other scalp problems, and as a wrinkle cream.

It contains many antioxidants, including tannins and flavonoids. Among the latter is the phytochemical kaempferol, which the *American Journal of Epidemiology* reports can reduce the risk of pancreatic cancer by 23 percent. Stevia helps to lower blood glucose levels by reducing the conversion of glycogen to glucose and decreasing the absorption of glucose in the gut. As a noncarbohydrate sweetener, stevia does not promote the growth of *Streptococcus mutans* inside the mouth, lowering the risk for dental caries and cavities. Certain compounds in stevia may actually curb the number of bacteria that cause caries.

In spite of widespread interest in the herbal sweetener, the Food and Drug Administration banned stevia in the 1990s and only recently granted GRAS status—"generally recognized as safe"—to a constituent of the leaf extract called rebiana. This food additive can now be found marketed under the name Truvia.

History and Lore

» Stevia is known as the "sweet herb," or *yerba dulce*, of Paraguay. Indian women once used the plant to make a contraceptive tea—and clinical tests have shown that stevia can impact fertility.

» Stevia is a naturally grown plant; therefore, the whole leaves cannot be patented nor can its name be trademarked.

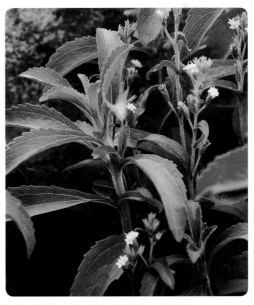

Lanky stevia produces tiny white flowers in late summer. Three to five plants will yield a year's supply of dried leaves.

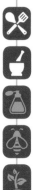

Sugar

Saccharum officinarum

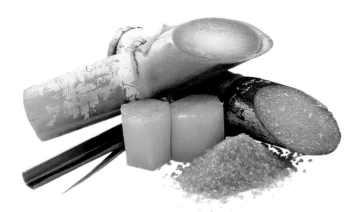

Most modern cooks take sugar for granted. Yet, for thousands of years, the sweet goodness of sugarcane was limited to Polynesia, and then India. It was not until the fifth century B.C., that Alexander the Great carried "the sacred reed" from India to the Mediterranean, where the Greeks and Romans began to use it as medicine. Meanwhile, the Arabs spread the plant to Egypt, Morocco, and Tunisia, and eventually to southern Spain.

European Crusaders may have tasted sugar in the Holy Land, but it was not used in Europe until the late 1200s, and then only by the wealthy.

Seafarers began seeking new regions to cultivate the plant, and when Columbus successfully introduced sugarcane to Santo Domingo in 1493, a New World industry was born. Growers from many nations set up plantations in Brazil, Cuba, Mexico, and the West Indies—and sugar at last became available to the masses. When demand necessitated a larger labor force to work the cane fields, slaves were brought over from Africa. The crop eventually became so lucrative that sugar was called "white gold."

After the British gained territories in the West Indies from Spain in 1655, they were suddenly sugar rich. During the Napoleonic Wars, however, European countries were denied British exports and turned to beets for sugar. By 1880, most of Europe relied on beet sugar alone. More recently, in America and Japan, high fructose corn syrup has replaced sugar in many products.

A reedy, tropical perennial, sugarcane is a member of the grass family, Poaceae—which includes corn, wheat, and rice—and grows from

Sugarcane plants are grasses, which produce only tiny flowers that appear as tassels of feathery inflorescences atop the tall stalks. It is best to harvest sugarcane before it blooms—it will stop producing sugar after flowering.

6 to 19 feet. The main product, sucrose, is found in the tubular stalks. The molasses-rich raw sugar can be processed into refined sugar or fermented to form ethanol, the alcohol used to make liquor.

Culinary Uses

When table sugar—including granulated, brown, and powdered sugars—is used in baking, it does more than add sweetness. In cake batter, sugar molecules form a tight bond with water molecules, providing moistness and ensuring tenderness by preventing the starches and proteins that add structure from becoming too stiff. Sugar also stabilizes meringues, leavens cakes and quick breads, deepens color and flavor through a reaction to heat called caramelizing, and adds crunch to baked goods as surface moisture evaporates in the oven and the sugar recrystallizes.

Healing Properties

The early Greeks and Romans used sugar for medicinal purposes—the physician Dioscorides prescribed it to treat digestive ailments and problems of the bladder and kidneys. In medieval Europe, it was used both as a flavoring and as a curative.

Alas, sugar contains no nutrients, and it can actually be harmful. Medical science blames the overconsumption of sugar for the disturbing rise in obesity and diabetes in the United States. Sugar is also addictive: it causes a massive release of dopamine—a neurotransmitter that heightens pleasure and energy—in the brain. In light of this, the American Heart Association recommends a maximum daily intake of nine teaspoons (37.5 grams or 150 calories—or one 12-ounce can of soda) for men, and six teaspoons (25 grams or 100 calories) for women.

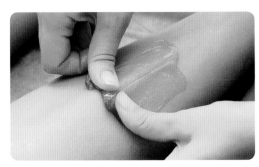

Combined with water and lemon juice, sugar makes a cheap alternative to wax hair removers offered at beauty salons.

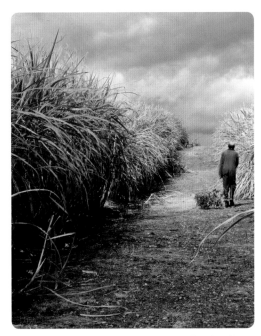

A worker in a sugarcane field at a Thai plantation. Growing sugar is a moneymaking business, and, by weight, it is the world's top crop. It is grown in 90 countries, with an annual harvest of almost two billion tons. The largest producers of sugar are Brazil, India, the European Union, China, and Thailand.

History and Lore

» Early Persians called sugarcane "the reed that gives honey without bees."
» Until the late 19th century, sugar was formed into a hard, conical "sugarloaf" that was typically stored in a locked cabinet.

Pour Some Sugar on Me

Sugar may not be the healthiest of foods, but it does have its beneficial uses. Since ancient times in the Middle East and Egypt, sugar has been used for hair removal. This method, known as sugaring, sugar waxing, or Persian waxing, is an inexpensive alternative to waxing or shaving. And, like waxing, sugaring removes hair by the root, so that when it grows back it will be softer and finer—and there will be less of it—than if you had shaved with a razor. These days, salons offer sugaring, but you can easily do it yourself. Check online for specifics: most recipes are simple—just combine sugar, water, and lemon juice, and then heat. The result will be a honey-like sugar paste that you can apply in strips and use again and again. ■

Tamarind

Tamarindus indica

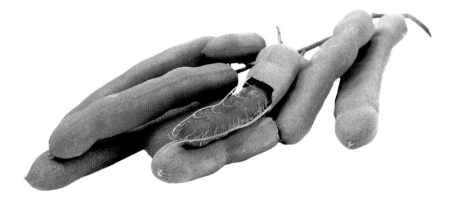

Tamarind's flavor is probably best known to Americans as the pungent kick found in Worcestershire sauce. Used around the world as a condiment and a souring agent, it is also valued as a medicine. The edible pulp is derived from the fruit, or pods, of the tamarind tree.

Originally native to tropical Africa, the tamarind still grows wild in parts of the Sudan. Often considered indigenous to India, it was actually introduced there many centuries ago. Europeans carried it to the New World in the 1500s, and it was eventually cultivated in Mexico and the Caribbean. Today, tamarind is grown in tropical regions across the globe.

> **DID YOU KNOW?**
>
> This tropical fruit tree, with it spreading boughs, yields a podlike fruit that is a much-prized ingredient in cookery and perfumery.

Valued as a shade tree in Asia, this sturdy evergreen is a member of the pea family, Fabaceae. A tamarind tree can live for 80 years or longer, and can reach heights of 80 or even 100 feet with a spread of 40 feet. The foliage is bright green and feathery, and the small flowers, which form racemes, are white with splashes of red or orange. The long brown fruit pods start out filled with a sour, juicy pulp. As they mature, the shell becomes brittle, and the pulp, the source of the seasoning, turns dense, sticky, and sweet.

The genus name comes from the Persian term *tamar-l-hind,* meaning "date of India."

Culinary Uses

Tamarind's fruity, tart flavor and its acidic taste—distinctly different from vinegar or lemon—go perfectly with Indian, Thai, and Asian cookery, such as curries, stir-fries, chutneys, sour soups, and lentil, rice, and noodle dishes. In the West, sweet-sour tamarind is used with meat, poultry, seafood, and vegetable dishes, in Worcestershire and HP sauces, in Mexican cuisine, and West Indian fruit drinks. It is also used to flavor desserts and candies; the pectin in the plant makes it useful for home canning jams and jellies.

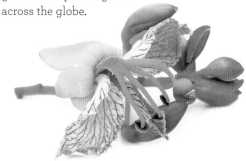

Tamarind flowers are tiny and inconspicuous, but lovely in form, with red and yellow five-petaled, elongated flowers.

Create a Signature Steak Sauce

Sure, you can buy prepared steak sauce, but nothing tastes as good as one you customize yourself, especially with tart tamarind as a secret weapon. Your T-bone will thank you.

Ingredients

- ⅛ to ¼ cup of tamarind pulp or paste
- 2 tablespoons dark brown sugar
- 2 cloves minced garlic
- ½ cup ketchup
- ¼ cup water
- ¼ cup white vinegar
- salt to taste

Directions

Mix the listed ingredients in a saucepan, and then try adding your favorite piquant or hot seasonings—diced onions, shallots, scallions, peppercorns, cayenne pepper, dry mustard, chili powder, cumin, or lemon juice. Bring to a boil, and then simmer for half an hour. Strain cooled mixture, pour into a lidded glass jar, and store in refrigerator; sauce will keep two to four weeks. Use on grilled steaks or as a marinade. ■

Tamarind pulp is normally sold in a dense, shrink-wrapped block, To cook with it, cut off a piece, cover it with a small amount of hot water for five minutes, and strain the seeds. The result should be a thin paste. In addition to the pulp, tamarind is also available in Asian groceries as a paste and a powder.

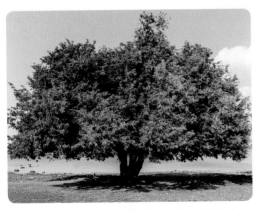

The magnificent tamarind is tall and spreading, with feathery foliage. It produces clusters of long, curved edible podlike fruit.

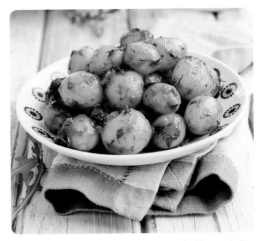

Tamarind paste gives a tangy taste layer to *imli iloo*, an Indian potato dish that blends many spices, such as garam masala.

Nutritionally, tamarind has beneficial amounts of vitamin A, thiamin, vitamin C, and dietary fiber, and contains calcium, copper, iron, magnesium, potassium, and phosphorus.

Healing Properties

Like many of the spices and seasonings known to ancient cultures, tamarind has a long medicinal history—as a laxative and digestion aid and for treating fevers, sore throats, rheumatism, inflammation, and sunstroke. The dried or boiled leaves and flowers were made into poultices for easing swollen joints, hemorrhoids, boils, and pink eye.

Tamarind contains tartaric acid, which not only adds zest to recipes, but it also supplies potent antioxidants that seek out and destroy free radicals in our systems. Tamarind is also employed as an emulsifying agent in a number of pharmaceutical syrups and decoctions.

Aromatic Qualities

The bouquet of tamarind has been compared to raisins, dates, guavas, and apricots. A number of perfumes contain piquant notes of tamarind.

History and Lore

» According to Hindu mythology, tamarind is associated with the wedding of the god Krishna, celebrated by a feast in November.

» To prevent scurvy, sailors once carried tamarind, a source of vitamin C, on long voyages.

» In some Asian countries, acidic tamarind pulp is used to polish brass.

Tamarind

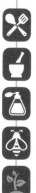

Wasabi

Wasabia japonica

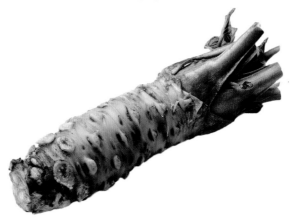

Many diners assume that they are eating wasabi whenever they order sushi or sashimi, but, in many sushi restaurants, that little plop of green sauce at the side of the plate is really a blend of mustard, horseradish, and food coloring. True wasabi, which the Japanese have enjoyed since at least the tenth century, is rare in most parts of the world. It is difficult to cultivate and, as a result, is quite pricey. It is worth searching out the real thing, however; it has a distinct taste and is not as harsh as the restaurant mixture.

Wasabi is native to the mountainous regions of Japan. It was likely first cultivated in the 16th century. Today it is grown commercially on the Izu peninsula in the Shizuoka, Nagano, and Iwate prefectures. The two most popular cultivars are *Wasabia japonica* 'Daruma'—dark green—and 'Mazuma'—pale and spicy. Due to increased worldwide demand, it is now also grown in New Zealand and California. In the wild, wasabi prefers cold streambeds at high altitudes, although some varieties will grow in moist soil.

A member of the Brassicaceae family, which includes cabbage, horseradish, and mustard, this evergreen perennial reaches a height of 18 inches and produces large, basal leaves, tall, narrow stems, and tiny white flowers. As the plant ages, the leaves fall off, leaving scars at the base of the stem, which becomes the rhizome-like source of wasabi.

Culinary Uses

Wasabi's taste has been described as horseradish with herbal notes. And while it makes the perfect complement to sushi and sashimi, it goes equally well with beef, seared seafood, teriyaki chicken, kebobs, rice, soba noodles, and avocados.

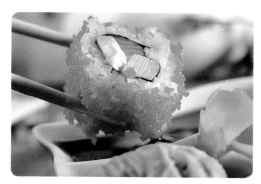

Wasabi is the natural complement to sushi, but be sure that the condiment you are served is the real thing. Many high-end restaurants will grate the fresh stem at tableside.

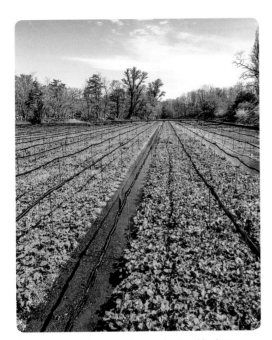

A wasabi farm in Nagano, Japan. Cultivating this plant requires meticulous care. Here, a network of small streams borders the rows of wasabi plants, providing them with the constant supply of fresh water that they must have to thrive.

Wasabi can be purchased in specialty food stores and online. It is available as a stem, ready for fine grating; as a dried powder; or as a premade paste. When using the dried product, mix equal parts powder with warm water or soy sauce until it turns a bright green, then let it sit for 15 minutes. This mixture makes a great addition to mashed potatoes, mayonnaise, dips, and vinaigrettes, and can be used in place of Dijon mustard in most recipes. Or create a zingy, crunchy snack food by coating roasted peanuts, soybeans, or peas with wasabi powder combined with sugar, salt, and olive oil. Freshly grated wasabi soon looses its flavor, so be sure to serve it quickly.

Nutritionally, wasabi contains high levels of vitamin C and B6, protein, dietary fiber, potassium, calcium, and magnesium.

Healing Properties

There is evidence that, even centuries ago, the Japanese understood the antimicrobial effects of wasabi when they served it with raw fish. In their folk medicine, it was used as an analgesic and as an antihistamine poultice to treat rheumatism, neuralgia, and bronchitis.

The plant contains the same cancer-fighting phytochemicals found in its Brassicaceae cousins cabbage, broccoli, and kale. The chemicals responsible for wasabi's taste and smell, called isothiocyanates, activate the body's critical antioxidant detoxifying systems. Studies also suggest that the plant may help prevent blood clots, obesity, asthma, and even tooth decay—wasabi can be lethal to *Streptococcus mutans,* a bacteria that causes plaque and cavities. And because wasabi is able to inhibit microbe growth, it has commercial potential as a preservative.

Aromatic Qualities

As with horseradish, the full aroma of wasabi is not released until the tissues are ruptured by grating, resulting in a complex mixture of chemicals that create both its smell and taste.

History and Lore

» The fiery taste of wasabi is not oil-based, like the heat caused by the capsaicin in peppers, so it quickly diminishes with additional food and drink.

» Wasabi is traditionally grated with a tool made of dried sharkskin. The abrasive surfaces, with fine scales on one side and coarser skin on the other breaks down the dense texture of the root, releasing its full flavor.

CURIOSITIES

An Olfactory Fire Alarm

Most people react quickly to the strident sound of a fire alarm. But the deaf cannot hear traditional alarms and must be alerted in other ways, especially when asleep and unable to see a flashing-light alarm. A group of researchers decided to address this problem and, based on wasabi's stinging nasal effect, came up with a wasabi vapor spray that successfully roused the deaf from sleep. One participant awoke ten seconds after the spray was released. Seven Japanese scientists received the 2011 Nobel Prize in chemistry for determining the optimum concentration of airborne wasabi that was required to alert sleepers. ▪

Wasabi

295

Grower's Guide

GARDENING TIPS FOR
GROWING HERBS AND SPICES

 ### Alfalfa
Medicago sativa

Alfalfa can be grown in a greenhouse, on a balcony, or in the garden. The plant requires light soil, mild sun exposure, and plenty of water. Seeds can be sown in the spring directly in the ground or in pots. They germinate within six days, and the plants are harvested once they reach the necessary height. Sprouts can be grown in special plastic sprouter boxes. Once established, alfalfa's extensive root system will nourish both plants and soil.

 ### Aloe
Aloe vera

It is best to buy young aloe plants from a garden shop. In warm climates, aloes can be kept outside; in regions with cold winters, bring them inside before temperatures drop. Indoors, they need a sunny spot; outdoors, they require full sun or partial shade. Fertilize once a year with a balanced liquid feed. In a pot, make sure that the root ball has plenty of room to grow. Keep watering to a minimum in winter; water more frequently in summer.

 ### Angelica
Angelica archangelica, A. sinensis

Welcome in the garden for its bright green foliage, angelica will grow from seeds in late autumn or early spring. Tamp seeds gently into the ground, and cover them with a light layer of soil. Variations of temperature, but not freezing, help the seeds to sprout. Plant seedlings in partial shade, near water, spaced at least 1 foot apart. Angelica will self-seed, and it will attract many beneficial pollinators.

 ### Aniseed
Pimpinella anisum

Aniseed plants prefer light, fertile, well-drained soil in semi-sun. Plant the seeds in May for harvesting in August. Cover seeds with about ⅛ inch of soil, and expect sprouts to appear in approximately four to six days. The plants have a taproot, so they do not transplant well after being established. Either start them in their final location or transplant them while the seedlings are still small.

 ### Arnica
Arnica montana

Yellow-flowering arnica can be raised from a nursery seedling or grown from a root cutting. The plant requires sandy alkaline soil, rich in humus, with good drainage. It will tolerate either full sun or partial shade. Keep soil moist and well-drained, but don't feel the need to fertilize. The flowers can be picked in midsummer and dried for decorating purposes. Note: Arnica plants can be toxic if ingested.

 ### Basil
Ocimum basilicum

Annual basil prefers rich, moist soil and six hours of sun a day, although it will grow in partial shade. It is easy to grow, but should be started indoors in flats, with seeds 6 to 10 inches apart. Transplant seedlings outdoors, again 6 to 10 inches apart, once risk of frost is past. Fertilize for more robust plants and pinch stem tips and flowers for fuller growth. Harvest before flowering. Note: Do not grow next to rue.

 ### Bay Leaf
Laurus nobilis

When bay leaf is grown in outdoor containers in USDA zones 8 to 11, this tall-growing conical evergreen will remain manageable and thrive in full sun to partial shade. It will grow indoors in cooler areas. Needs well-drained soil—half cactus soil, half potting mix or one part sand, two parts potting mix. Allow soil to dry between watering. It is a slow growing tree; it flowers after ten years or more.

 ### Bee Balm
Monarda spp.

Bee balm enjoys moist, light soil, and a location where it receives only the morning sun, because this increases flowering compared to plants in full sun, which can get leggy. It is easily propagated by its creeping roots and by slips or cuttings. If using cuttings, place them in a shady spot in May, and plants will take root just like other mints. Butterflies, hummingbirds, bees, and other nectar-seeking creatures love bee balm flowers.

 ### Bergamot Orange
Citrus bergamia

Bergamot orange can be grown in regions that rarely see freezing temperatures, from USDA zones 9 to 11. It prefers full sun throughout the day and acidic to neutral soil. It is hardy, but certain conditions can stress it. It can withstand only short periods of frost before damage occurs. A bergamot orange tree needs a steady supply of water during dry summer months, and it should also be protected from high winds.

 ### Borage
Borago officinalis

Borage is a hardy pant that flourishes in ordinary soil, in sun or shade, with moderate water. It can be grown from seeds sown in autumn or early spring, or grown indoors in late winter or early spring. Plant seeds ½ inch deep and 4 inches apart. As seedlings mature, thin to 15 inches apart. Seeds may be sown in autumn for flowering in May; spring plantings will flower in June. Borage self-seeds.

Burdock
Arctium spp.

Burdock will adapt from partial shade to full sun. It prefers light, sandy soil, which also makes harvesting the deep roots easier. Sow seeds in fall or start indoors in spring—start 4 weeks before final frost, cover lightly with soil, and keep moist. Transplant burdock to pots when leaves first show, and then to ground after final frost. Harvest root in 8 to 12 weeks. Mature burdock is hardy and will self-seed.

Calendula
Calendula officinalis

Calendulas grow best in sunny locations in most types of soil, though they prefer rich, well-drained soil. Seeds sown in April will germinate freely. Keep seedlings free from weeds, and thin out to 9 or 10 inches apart. Plants begin to flower in June and continue until frost kills them. The seeds ripen in August and September; plant will self-seed and increase from year to year. Calendulas deter some tomato pests.

Capers
Capparis spinosa

Capers require dry heat and strong sunlight to flourish. They do grow readily from seeds gathered from ripe fruit if they are planted in well-drained seed starter mix, but seedlings may take as many as three months to germinate. Plants can also be propagated from cuttings, although these are at greater risk of damage from drought during the first year or two. An added bonus of caper bushes? They are deer resistant.

Caraway Seed
Carum carvi

Caraway seeds like cool weather, and they can be sown ½ inch deep in the autumn, as soon as they ripen, or in March. Sow in drills, and then thin seedlings to 1 foot apart in well-drained, sandy soil in an area with full sun to partial shade. Can also be started from cuttings. Plants put down a taproot, so they should not be transplanted once established. Water well during the first year. Caraway easily reseeds.

Cardamom
Elettaria cardamomum, Amomum spp.

Cardamom is native to tropical regions, and should only be grown outdoors in USDA zones 10 to 13, where minimum temperature is 35 degrees or higher. Prefers a rich, loamy, slightly acidic soil. For best results, fertilize soil with phosphorus and potassium. Can also be grown indoors or in a greenhouse in zones 9 and lower, or overwintered in a large, deep container that can be moved indoors as needed.

Catnip
Nepeta cataria

Catnip, like most mints, is easy to cultivate in the garden. The seeds are slow germinators, so nursery seedlings work best. Plant in light, sandy soil in full sun, water well, and pinch top growth as the herb matures to encourage bushiness. If you have a cat, leave space around the plant for your pet to roll in the leaves. It is also easy to grow on a windowsill so that your cats will always have a fresh supply.

Cayenne
Capsicum annuum

Cayenne prefers well-drained, sandy, acidic soil and a warm climate. Soak seeds overnight, then plant indoors in a peat pack if outdoor temperature is below 75 degrees. Place a few seeds in pack, cover with ¼ inch of soil. Keep soil damp. After risk of frost, transplant seedlings to composted bed with eight hours of sun daily. Space 18 to 24 inches, in rows 24 to 36 inches apart and mulch. Most varieties need 100 days to mature.

Celery Seed
Apium graveolens

Celery can be tricky to grow. It is a heavy feeder that requires fertilizer and a lot of water or the stalks will be small and dry. Soak seeds overnight, and start indoors eight to ten weeks before last frost. Harden off seedlings before transplanting by decreasing water and keeping outdoors a few hours every day. Transplant 10 to 12 inches apart, then mulch and water. To keep maturing stalks from sprawling, tie them together.

Chamomile
M. chamomilla, C. nobile

German chamomile can be seeded indoors six weeks before final frost or outdoors in the fall or early spring in partial sun, and in soil that is not too rich. Will self-seed in the fall. Its flopping flowers make it a better underplanting than a feature plant. Perennial Roman chamomile can be grown from seeds, root cuttings, or division. Space 6 to 12 inches apart in full sun. Perfect as a ground cover between stones or pavers.

Chervil
Allium schoenoprasum

Chervil is easy to grow in a cool, moist, secluded spot, but it should be seeded in place, because its long taproot makes it difficult to transplant once it is established. This cool-weather herb should be planted in early spring or late fall in USDA zones 2 to 10. Plants can easily go to seed, or "bolt," and stop producing new greens in hot midsummer weather. Protect from full summer sun. Chervil is an excellent companion for brassicas.

Chives
Allium schoenoprasum

Chives are hardy perennial herbs that will thrive in a sunny spot in rich, moist, well-drained soil. This cool-season, cold-tolerant perennial (USDA zones 3 to 9) should be planted in early spring. Add aged compost to the soil before planting. Seeds can be started indoors eight to ten weeks before the last frost. If the flowers ripen and the seeds disperse, chives can pop up in random moist spots. Weed between clumps.

Cilantro/Coriander
Coriandrum sativum

Coriandrum sativum is a sun-loving, frilly-leafed, aromatic annual that yields both the herb cilantro and the spice coriander. It grows quickly in fertile, well-drained soil during the cooler months in the spring and fall. After flowering, the seeds (coriander) can be gathered and dried, and it will reseed if given its own corner of the garden. The leaves (cilantro) can withstand a light frost.

Clary Sage
Salvia sclarea

Easy to grow, biennial clary sage provides a generous floral display. It can tolerate some cold, but it is only hardy to USDA zone 6. Start from seeds, cuttings, or layering; plant in early spring in full sun and well-drained soil. Transplant seedlings to open ground, 1 foot apart each way. A rosette appears the first year, followed by mature growth the next. The plant should die off at the end of the second summer; there is minimal self-seeding.

Comfrey
Symphytum spp.

Prepare the comfrey bed by weeding thoroughly and dressing with manure. Plant seeds or cuttings in permanent positions, because the roots go deep and the plants are long-lived. Situate in sun or partial shade in enriched, slightly alkaline, loosened soil; water regularly. Do not harvest leaves in first season; allow plant to become established. Flowering stems weaken plant for healing use and should be removed.

Cretan Dittany
Origanum dictamnus

Cretan dittany enjoys sunny locations and well-drained mildly alkaline soil conditions. It also does well in containers. Can be propagated by seed, division in spring or fall, or stem cuttings. Seed germination takes about two weeks indoors if sown before last frost. Be sure to provide light shade in garden until plants get established. Cretan dittany be used as a border or edging plant, in hanging baskets or rock gardens.

Cumin
Cuminum cyminum

Cumin has a long growing season. Start seeds indoors four weeks before final frost. Sow them ¼ inch below soil, and water moderately until germination. Transplant outdoors to well-drained, rich soil in full sun once temperature lows reach 60 degrees. Seedlings should be 4 to 6 inches apart. Harvest when seed pods turn brown; allow them to dry before harvesting seeds. Plant will produce for two years.

Dandelion
Taraxacum officinale

These edible wildflowers abound in lawn and verge, but by cultivating dandelions, you will know exactly when to pick tender young greens and know they are free of any toxic chemicals. Plant does well in all hardiness zones. Sow seeds in early spring, directly in garden, ¼ inch deep and 8 inches apart. Harvest greens throughout growing season. Harvest edible root second year. Deadhead before clocks appear to avoid escapees.

Dill
Anethum graveolens

Dill thrives in loamy soil and full sun. Sow seeds ¼-inch deep and 18 inches apart, and then gently rake seeds into the soil. Dill does not like being transplanted, so start seeds in early summer—soil temperature should be 60 to 70 degrees. Plants will appear in 10 to 14 days. After another 10 to 14 days, thin to 12 to 18 inches apart. Do not plant dill near fennel: the two species will cross-pollinate and produce bad-tasting herbs.

Echinacea
Echinacea spp.

This flower thrives when temperatures fluctuate, so get them into the ground before spring fully turns to summer. Start from seeds (species only, hybrids are sterile) in the fall or nursery plants in spring. Choose a sunny location (at least five hours of sun daily) with rich soil. Water regularly and fertilize lightly—too much can makes plants leggy. Seed heads feed small birds all winter. Note that hybrids need more care.

Elder
Sambucus nigra

Elder is a hardy, easy-to-grow shrub. It tolerates most soils—just not dry soil. Loamy, moist soil in a sunny location is best. Elder comes as bare-root plant or potted plant; place into a bushel basket–sized hole, adding compost as you backfill. Plant two or more cultivars to ensure cross-pollination—ideally 5 feet apart. Berries appear the first year, but the second-year crop will be better. Do not prune until the third year.

Evening Primrose
Oenothera biennis

Hardy, biennial evening primrose grows easily on dry stony ground or in well-drained sandy soil. Sow seeds in late spring, and keep watered until established. The blooms are a vibrant yellow, and the seeds are small and brown-black in color. The plant seeds readily and you will never be without it unless you snap off blooms past their prime to prevent reseeding. It can spread enthusiastically, so keep it under control.

Fennel
Foeniculum vulgare

Fennel is a perennial herb that will grow well in warmer climates where there is plenty of sun, and it can continue to produce for years. Sow seeds in early April in ordinary soil, in drills 15 inches apart, lightly covered with soil. Then, separate seedlings to the same distance. If sowed in April, the plant will be in full flower by July. Do not plant fennel near dill: the two species will cross-pollinate and produce bad-tasting herbs.

Fenugreek
Trigonella foenum-graecum

Fenugreek is an annual of the Mediterranean that needs full sunlight and well-drained, neutral to slightly acidic soil. Start seeds after the last frost, planted about ¼ inch deep. The seedlings do not like to be transplanted, so sow 5 to 6 inches apart to allow for growth. Add compost to keep the soil rich. Harvest seed pods from early to mid fall. To enjoy the seeds all year, dry the pods, and store them in airtight containers in a dry, dark spot.

Feverfew
Tanacetum parthenium

Perennial feverfew is propagated by seed, division of roots, or by cuttings. Seeds should be sown indoors in March, transplanted in late spring with 1 foot or more between plants and 2 feet between rows. Feverfew enjoys full sun and well-drained soil of any consistency. It is hardy to USDA zone 5, and it should be cut back to the ground in the autumn. Cultivars include double flowers, pom-poms, and yellow flower heads.

Garlic
Allium sativum

Garlic requires highly fertile soil in a sunny location. Sow in fall—garlic prefers cool weather for growing foliage, then warm weather for bu*lb* production. (Old-timers say plant by Columbus Day.) Use agricultural bulbs, not cloves from the grocery store. Plant cloves with tips up, 2 inches deep, 5 inches apart, in rows 15 to 24 inches apart. Mulch heavily, but lessen in spring, as greens show. Bulblets at top of scapes can be cooked.

Ginger
Zingiber officinale

Ginger likes warmth, partial shade, and rich soil. Start with an organic ginger rhizome from the grocery store that shows "eye buds." Cut off buds and plant them 1 or 2 inches below the surface of the soil—either in garden plot or in 12-inch plastic pots—with the eyes facing up. Water and wait . . . ginger is a slow grower, but plant may reach 2 feet. The longer you wait to harvest your root, the larger it will be. Overwinter pots indoors.

Ginkgo
Ginkgo biloba

A native of China, the ginkgo grows best in USDA zones 3 to 8. It prefers moist, well-drained soil in full to partial sun. Slow-growing, slender at first, with sparse branches, mature trees can reach over 100 high and 60 feet wide, with pyramidal, irregular crowns. The 3-inch fan-shaped green leaves turn bright yellow in autumn. Male catkins and female ovules appear in March or April, with smelly seedpods appearing in fall.

Ginseng
Panax ginseng, P. quinquefolius

This herb will only grow in conditions that mimic its native range—a cool climate with 75 percent shade and 20 to 40 inches of rainfall. Can be grown from seeds, root division, or cuttings, but seeds are iffy and can take 18 months to germinate. Rootlets purchased online are the best course, and they can be planted in fall or spring in rich, loamy soil. Root is best left to mature for five to ten years.

Goldenseal
Hydrastis canadensis

Goldenseal is a woodland herb that is propagated from seeds, rhizome division, or cuttings. For rhizome division, dig up a mature plant, rinse root ball, and cut off an inch or so that shows a root bud and filament roots. Place root in prepared soil of loam, peat, and sand in descending proportions; spread out roots, then cover with 2 to 3 inches of soil. Roots can be dug up and dried for medicine in the autumn of the third year.

Heartsease
Viola tricolor

Grow heartsease for its medicinal uses or for its long season of pretty pansy flowers. It is a small, clumping plant that appreciates partial shade, but, other than that, it is easy to grow in moist soil. Makes a good project for young or beginning gardeners. Sow indoors in March, outdoors in fall or April. Replant seedlings about 6 inches apart. This plant is hermaphroditic—it can fertilize itself and will self-sow. Also pollinated by bees.

Hibiscus
Hibiscus sabdariffa

Plant hibiscus in full or partial sun in tropic or warm-temperate regions; water regularly to ensure blossoms; do not let soil dry out. Can be grown in containers; but make sure to use a pot that is wider but not much deeper than a nursery pot. Requires regular feeding, using a diluted liquid fish emulsion–seaweed combination. In areas with cold winters, plants should be brought indoors to overwinter.

Hops
Humulus lupulus

Gardeners preach that "hops like what potatoes like"—especially moist, temperate locations and sunlight. In cooler climates, start rhizomes indoors in pots, and then transplant after last frost. Plant rhizomes with buds facing up, 2 inches below surface, at least 5 feet apart. Train vines up tripods, twine fences, or walls. Water sparingly during first season. Harvest cones for beer-making in September and October of second year.

Horseradish
Armoracia rusticana

Horseradish is a cold-hardy perennial, easy to grow in sun or partial shade. In spring, set out roots a few weeks before last frost in moist, rich soil; enriched clay or sandy loam with a near neutral pH is also acceptable. Harvest in late fall, after several frosts have damaged the leaves, using a digging fork to loosen the soil around the root. Grow near the outer edge of garden in a permanent patch, becasue it is difficult to eradicate once established.

Hyssop
Hyssopus officinalis

Perennial hyssop enjoys full sun to partial shade and light, dry soil. Sow seeds indoors 8 to 10 weeks before last frost, close to surface of soil. Hyssop seeds usually take between 14 and 21 days to germinate. Transplant after risk of frost is past, 12 to 24 inches apart, in composted bed. Plants can also be propagated by root division in autumn. Prune to first set of leaves after flowering for better blossoms the following year.

Jasmine
Jasminum spp.

Tropical jasmine can be grown in USDA zones 6 to 8. Check requirements for the cultivar you have chosen for level of sun, type of soil, and growing needs—does it vine up or sprawl along the ground? Some cultivars do best wintering indoors or strictly as houseplants. Compost soil to ensure healthy blossoms, move plant from container into a hole the size of the root ball, and press soil firmly until plant is erect; water to settle soil.

Juniper Berry
Juniperus communis

Purchase young juniper trees from a reliable garden shop. Water thoroughly before planting. Prepare generous hole; ensure drainage by adding gravel or grit and organic matter and mixing with soil from hole. Remove root ball from pot, tease out larger roots, and place in hole, matching surrounding soil level to level in the pot. Backfill with organic matter, pat down firmly. Water well during first year. Juniper also thrives as container plant.

Lavender
Lavandula angustifolia

Lavender enjoys dry, sandy soil and full sun. Seeds should be started early indoors, 8 to 10 weeks before the final frost. The small seeds need light to germinate, so cover finely with soil. Transplant seedling to pots as they grow; once all risk of frost is past, place seedlings in garden, 12 inches apart. Keep roots near surface, barely covered with soil. Do not cut lavender branches, only flower stems; massage stems to remove any dead matter.

Lemon Balm
Melissa officinalis

Start lemon balm seeds indoors—they need light and warmth, at least 70 degrees, to germinate—then place outside after last frost. Plant seedlings 20 to 24 inches apart. Lemon balm grows in clumps and spreads vegetatively, as well as by seed. Trim back to encourage bushy growth. In temperate zones, the stems die off in winter, but shoot up again in spring. Lemon balm grows vigorously and will spread if not curbed.

Lemon Verbena
Aloysia citrodora

Lemon verbena does well in loose, loamy soil. Good drainage and warm weather are critical. Plant in full sun or light shade. Lemon verbena also does well in a pot at least 1 foot in diameter to allow its roots to spread. Trim leaves to keep the shrub tidy. In cooler climates, plant near a white or pale wall to afford reflected light. Bring plant indoors to overwinter, although most leaves will drop off.

Lemongrass
Cymbopogon citratus, C. flexuosus

In harsher climates, lemongrass can be grown outdoors as an annual or taken indoors during cold weather. Sow seeds indoors from January to March on the surface of rich soil; cover with thin layer of vermiculite or compost. Plants germinate in 20 to 40 days. Separate seedlings into 3-inch pots. Acclimate outdoors in late spring after final frost; plant in sunny location and liquid feed occasionally.

Licorice
Glycyrrhiza glabra

Technically a weed, the shrubby licorice plant can still be a part of a kitchen herb garden. A member of the pea family, it can be grown in most sunny locations in moist, fertile soil. The plant can tolerate strong winds, but it is not suitable in coastal, maritime environments. Scarify seeds before sowing. Seedlings should be set two to three feet apart. As a garden ornamental, the plant flowers in August and September.

Lovage
Levisticum officinale

Lovage can be started from seed or from nursery stock. It will grow in full sun or partial shade, but chose its site with care, for lovage is a long-lived perennial. Keep seedlings a minimum of 24 inches apart. Harvest leaves before flowering. Seeds mature for picking in August. Lay branches out flat to dry. Afterward, place in a large bag and shake to remove the "nutlets." Caution: The sap on cut stalks may burn skin.

Marjoram
Origanum majorana

Marjoram can be grown indoors as a windowsill herb or started in pots and transferred to the garden in full sun. Seeds are "dustlike," so handle them carefully—sprinkle them over soil and water gently. Thin seedlings to 10 inches apart. Harvest leaves just before flowering, and then cut back to prevent stragglers. Stem cuttings can be taken in summer and propagated in a starter mix to overwinter until spring.

Milk Thistle
Silybum marianum

Milk thistle is hardy in USDA zones 5 to 9; it prefers sunny or slightly shady areas, and average soil. Sow seeds after the last chance of frost, 3 to 5 seeds per hole at a depth of 1 inch, planted 12 to 15 inches apart. Seeds should germinate in three weeks. Pull out the weaker seedlings at each spot when they reach 2 inches in height. Seeds can be harvested in fall or left for the finches. New plants will also grow from buds on the root system.

Mugwort
Artemisia vulgaris

Mugwort is easy to grow, even in ordinary garden soil. The plant is propagated by cuttings taken in the spring or by root division of an established plant during autumn or spring. The leaves and flowering tips are used for medicinal purposes—leaves should be gathered for drying before the flowers appear, and the flowering tips should be gathered while they are still in bud. It can be invasive, so take extra care to keep in under control.

Mullein
Verbascum thapsus

Mullein does best in sandy, well-drained soil and full sun. Seeds can be directly sown in the fall, covered with a thin layer of dirt, and then mulched. Or start seeds indoors in spring after cold stratification—30 days in refrigerator in a plastic bag with loose potting medium. Then place seeds in flats, just below surface, and keep moist. Once seedlings have leaves, transplant them outdoors, about 16 inches apart in dryish soil.

Mustard
Brassica spp., *Sinapis* spp.

Mustard is easy to grow, and in addition to seeds for spice, the greens are tasty and nutritious. Plant seeds 1 inch apart, three weeks before final frost. Thin seedlings to 6 inches apart, and add a balanced fertilizer. The plant enjoys cool weather and will flower more quickly in warmer weather. Once the seed pods turn brown, the seeds are ready for harvesting. Place pods in a bag, and wait for seeds to burst from the pods.

Nasturtium
Tropaeolum majus, T. minus

Nasturtium seeds are large and easy to handle; sow outdoors, 10 to 12 inches apart, a week before the last frost. Seedlings can be started indoors, but their taproots make them difficult to transplant, so use peat pots that can go straight into the garden. Nasturtiums like full sun, but grow well in part shade. They prefer cool, damp, well-drained soil. Cut back in the heat of summer, for new blossoms when cooler weather arrives.

Nettle

Urtica dioica

Nettles do well in moist, rich soil, especially near streams, with full or partial sun. The tiny, light-dependent seeds can be started indoors in flats in late winter, or outdoors after the last frost. Tamp seeds down, then cover with a thin layer of soil. (Stratification of seeds can help germination.) Seedlings should be thinned to 8 inches apart. Nettles prefer their own spot, slightly away from other herbs.

Onion

Allium cepa

Biennial onions like fertile, well-drained soil and full sun. Grow from seeds, indoor transplants, or bulb sets. Seed in spring when soil reaches 50 degrees. Plant ¼ inch deep, ½ inch apart, in rows 18 inches apart. Thin seedlings to 4 inches. Start seeds indoors eight to ten weeks before final frost. Harden off; plant outside two weeks before final frost. Plant sets 1 inch deep before final frost. Avoid spots where other alliums grew for at least three years.

Oregano

Origanum vulgare

Oregano prefers loamy soil and full sun. Start from seeds or take cuttings from an established plant. Plant seedling 10 inches apart; pinch tops for fuller growth. Plant does not mind being a little dry. Thin out older plants after three years; the self-seeding oregano will fill in the gaps. Harvest leaves as needed. An extremely variable species, there are many subspecies and cultivars grown for ornamental, culinary, and medicinal uses.

Paprika

Capsicum annuum

Paprika peppers like well-drained soil in full sun. Start seeds indoors eight weeks before final frost. Sow ¼ inches deep in starting medium. Keep warm with heating mat and artificial light. Set plants out two to three weeks after last frost, when nights are warm, above 60 degrees. Plant seedlings 12 to 24 inches apart, in rows 36 inches apart. Select a location that has not been used for tomatoes, potatoes, or alliums.

Parsley

Petroselinum spp.

Parsley prefers loamy soil, and full or partial sun. Plant seeds (after soaking overnight) indoors in small pots 10 or 12 weeks before final frost, or plant them in the ground 3 weeks before final frost. Plant seedlings 6 to 8 inches apart, near asparagus, corn, and tomatoes. Keep well watered. Harvest when leaf stems have three segments; trim outer leaves first. Will grow indoors in cold weather.

Passionflower

Passiflora incarnata

Passionflowers are hardy in USDA zones 5 to 9. They are easy to grow in partial to full sun and adapt to most well-drained soils. They need a protected location and heavy mulching if severe cold is a risk. Plant early in spring, and add compost to the hole. Apply a 10-5-20 fertilizer in early spring, and then again six weeks later. Keep the soil evenly moist to ensure good flowering and growth.

Patchouli

Pogostemon cablin

Tropical patchouli will grow in temperate zones as an annual from either seeds or cuttings first rooted in water. This herb likes rich, moist soil and indirect sunlight. Water frequently during dry weather, although a withered plant will usually bounce back. The fragrant flowers blossom in late fall. Bring potted plants indoors during the winter. For drying, trim leaves several times during the growing season.

Peppermint

Mentha x piperita

Peppermint requires minimal care. Plant seeds in fall before the first frost of winter, or after the final frost of spring in fertile, moist soil. Space out seedlings 18 to 24 inches apart. Peppermint prefers full sun or partial shade. The plant can send out runners both above and below the ground—in a small garden, it is best to keep it in containers. Peppermint is a great companion plant for tomatoes and cabbage.

Poppy Seed

Papaver somniferum

Opium poppies need tilled soil augmented with organic fertilizer. The seeds of this cold-hardy plant can be sown in the ground in fall or in spring close after the last snowfall. Sprinkle seeds over prepared bed and water regularly. Seeds will germinate in a week to 25 days. When seedlings reach 6 inches, thin to 10 inches apart. At 10 inches, add liquid fertilizer. Harvest seeds after flowers fall off and seed-pod vents open.

Ramps

Allium tricoccum

Ramps are a woodland plant that still grows wild in many states; they can be difficult to cultivate in gardens. It is best to propagate from bulbs or young plants. Plant bulbs 3 inches deep, 4 to 6 inches apart, burying roots and keeping just the tip of the bulb above the surface. Transplant young plants to the same depth they were growing, 6 inches apart. Mulch with hardwood leaf litter, not pinebark. Harvest in spring.

Rose Hips

Rosa spp.

Roses have a reputation for being a challenge, but many new varieties are hardy and insect- and disease-resistant. Bare-root roses should be planted in early spring; potted roses can go in any time from early spring to early fall. For obtaining hips, the best cultivars are wild roses like *Rosa canina* and *Rosa rugosa*. Most roses require a minimum of five hours of sunlight, loamy soil, and frequent feeding during the blooming season.

Rosemary

Rosmarinus officinalis

Rosemary is easy to grow and does not like fussing. Start with a nursery plant (rosemary is propagated through cuttings), and situate it in a sunny spot with good drainage and circulation. Fertilize in spring with fish-kelp emulsion. In colder climates, the plant can winter indoors in a sunny window (or under artificial light). Harvest sprigs above the woody growth. Dry using a rack or by hanging upside down in bunches.

Rue
Ruta graveolens

Rue is a popular landscape plant that prefers well-drained soil, and it will thrive in rocky, dry gardens where little else will grow, as long as there is full sun. Start from surface-sown seeds, because they need light to germinate. Seedlings will appear in one to four weeks; transplant to warm, sunny location. Rue does well in USDA zones 4 to 9. Mulch heavily to overwinter in colder zones. Do not cut back.

Safflower
Carthamus tinctorius

Safflower plants furnish seeds for songbirds like cardinals and chickadees. They grow best when rainfall is less than 15 inches per year. Sow seeds 1 to 1½ inches deep, 6 to 10 inches apart in April or May after last frost. Mature plants have prickly spines, so do not attempt to transplant. To harvest seeds, allow heads to mature for one month after flowering ends. Use gloves to collect flower heads; crush to remove seeds.

Saffron
Crocus sativus

The exotic saffron crocus is relatively easy to grow. Starter kits are even available from gardening centers. Plant the bulbs, or corms, in summer 6 inches apart and 3 inches deep in rich, well-drained soil. Plants will bloom—and stigmas can be picked—in the fall. Divide plants every four years. Initially, the saffron harvest will be low, but the plants will keep adding blooms. Overplant your crocus bed with summer annuals.

Sage
Salvia officinalis

The silvery hue of sage leaves makes it a favorite with gardeners, both for ornamental borders and herb gardens. It grows best in a warm, rather dry border, but this hardy perennial (USDA zones 5 to 8) will take root almost anywhere in slightly alkaline soil. Use cuttings to propagate rather than seeds. Sage also makes an excellent pot herb. It thrives in semishade, rather than full sun. Harvest leaves any time before plant flowers.

Salad Burnet
Sanguisorba minor

Salad burnet grows well in arid conditions, even in limestone, and it will produce all year long in the right climate. It appears in the early spring, but it will hold up well in the heat. This perennial spreads through rhizomes, but it might self-seed. Plant in full sun to partial shade. It forms a clump, growing in a loose, well-contained rosette. Start harvesting leaves when plants are 4 inches tall. Trim buds to encourage leaf growth.

Scallion
Allium fistulosum

Scallions like fertile, well-drained soil and full sun. Can be grown from seed, indoor transplants, or sets—small bulbs from the previous season. Plant seeds after soil reaches 50 degrees, ¼ inch deep, ½ inch apart in rows 1 foot apart. Thin seedlings to 4 inches. You can also start seeds indoors eight to ten weeks before final frost. Harden off, then plant outside two weeks before final frost. Maintain moisture.

Sesame Seed
Sesamum indicum

The sesame plant is an annual that likes full sun and well-drained soil. Start seeds indoors at least 4 weeks before final frost. Sow in light potting medium, ¼ inch below surface, and make sure to keep plants moist. Transplant seedlings outdoors after last risk of frost, when temperatures range in the 60s. Place seedlings 10 to 12 inches apart. Seeds will be ready for harvest in three months.

Sorrel
Rumex acetosa, R. scutatus

Garden sorrel, *Rumex acetosa,* likes moist soil in sun or partial shade, while French sorrel, *R. scutatus,* prefers dry soil and a sunny, open situation. Sow seeds in March in drills 6 inches apart, and then thin to 18 inches apart when the plants reach 2 inches in height. In July, cut stalks back to force the growth of new, tender leaves. Both varieties of culinary sorrel are propagated via root division.

Spearmint
Mentha spicata

Spearmint grows easily in moist, fertile soil with partial shade. Plant seedlings 24 inches apart. Because the plant sends out aggressive underground runners, some gardeners prefer to keep spearmint confined to containers. It can also be grown indoors, making a great addition to a windowsill herb garden. Leaves should be harvested for drying just before flowering; they lose their potent scent after that.

Spikenard
Nardostachys jatamansi

Perennial spikenard prefers moist, rich soil and full sun or partial shade in USDA zones 5 to 8. The small seeds are difficult to grow, so it is best to scarify—scratch the surface—and cold stratify them—place in sandy soil and store in refrigerator for a month or two—in mid to late winter. Then, sow indoors or in warm location. Tamp seeds and cover lightly with soil. Seedlings germinate in four weeks; transplant 4 inches apart when full leaves appear.

St. John's Wort
Hypericum perforatum

St. John's wort is a bushy perennial that grows well in USDA zones 5 to 9. It can reproduce vegetatively or sexually. The seeds need a short frost period to germinate, so they are best sown in late fall. In spring, place them in a freezer for a short time. The plants prefer a sunny or partial shade location, in dry, slightly alkaline soil, but will adapt to almost any conditions. Harvest when flowers are in full bloom.

Star Anise
Illicium verum

Star anise cannot handle temperatures lower than 23 degrees (hardy to USDA zones 7 to 9), so it should be grown indoors or in a greenhouse. It is content in a container with well-drained soil and a partial-shade location. The tree can be propagated by seeds sown in the spring or by semi-ripe cuttings in summer. It grows slowly and can take 15 years to grow fruit, but it may continue to produce for a hundred years.

Stevia
Stevia rebaudiana

Stevia prefers rich, well-drained soil; full sun; warm temps. Start seeds indoors in peat pack, 8 weeks before final frost. Cover with ⅛ inch potting soil and mist. Grow under plastic with fluorescent light, 24 hours a day for three weeks, then 15 hours. Remove plastic when plants emerge and leaf out; cut off tip to force branching. Place seedlings in 5-inch pots and harden off outdoors before planting in garden. Winter stevia indoors.

Summer Savory
Satureja hortensis

Summer savory prefers full sun and rich soil. Plant seeds indoors six weeks before final frost or outdoors around the time of last frost. Cover with a thin layer of soil so that light reaches them. Keep moist. Transplant seedlings of 4 inches on a cloudy day, and place 10 inches apart. Harvest tender shoot tips continuously after plant reaches 6 inches. Harvested seeds need to be used by next season, or they lose viability.

Sweet Woodruff
Galium odoratum

Sweet woodruff is easily grown in medium-to-wet soils in partial shade to full shade. It spreads by creeping roots or by division to form an attractive ground cover. It makes a lovely edging plant. If sweet woodruff become aggressive, it can be mowed with a rotary mower set on high. Plants in dry sunny spots may go dormant by midsummer. In the spring, cut back any old growth to keep plants full and healthy.

Tansy
Tanacetum vulgare

Perennial tansy does well in moderately fertile, well-drained soil when planted in full sun. Hardy in USDA zones 4 to 8. Propagates from cuttings, division, or seeds. Seeds may require a month of cold stratification to germinate. Start potted seeds indoors at shallow depth, in winter or spring; keep moist. Transfer outside only when well established. Stake leggy stems. Tansy self-seeds if not deadheaded.

Tarragon
Artemisia dracunculus

Tarragon is sterile and does not grow from seeds; propagation is from cuttings or by root division in early spring. It does well in warm, sunny, slightly dry locations. Fertilize established plants with fish emulsion. Folklore says the fresh leaves can be picked between Midsummer's Eve—late June—and Michaelmas—the end of September. Harvest stems in August for drying. If not thinned regularly, the plant can strangle itself.

Thyme
Thymus vulgaris

Evergreen thyme attracts pollinators like bees and butterflies to your garden, and it also attracts wildlife. It prefers a location in full sun. Start seeds indoors, set out seedlings after the last frost in well-drained, slightly alkaline soil. Add lime if needed. Use slow-release fertilizer when planting, then again each spring. Prune lightly after the first year. Allow several months of growth before snipping off sprigs for cooking.

Turmeric
Curcuma longa

Turmeric grows from root or rhizome cuttings, not seeds, in full sun or slight shade. The plant does well in a large, deep container that can be brought inside in cooler weather. Plant cuttings 2 inches down in well-drained potting soil; sprouts should appear in a month or two. Keep moist and feed biweekly with liquid fertilizer. It can take eight or ten months for a new crop of roots to develop.

Valerian
Valeriana officinalis

Valerian can be propagated from seeds, but it can be temperamental. Opt for root division or for rooting the volunteer runners, or "daughters," of existing plants. Space new plants 3 feet apart on all sides. Valerian is hardy in USDA zones 4 to 9, but requires at least six hours of full sun. Add a layer of mulch in spring and fall. Once it takes hold in your garden, valerian will return year after year.

Watercress
Nasturtium officinale

Watercress, a perennial semiaquatic plant, prefers clean, moving water or boggy wetlands to thrive. If grown in merely moist soil, it looses flavor, although it gains nutrients. It can be grown from seeds or cuttings, which will readily sprout roots when grown in any garden pond or bog garden. Harvesting of the greens can begin 30 to 40 days after sprouting. Seeds can be harvested from midsummer through autumn.

Winter Savory
Satureja montana

Winter savory is a hardy perennial that can be propagated from seeds (plant in April, roughly 9 inches apart), cuttings, or by root division. Plant does well in poor, stony soil; otherwise it takes in too much moisture, which can harm it in winter. Harvest leaves for cooking before plant flowers to avoid a bitter taste. Harvest leaves for drying after the plant has flowered. With its mounded growth, it makes an attractive border plant.

Wormwood
Artemisia absinthium

Wormwood is an attractive landscape plant with silvery gray, aromatic foliage, and it can be easily cultivated in dry soil. This woody perennial prefers fertile, midweight, nitrogen-rich soil and a spot with shade or partial sun. It can be propagated by root division, cuttings taken in spring or autumn, or by seeds sown in the fall. Plant seedlings 2 feet apart. Wormwood will also self-seed generously if not deadheaded.

Yarrow
Achillea millefolium

Yarrow is easy to grow and makes a striking rock garden addition, perfect for cutting or drying. It is hardy in USDA zones 3 to 9 and prefers full sun. Plant seeds in spring in well-drained, average-to-poor soil with a thin layer of compost. Thin out seedlings to two feet apart. Yarrow can be an invasive plant, so keep an eye on it. Divide plants every three to five years in early spring or fall.

Glossary

ALKALOID Any of numerous usually colorless, complex, and bitter organic bases (such as morphine or codeine) containing nitrogen and usually oxygen that occur especially in seed plants. An alkaloid is a basic organic compound with alkaline properties and generally a marked physiological effect on the nervous and circulatory systems. Alkaloids show varying pharmacological effects; for example, they can act as analgesics, local anesthetics, tranquilizers, vasoconstrictors, antispasmodics, and hallucinatory agents.

AMINO ACID Any of a class of 20 molecules that are combined to form proteins in living organisms. The sequence of amino acids in a protein—and hence protein function—is determined by the genetic code.

ANALGESIC A medication used to relieve pain.

ANESTHETIC A drug that causes anesthesia, or a reversible loss of sensation.

ANNUAL A plant that grows for only one season, produces seeds, and then dies in the winter.

ANTIALLERGENIC A substance that does not aggravate an allergy.

ANTIFUNGAL An agent that is destructive to fungi, suppressing their reproduction or growth.

ANTIHISTAMINE A drug that blocks histamine, typically used to treat allergic reactions.

ANTI-INFLAMMATORY An agent that reduces the heat, redness, and swelling of inflammation.

ANTIMICROBIAL An agent that kills microorganisms or inhibits their growth.

ANTIOXIDANT A chemical compound that protects against cell damage from molecules called oxygen-free radicals, which are major causes of disease and aging.

ANTISCORBUTIC A drug or substance having the effect of preventing the disease scorbutus, or scurvy.

ANTISEPTIC A substance that discourages the growth of microorganisms.

ANTISPASMODIC A drug or substance that is used to relieve spasm of the involuntary muscles.

ANTIVIRAL A drug or treatment that is effective against viruses.

ASTRINGENT An agent that causes contraction or shrinkage of tissues; it is used to decrease secretions or control bleeding.

AYURVEDIC MEDICINE The ancient Indian medical system of sustaining health and fighting disease based on equilibrium with nature. Ayurvedic medicine uses thousands of plants.

BIENNIAL A plant whose life cycle extends over two growing seasons.

BRACT A modified leaf or scale with a flower or flower cluster in its axil. Bracts can be larger and more colorful than the actual flower, as with a poinsettia.

CARMINATIVE An agent that relieves and removes gas from the digestive system.

CAROTENOID The natural, fat-soluble pigments found in certain plants that provide the bright red, orange, or yellow coloration of many fruits and vegetables.

COMPOUND A substance formed by the chemical union of two or more elements.

CULTIVAR A plant variety that has been created in cultivation by selective breeding.

DECIDUOUS Shedding leaves annually.

DECOCTION A preparation made by simmering tough plant parts in water.

DECONGESTANT A drug or substance that shrinks the swollen membranes in the nose, making it easier to breathe.

DIURETIC A substance that increases the flow of urine from the body.

DOUBLE-BLIND A clinical trial in which neither the doctor nor the patient knows whether the patient is being administered a placebo or the test drug.

ENZYME Proteins that accelerate chemical reactions in organic substances by catalytic action.

ESSENTIAL OIL (Also called *volatile oil*) A hydrophobid, aromatic volatile oil found in specialized glands of plants (as in the mint family). Many plants containing essential oils are known for their fragrance and cultivated for the food and perfume industries.

ESTROGEN A group of hormones produced mainly in the mammalian ovaries that are necessary for female sexual development and reproductive functioning.

EVERGREEN A plant that retains its green foliage throughout the year.

EXPECTORANT A substance that stimulates removal of mucus from the lungs.

EXTRACT A concentrated active constituent that is obtained from a plant using a solvent, such as ethanol or water.

FAMILY A level of classification in the plant kingdom above genus and species, with technical family names usually ending in the suffix "-aceae."

FLAVONOID A group of chemical compounds—low-molecular-weight phenylbenzopyrones—occurring in all vascular plants. In the diet, flavonoids are found in many fruits, vegetables, teas, wines, nuts, seeds, and roots. Many of the medicinal actions of foods, juices, and herbs are directly related to their flavonoid content. They exhibit antioxidant properties and other effects.

FREE RADICAL A chemical that is highly reactive and can oxidize other molecules. When produced within cells, free radicals can react with membranes and genetic material to damage or destroy cells and tissues.

GENUS A level of classification in the plant kingdom that falls directly below family; the first word of the two-name Latin binomial, which is always capitalized.

GLUCOSIDE A glucoside is a glycoside that is derived from sugar; they are common in plants, rare in animals.

GLYCOSIDE A product of secondary metabolism in plants. Glycosides break down into two parts—the glycone component, or sugar, and the nonsugar, or aglycone component. The therapeutically active constituent is the aglycone, which can selectively affect a particular organ in the body. Glycosides include some of the most effective plant drugs, but some plants containing them are highly toxic.

HERBACEOUS A type of plant with little or no woody tissue, usually living a single season.

HIGH-DENSITY LIPOPROTEIN (HDL) Lipoprotein that contains a small amount of cholesterol and carries cholesterol away from body cells and tissues to the liver for excretion from the body. Lower levels of HDL increase the risk of heart disease, so the higher the level of HDL in the bloodstream, the better. The HDL component normally contains 20 to 30 percent of total cholesterol.

HOMEOPATHY A form of alternative medicine that treats patients using preparations containing infinitesimal doses of a substance that, in normal doses, would produce symptoms of the disease it is intended to treat.

INFLAMMATION The immune system's response to tissue injury or harmful stimulation caused by physical or chemical substances. Release of inflammatory chemicals and increased blood flow to affected areas results in swelling, redness, and pain.

INFLORESCENCE Group or cluster forming the flowering part of a plant.

INFUSED OIL The result of an herb or plant part being soaked or macerated in oil and heated. The infused oil is then strained out.

INFUSION Tea made by steeping an herb or plant part in hot water.

INSULIN A hormone that is needed to convert sugar, starches, and other food into glucose (blood sugar); excessively high blood glucose levels could lead to diabetes.

LINIMENT A thin medicinal fluid rubbed on the skin to reduce pain.

LOW-DENISITY LIPOPROTEIN (LDL) The major cholesterol carrier in the blood. LDL transports cholesterol from the liver and intestines to various tissues. LDL is known as bad cholesterol because high levels are linked to coronary artery disease.

MUCILAGE A gelatinous substance produced by some plants that is often used in herbal medicine as a soothing agent.

NATURALIZED In botany, any process when a non-native plant escapes into the wild and survives. Cultivated plants are a major source of adventive populations.

NATUROPATHY/IC A system of therapy that avoids drugs and surgery and emphasizes the use of natural remedies.

PECTIN A polysaccharide extracted from the cell walls of plants, used in making jellies and jams.

PERENNIAL Any plant that has a life cycle of more than two years.

PHARMACOPOEIA A book containing an official list of medicinal drugs together with articles on their preparation, usually produced by legislative authority. Also, a stock of medicinal drugs.

PHENOLICS OR POLYPHENOLS A large group of chemicals derived from phenol (a benzene ring with one hydroxyl group attached) that contribute to the color, taste, flavor, and medicinal actions of many plants. In wine grapes, phenolics are found widely in the skin, stems, and seeds.

PHYTOCHEMICAL A chemical found naturally in plants that has metabolically active qualities.

PHYTOMEDICAL Pertaining to medicine based on active ingredients within an herbal base, sometimes used to describe all plant-based medicines.

PHYTONUTRIENT A substance found in many plants that is believed to be beneficial to human health and to help prevent certain diseases.

PINNATE An arrangement of leaflets, found on either side of a stem, typically in pairs opposite each other.

PLACEBO An inactive pill, liquid, or powder that has no treatment value but is used in tests to determine whether the effects of a drug are real or brought on by the patient's desire to be cured.

POULTICE A preparation of fresh, moistened, or crushed dried herbs or spices, which is applied externally to treat ailments.

RHIZOME A somewhat elongated, usually horizontal, subterranean plant stem, often thickened by deposits of reserve food material, that produces shoots above and roots below; distinguished from a true root in having buds, nodes, and usually scalelike leaves.

SAPONIN Any of several glycosides in plants that make a soapy lather if mixed with water.

SEPAL One of the separate, green parts that surround and protect the bud of a flower and extend from the base of a flower after it has opened. Sepals tend to occur in the same number as the petals and to be centered over the petal divisions.

SESQUITERPENE A terpene-based compound that, when taken from a plant, can stimulate glands in the liver. Sesquiterpenes may have antiallergenic, antispasmodic, and anti-inflammatory properties.

SESQUITERPENE LACTONE A class of chemicals found in many plants that can cause allergic reactions and toxicity if overdosed, particularly in grazing livestock. In moderate amounts, such chemicals can have anti-inflammatory, antibacterial, antiparasitic, anticancer, and antispasmodic properties.

SPECIES A level of classification in the plant kingdom below genus; second name in the Latin binomial, designating organisms in a genus.

STAMEN The pollen-bearing organ of a plant, consisting of the filament and the anther.

STIGMA The receptive tip of a carpel or several fused carpels in the female reproductive parts of a flower.

STOLON Stems that grow at the soil surface level or just below ground that form adventitious roots at the nodes, and new plants from the buds; often called runners.

SUBSPECIES A level of classification in the plant kingdom below species, recognizing differences in a species not great enough to warrant classification as a species; designated, following the species name, by the abbreviation subsp.

TANNIN A group of simple and complex phenol, polyphenol, and flavonoid compounds bound with starches. Aside from their astringent, mouth-puckering properties, these chemicals can help stanch bleeding from small wounds, slow uterine bleeding, reduce inflammation and swelling, dry out weepy mucous membranes, and relieve diarrhea.

TINCTURE A plant medicine prepared by soaking an herb in water and ethanol (never isopropyl alcohol); traditional herbal preparations are dispensed as alcohol-based liquid medicines.

UMBEL An inflorescence that consists of a number of short flowers stalks, or pedicels, that spread from a common point; appearance is similar to umbrella ribs.

VARIETY In botany, a type of plant that arose in nature, as opposed to a cultivar, which is a variation of a species deliberately bred by humans. *Also see* cultivar.

VOLATILE OIL *See* essential oil.

Contributors

NANCY J. HAJESKI writes adult and young adult nonfiction under her own name; recent titles include *Ali: The Official Portrait of the Greatest of All Time* and *The Beatles: Here, There and Everywhere*. Writing as Nancy Butler, she focuses on romantic fiction and has produced 12 Signet Regencies, two of which won the RITA award from the Romance Writers of America. She also adapted four of Jane Austen's books as graphic novels for Marvel Entertainment. Her *Pride and Prejudice* made the *New York Times* bestseller list and remained there for 13 weeks. An avid gardener who grows her own herbs, Hajeski lives in the Catskill Mountains next to a world-class trout stream.

KELLEY EDKINS (consultant) is the owner of Gardens by Kelley, a sustainable, organic landscape design company. The facilitator and operator of the first DEC compost facility site in Sullivan County, New York—a static-pile vermi-compost called The Bee Green Community Garden—Kelley has been cultivating medicinal herbs, native plants, and endangered species for 20 years. Her organic farm, Honeybee Herbs, focuses on plants that provide food for honeybees, and she sells herbal and honeybee products at farmer's markets and festivals. Kelley is a Master Gardener, holistic beekeeper, and compost expert who shares her knowledge with school students, politicians, and clients.

GUDRUN FEIGL (consultant) is the founder of Mount Pleasant Herbary—a small producer of botanical soaps, herbal tea blends, salves, and other related items made from homegrown herbs. Gudrun has been studying herbalism since starting her business in 2009. She sells her products at local farmer's markets and also teaches workshops on herbs. Gudrun grew up in Germany, close to the border of Switzerland. She now lives in northeast Pennsylvania with her husband and daughter.

Image Credits

Front cover: Top (left to right), Diana Taliun/Shutterstock; Roberto A Sanchez/iStockphoto; stockcreations/Shutterstock; bottom (left to right), Dream79/Shutterstock; (above), Dream79/Shutterstock; (below), SOPA/eStock Photo; Elena Elisseeva/age fotostock. **Front flap:** Preto Perola/Shutterstock. **Back cover:** Top (left to right), Andris Tkacenko/Shutterstock; Sebastian Duda/Shutterstock; bottom (left to right), freya-photographer/Shutterstock; Jiri Vaclavek/Shutterstock; science photo/Shutterstock. **Back flap:** Brian Balster/Shutterstock.

Icons: Culinary—puruan/SS; Medicinal—Kapreski/SS; Aromatic—Visual Idiot/SS; Pollinator—tereez/SS; Grower's Guide— justone/SS

Introduction: 1 Andrii Gorulko/SS; 2–3 Krzysztof Slusarczyk/SS; 5 Elena Schweitzer/SS; 6 "Physician Preparing an Elixir" *De Materia Medica* by Dioscorides/Rogers Fund, 1913; 7*b*Vilor/SS; 7*t* racorn/SS; 8 Sadik Gulec/SS; 9*l* Only Fabrizio/SS; 9*r* Robert Crow/SS

Chapter One: 12*t1* bepsy/SS; 12*t2* Blend Images/SS; 12*c1* michaeljung/SS; 12*c2* miropink/SS; 12*b1* blueeyes/SS; 12*b2* Dani Vincek/SS; 13*t1* angelakatharina/SS; 13*t2* Sunny studio/SS; 13*c1* sarsmis/SS; 13*c2* Goodluz/SS; 13*c3* Natalia Klenova/SS; 13*b1* Katie Smith Photography/SS; 13*b2* Natalia Klenova/SS; 15 Dream79/SS; 16 Beata Becla/DT; 17 Andris Tkacenko/SS; 18*b*govindji/SS; 18*t* Dionisvera/SS; 19*s* Patricia Hofmeester/SS; 19*l* Magdalena Kucova/SS; 20*b* ksena2you/SS; 20*t* Karl Allgaeuer/SS; 21*s* *Pallas and the Centaur* by Botticelli (c. 1482); 21*l* Gabriela Insuratelu/SS; 22*b* Barbro Rutgersson/DT; 22*t* Catherine311/SS; 23*r* Bochkarev Photography/SS; 24*b* Africa Studio/SS; 24*t* Tim UR/SS; 25*s* David Woolfenden/SS; 26*b* Alexander Kuguchin/SS; 26*t* eye-blink/SS; 27*l* Dream79/SS; 27*r* Marilyn Barbone/DT; 28*b* Piotr Marcinski/SS; 28*t* Jiang Hongyan/SS; 29*s* racorn/SS; 29*l* Kati Molin/DT; 30*b* picturepartners/SS; 30*t* Odua Images/SS; 31*s1* marylooo/SS; 31*s2* ksena2you/SS; 31*s3* David Iushewitz/DT; 31*s4* Fablok/SS; 31*s5* Elena Schweitzer/SS; 31*s6* BW Folsom/SS; 31*s7* Elena Schweitzer/SS; 31*s8* Maks M/SS; 31*s9* NinaM/SS; 31*s10* HandmadePictures/SS; 31*s11* HandmadePictures/SS; 31*s12* Linda Vostrovska/SS; 32*b* Swapan Photography/SS; 32*t* Swapan Photography/SS; 33*l* Olga Nayashkova/SS; 33*r* Swapan Photography/SS; 34*b* Lcswart/DT; 34*t* LalithHerath/SS; 35*s* Duskbabe/DT; 35*l* Mokkie/Wikipedia 36*b* KPG_Payless/SS; 36*t* Scisetti Alfio/SS; 37*s* Ian 2010/SS; 37*r* sonsam/SS; 38*b* Andrey Starostin/SS; 38*t* Dionisvera/SS; 39*s* vanillaechoes/SS; 39*r* alexsol/SS; 40*b* ra3rn/SS; 40*t* Kelvin Wong/SS; 41*l* Vladf/SS; 41*r* Andrii Gorulko/SS; 41*t* Heike Rau/SS; 42*b* Monkey Business Images/SS; 42*t* bonchan/SS; 43*s* iko/SS; 43*l* TAGSTOCK1/SS; 43*r* picturepartners/SS; 44*b* wasanajai/SS; 44*t* noppharat/SS; 45*s* wonderisland/SS; 45*r* stoonn/SS; 46*b* Paul J Martin/SS; 46*t* Africa Studio/SS; 47*s* indigolotos/SS; 47*l* Vaclav Mach/SS; 48*b* LittleStocker/SS; 48*t* nednapa/SS; 49*s* ImagePost/SS; 49*l* Banprik/SS; 50*b* dabjola/SS; 50*t* enzo4/SS; 51*s* Image Point Fr/SS; 51*r* SS; 52 Elena Schweitzer/SS; 53*s* Irina Bg/SS; 53*l* Mersant/DT; 53*r* Krzycho/SS; 54*b* Tamara Souchko/DT; 54*t* Jamie Hooper/SS; 55 Tuan Nguyen/DT; 56*b* Galina Ermolaeva/DT; 56*t* Madlen/SS; 57*s* AndiPu/SS; 57*l* BestPhotoPlus/SS; 57*r* Madlen/SS; 58*b* Stargazer/SS; 58*t* Alexander Raths/SS; 59*s* Mona Makela/SS; 59*l* MarkMirror/SS; 59*r* KPG_Payless2/SS; 60*b* Oliver Hoffmann/SS; 60*t* Maks Narodenko/SS; 61*s* Brent Hofacker/SS; 61*l* Lithiumphoto/SS; 62*b* Swetlana Wall/SS; 62*t* Alfio Scisetti/DT; 63*s* Patricia Hofmeester/SS; 63*l* Startdesign/DT; 64*b* eAlisa/SS; 64*t* Givaga/SS; 65*s* Heike Rau/SS; 65*r* Goodluz/SS; 66*b* Voraorn Ratanakorn/SS; 66*t* Tamara Kulikova/SS; 67*s* Goodluz/SS; 67*l* schankz/SS; 68*b* Irina Fischer/SS; 68*t* Robyn Mackenzie/SS; 69*l* mirabile/SS; 69*r* Jorge Salcedo/SS; 70 Teresa Kasprzycka/SS; 71 teleginatania/SS; 72 picturepartners/SS; 73*l* Roger Meerts/SS; 73*r* Bildagentur Zoonar GmbH/SS; 74*b* ksena2you/SS; 74*t* Imageman/SS; 75*s* Serg Zastavkin/SS; 75*l* Heike Rau/SS; 76*b* Hurst Photo/SS; 76*t* Melinda Fawver/SS; 77*s* Ppy2010ha/DT; 77*b* Wollertz/SS; 77*t* Lidara/SS; 78*b* Zerbor/SS; 78*t* Teresa Azevedo/SS; 79*s* U.S. Dept. of Agriculture; 79*r* Studio 37/SS; 90*b* artcasta/SS; 80*t* Volosina/SS; 81*s* picturepartners/SS; 81*l* kostrez/SS; 81*r* Tobias Arhelge/SS; 82*b* KPG_Payless/SS; 82*t* Scisetti Alfio/SS; 83*t1* Madlen/SS; 83*t2* Nataliia Pyzhova/SS; 83*t3* Nataliia Pyzhova/SS; 83*t4* eAlisa/SS; 83*r* SurangaSL/SS; 84*b* Vladimira/SS; 84*t* haraldmuc/SS; 85*l* auremar/SS; 85*r* Tadas_Jucys/SS; 86*b* allou/SS; 86*t* cynoclub/SS; 87*s* Heike Rau/DT; 87*r* Heathse/DT; 88*t* Irina Fischer/SS; 89*b* Alexander Mychko/DT; 89*l* HandmadePictures/SS; 89*r* fotolinchen/Getty Images

Chapter Two: 90 Laura Bartlett/SS; 92 Lopatin Anton/SS; 93 Svetlana Lukienko/SS; 94*b* wjarek/SS; 94*t* Kazakov Maksim/SS; 95*l* Tim Belyk/SS; 95*r* Pictureguy/SS; 96*b* Piotr Marcinski/SS; 96*t* kedrov/SS; 97*l* science photo/SS; 97*r* successo images/SS; 98*b* KENNY TONG/SS; 98*t* marilyn barbone/SS; 99*s* Library of Congress; 99*l* magnetix/SS; 100*b* Dr. Morley Read/SS; 100*t* wasanajai/SS; 101*s* rsfatt/SS; 101*b* hjschneider/SS; 101*t* Christian Vinces/SS; 102 Scisetti Alfio/SS; 103*s* Szasz-Fabian Ilka Erika/SS; 103*l* indykb/SS; 104*b* valzan/SS; 104*t* honobono/SS; 105*s* Stocksnapper/SS; 105*l* zprecech/SS; 106*t* Lianem/DT;107*l* Heike Rau/SS; 107*r* *Köhler's Medicinal Plants* (1887); 108*b* Vic and Julie Pigula/SS; 108*t* bonchan/SS; 109*s* Lubava/SS; 109*b* Oksana Kuzmina/SS; 109*l* Feldarbeit/DT; 109*r* SS; 110 Chamille White/SS; 111*s1* Marilyn Barbone/DT;111*s2* BW Folsom 111*s3* NinaM/SS; 111*s4* Marilyn Barbone/DT; 111*s5* Elena Schweitzer/SS; 111*s6* matka_Wariatka/SS; 111*s7* matka_Wariatka/SS; 111*s8* ribeiroantonio/SS; 111*s9* matka_Wariatka/SS;111*s10* Discovod/SS;111*s11* Fablok/SS; 111*s12* Elena Schweitzer/SS; 112*b* Robert Biedermann/SS; 112*t* oksana2010/SS; 113*s* daffodilred/SS; 113*l* Botamochy/SS; 114*b* picturepartners/SS; 114*t* picturepartners/SS; 115*s* Image Point Fr/SS; 115*r* Wil Tilroe-Otte/SS; 116*b* marilyn barbone/SS; 116*t* marilyn barbone/SS; 117*l* Kelly Marken/SS; 117*r* Ruud Morijn Photographer/SS; 118*b* PathDoc/SS; 118*t* oksana2010/SS; 119*l* LorraineHudgins/SS; 119*r* Elena Elisseeva/SS; 120*b* Kletr/SS; 120*t* Bildagentur Zoonar GmbH/SS; 121*s* photo-oasis/SS; 121*l* Christa Eder/DT; 122*b* D. Kucharski K. Kucharska/SS; 122*t* Emberiza/DT; 123*l* Stocksnapper/DT; 123*r* Hiroshi Ichikawa/SS; 124 Gita Kulinica/DT;125 Pixelrobot/DT;126*b* Vic and Julie Pigula/SS; 126*y* Sandra Caldwell/SS; 127*l* Blend Images/SS; 127*r* BONNIE WATTON/SS; 128*b* sima/SS; 128*t* Scisetti Alfio/SS; 129*b* cowardlion/SS; 129*r* JPRichard/SS; 130*b* Valeriy Kirsanov/DT; 130*t* sunsetman/SS; 131*l* Lcc54613/DT;131*r* Chinaview/SS; 132*t* StevenRussellSmithPhotos/SS; 132*b* Steven Foster, Steven Foster Group, Inc.; 133 *Curtis's Botanical Magazine* (1833); 134*b* MarkMirror/SS; 134*t*

Index

National Geographic Complete Guide to Herbs & Spices

Published by the National Geographic Society

Gary E. Knell, *President and Chief Executive Officer*
John M. Fahey, *Chairman of the Board*
Declan Moore, *Chief Media Officer*
Chris Johns, *Chief Content Officer*

Prepared by the Book Division

Hector Sierra, *Senior Vice President and General Manager*
Janet Goldstein, *Senior Vice President and Editorial Director*
Jonathan Halling, *Creative Director*
Marianne R. Koszorus, *Design Director*
Susan Tyler Hitchcock, *Senior Editor*
R. Gary Colbert, *Production Director*
Jennifer A. Thornton, *Director of Managing Editorial*
Susan S. Blair, *Director of Photography*
Meredith C. Wilcox, *Director, Administration and Rights Clearance*

Staff for This Book

Sanaa Akkach, *Art Director*
Michelle Cassidy, *Editorial Assistant*
Moseley Road Inc., *Design and Production*
Marshall Kiker, *Associate Managing Editor*
Judith Klein, *Production Editor*
Galen Young, *Rights Clearance Specialist*
Katie Olsen, *Design Production Specialist*
Nicole Miller, *Design Production Assistant*
Darrick McRae, *Manager, Production Services*
Wendy Smith, *Imaging*

MOSELEY ROAD Inc., www.moseleyroad.com
Sean Moore, *President*
Karen Prince, *General Manager*
Lisa Purcell, *Art Director*
Gudrun Feigi, Kelley Edkins, *Editorial Consultants*
Connie Binder, *Index*
Adam Moore, *Production Director*

The National Geographic Society is one of the world's largest nonprofit scientific and educational organizations. Founded in 1888 to "increase and diffuse geographic knowledge," the member-supported Society works to inspire people to care about the planet. Through its online community, members can get closer to explorers and photographers, connect with other members around the world, and help make a difference. National Geographic reflects the world through its magazines, television programs, films, music and radio, books, DVDs, maps, exhibitions, live events, school publishing programs, interactive media, and merchandise. *National Geographic* magazine, the Society's official journal, published in English and 38 local-language editions, is read by more than 60 million people each month. The National Geographic Channel reaches 440 million households in 171 countries in 38 languages. National Geographic Digital Media receives more than 25 million visitors a month. National Geographic has funded more than 10,000 scientific research, conservation, and exploration projects and supports an education program promoting geography literacy. For more information, visit www.nationalgeographic.com.

For more information, please call 1-800-NGS LINE (647-5463) or write to the following address:

National Geographic Society
1145 17th Street NW
Washington, D.C. 20036-4688 U.S.A.

For information about special discounts for bulk purchases, please contact National Geographic Books Special Sales: ngspecsales@ngs.org

For rights or permissions inquiries, please contact National Geographic Books Subsidiary Rights: ngbookrights@ngs.org

ISBN: 978-1-4262-1586-5
ISBN: 978-1-4262-1587-2 (deluxe)

Printed in the United States of America

15/QGT-CML/1

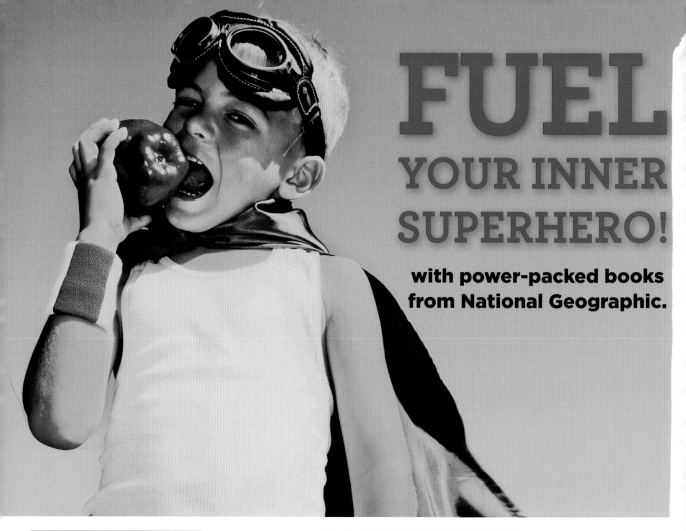
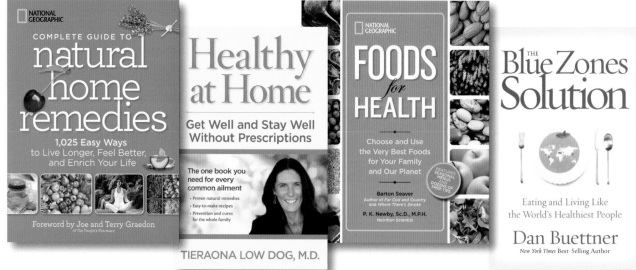
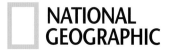